From Microbe to Man

Biological Responses in Microbes, Animals, and Humans upon Exposure to Artificial Static Magnetic Fields

Authored by

János F. László
Faculty of Informatics
University of Debrecen,
Hungary

From Microbe to Man

Biological Responses in Microbes, Animals, and Humans upon Exposure to Artificial Static Magnetic Fields

Author: János F. László

ISBN (eBook): 978-1-68108-102-1

ISBN (Print): 978-1-68108-103-8

First published in 2016.

Bentham Science Publishers Ltd.
Executive Suite Y - 2
PO Box 7917, Saif Zone
Sharjah, U.A.E.
Email: subscriptions@benthamscience.org

BENTHAM
SCIENCE

CONTENTS

Foreword

Dear highly distinguished reader,

Writing a foreword to a unique, fascinating, and excellent book is a great honor. The honor is combined with the feeling of pleasure and satisfaction as the whole creative process, the original concept, the brilliant ideas, as well as the experimental work I have known from the very beginning. The execution of original ideas needs enthusiasm, insistence, hard work, and first of all belief in that the concept is correct.

Dr. János F. László had original ideas, optimism, enthusiasm, and belief. He was a highly qualified physicist who approached the question of biological effects of static magnetic fields from the physicist's point of view. He aimed at obtaining legitimate evidence on the biological effects of static magnetic field under both *in vitro* and *in vivo* circumstances. In addition, he and his coworkers, collaborators, colleagues were not satisfied with providing merely a description of the effect of static magnetic field, but tried to clarify the mechanism of action, the time-dependency of the effect, and the "dose-dependency" of the SMF-induced action. Why is this important? Static magnetic field (SMF) therapy is used by large numbers of people for self-care all over the world; however, the SMF dosage, treatment regimens, and mechanism of action have not yet been established. Therefore, it is of utmost importance to elucidate, first under experimental conditions, the mechanism of action, the optimal duration to SMF exposure, and the effective dosage. The research initiated, carried out, and permanently stimulated by János László focused on these unanswered questions.

As the book quite adequately reflects, the analysis and examination of the biological actions of SMF were based on a well-designed systemic study. Experiments were carried out first in microorganisms (bacteria) than in mollusks, followed by mammals (mice and rats), and finally in humans. Thus, the book synthetizes the biological effects obtained from both animal and human subjects – and what is exceptional is that the outcome and conclusion were based on the author's own results – as opposed to the data in the literature. The final goal of all the studies was to establish the potency, efficacy, and safety of SMF which are the basis of its human application. Consequently, the results summarized in the present book have not only importance for basic science but also for clinical practice.

To my greatest sorrow, the preface cannot be finished by wishing the author further successful research and encouraging him to write the next volume about his newest findings. János László, shortly after finishing his excellent book, passed away leaving behind him many unanswered questions and unresolved problems. The present volume, however, will convince everyone that his oeuvre is complete, and this book which is based on wide collaboration of different fields of science will certainly constitute a determinant reference book for a long time in the field of magnetic field research.

February 24, 2015. **Prof. Dr. Klara Gyires MD, Phd, DSc**

Preface

I am fully aware of the risk I undertook when, accepting the challenge; I decided to write this book. The challenge appeared in a crystal clear form of a kind request from Bentham Science. This very distinguished publishing company expressed their feeling that my experience with static magnetic fields (SMF) may be of interest to a broader audience. I hope they were right…

I spent almost 2 decades in the research field of controlled thermonuclear fusion, while being employed at the Technical University of Budapest, Hungary. Stellarators use very complex external SMF to keep the plasma focused inside the vacuum vessel. When facing the problem of SMF-exposure on living organisms, I felt predestined to contribute to this unique and challenging exploration.

What do I mean when I say I undertook some risk? The effect of SMF-exposure on living tissues is namely like sport. Few have adequate knowledge about it, while many have opinion or prejudice. It is also not widely acknowledged that in the past 60 years, parallel with the discovery and development of nuclear magnetic resonance spectroscopy (NMRS) and its entry to medical diagnosis (as magnetic resonance imaging or MRI), serious research has been done resulting in 7 Nobel Prize winners. This made it all the more important to clarify whether the result of the diagnosis of MRI would have a correlation with the SMF-exposure itself. Let us immediately clear some points:

- An SMF exists that has a clinically significant analgesic and anti-inflammatory effect,
- This response relies in the biology of the subject itself mobilizing its own defense systems in overcoming pathological conditions.

Taking risks happens when strong motivation is at hand. I happen to have several. I wrote this book, because (i) I wanted to overview what we have done in the past 7 years in a concise form, (ii) I want to encourage fellow scientists to join us and share our efforts and victories, (iii) I am looking for sponsors who would provide sources for research but leave research independent.

I am often asked by laypeople as well as professionals whether this or that jewelry, band, mattress, pillow, or disk including permanent magnets, available in the market would really "act" as pain-killer or anti-inflammatory device. Well, my best answer to that query is "I don't know. They may." My experience tells me that there are some arrangements, structures of permanent magnets that exert measurable (patho)physiological effects when living tissues are exposed to it. Such arrangements are discussed in this book, which makes up for the evidence-based part of it. The scientifically non-evaluated and/or non-reproducible experiments with other arrangements "may still act". They certainly "act" at the psychosomatic level. The placebo effect induced by magnetic fields can rise up to 60%. Is this good or bad news? Placebo effect itself has a good reputation and an evidence-based foundation in medicine, and serves as one of the most effective therapeutical strategies in otherwise unmanageable diseases. It is inexpensive, it acts immediately, and it can have a long lasting beneficial effect. However, placebo also has side effects. Unfortunately, there's no such thing as a free lunch.

A well-founded hope is slowly evolving that we might create a method for analgesia and anti-inflammation that is at least as effective as conservative options but may have fewer side effects and interactions.

Is it really a surprise for the respected Reader that static magnetic fields (SMF) can affect a living object? An ever increasing annual number of publications reporting about evidence-based medical research prove that living objects respond to external magnetic fields in a wide range of frequencies. These results are briefly reviewed in the preliminaries of the chapters. However, I feel encouraged to concentrate on our own studies which provide the first pieces of evidence in some fundamental aspects of research that exposure to an external, artificial SMF can induce or assist certain (patho)physiological effects.

This book basically covers all phases of studies regarding the effect of SMF-exposure on living matters starting from *in vitro* assays, through *in vivo* experimental tests, ending with human trials. In the beginning, though, I must be a little more technical in order to introduce the fundamental steps of medical device development to the Reader. Most of the developmental steps follow the rule: The stronger, the longer lasting, and the more prompt the beneficial response to SMF-exposure compared to sham-exposure, the further we got with the optimization of the SMF-producing generator.

In all honesty, I must admit that not all experiments provided evidence for the beneficial effect of SMF-exposure on the specific biological response tested. Even if a positive response was found, we were not always convinced that it was the exclusive action of SMF-exposure. Therefore, we had to differentiate between several options to the best of our knowledge.

1. Is there really no effect that can be measured?
2. Would there be an effect if we chose a more appropriate model?
3. Can we still miss observability of an effect in a perfect model by superficial execution?

These are concerns probably every researcher must deal with. However, we have never encountered a situation in which the exposure in the applied magnetic induction range and the applied short periods of time would have caused negative (that is harmful) main or side effects.

Although the viability of a number of healthy microorganisms was tested *in vitro*, human lymphocytes and macrophages resulted in more interesting insight when SMF-exposure followed gamma-irradiation or lipopolysaccharide-activation. The Reader will soon realize that we spent most of our time with *in vivo* experimental research. The reason for this is that these tests have provided the most positive results; consequently, they were more applicable for device development. Within *in vivo* animal tests, we selected pain models in invertebrates and also in mammals, further divided into acute and chronic pain models, inflammation tests is mammals, as well as an allergy test. The human trials presented here must be considered incidental; nevertheless, they still open up new vistas of future research and development.

I am personally proud to have succeeded in getting a little beyond the level of phenomenology by revealing some of the possible background mechanisms in action. It seems obvious today that a living object that has self-motion in an external SMF is subject to an induced time-dependent magnetic flux and, consequently, to internal electric potential differences; however, the point whether these changes can be scientifically measured in the biological response is still open for discussion. A model is presented to physically correctly simulate and thus assess the generated magnetic potentials in rodents that move in an inhomogeneous SMF within geometric restraints.

When designing a model to test SMF-exposure, the first consideration, contrary to therapy, is (i) to expect a positive result. This condition was unfortunately very effective in limiting the number of models. (ii) Science in general must advance Based on experimental results; such results have either not yet existed or if existed, were ambiguous. (iii) The result should have a clinical relevance. Other factors that have also played a restricting role were (iv) time- and budget-restrictions. (v) Also, a laboratory should be picked for the measurement that has a traditional practice in the field of the model. This choice provided further advantages: The experience in the lab furnished us with immediately comparable results to those achieved with other (mostly chemical) agents in the same model. (vi) We started with *in vitro* and *in vivo* measurements where the role of placebo (and other psychosomatic) effects could be minimized. (vii) We always aimed at (but were not always successful in) repeating the experiment in another laboratory in order to check reproducibility. Another important point in the choice of experiment was the (viii) level of hospitality of the host institute for a new and important research field. I have astonishingly positive experiences with this latter factor.

Research in the field of SMF-induced or -assisted biological responses is a rather new, but very important and promising field with high expectations from both the research society as well as the average man. On one side of the topic is the knowledge we can gain from natural sciences: The method of nuclear core and electron resonance, the spectroscopy methods of molecular, even atomic resolution, and the quantum mechanics describing their operation. On the other side there is the knowledge we obtain from life sciences, where explanation is given on the level of receptors and enzymes. The imaginary tunnel of scientific cognition is bored from both sides. Although we are unfortunately far from joining the 2 bores, the present book hopefully serves as a step from the direction of receptors toward magnetic spins.

The manuscript of this book is based on materials published in 2 book chapters:

Series in Mathematics and Life Sciences 1 (Antoniouk AV, Melnik RVN Eds.), De Gruyter, Berlin, Germany, 2013, *pp*. 247-275.

Recent Developments in Brain Research 1 (Pandalai SG Ed.), Research Signpost, Kerala, India, 2012, *pp*. 1-43.

and in the following papers (in anti-chronologic order and alphabetic order of journal name within):

Authors	**Article title**	**External reference**	**Year**	**Reference page number in this book**	**Publisher**
Kiss B, Gyires K, Kellermayer M, László JF	Lateral gradients significantly enhance static magnetic field-induced inhibition of pain responses in mice—a double blind experimental study	Bioelectromagnetics 34:385-396		79, 97	Wiley
Mészáros Sz, Tabák AG, Horváth Cs, Szathmári M, László JF	Influence of local exposure to static magnetic field on pain perception and bone turnover of osteoporotic patients with vertebral deformity—a randomized controlled trial	International Journal of Radiation Biology 89:877-885	2013	241	Informa Healthcare
Vergallo C, Dini L, Szamosvölgyi Zs, Tenuzzo BA, Carata E, Panzarini E, László JF	*In vitro* analysis of the anti-inflammatory effect of inhomogeneous static magnetic field-exposure on human macrophages and lymphocytes	PLOS ONE 8:e72374		183	PLOS

Authors	Article title	External reference	Year	Reference page number in this book	Publisher
László JF, Hernádi L	Whole body static magnetic field exposure increases thermal nociceptive threshold in the snail, Helix pomatia	Acta Biologica Hungarica 63:441-452	2012	51	Akadémiai
László JF, Farkas P, Reiczigel J, Vágó P	Effect of local exposure to inhomogeneous static magnetic field on stomatological pain sensation a double-blind, randomized, placebo-controlled study	International Journal of Radiation Biology 88:430-438		215	Informa Healthcare
László JF, Pórszász R	Exposure to static magnetic field delays induced preterm birth occurrence in mice	American Journal of Obstetrics and Gynecology 205(4):362.e26-e31	2011	145	Elsevier
László JF, Szilvási J, Fényi A, Szalai A, Gyires K, Pórszász R	Daily exposure to inhomogeneous static magnetic field significantly reduces blood glucose level in diabetic mice	International Journal of Radiation Biology 87:36-45		133	Informa Healthcare
Kovács-Bálint Zs, Csathó Á, László JF, Juhász P, Hernádi I	Exposure to an inhomogeneous static magnetic field increases thermal pain threshold in healthy human volunteers	Bioelectromagnetics 32:131-139		197	Wiley
László JF, Kutasi J	Static magnetic field exposure fails to affect the viability of different bacteria strains	Bioelectromagnetics 31:220-225	2010	41	
Kubinyi Gy, Zeitler Zs, Thuróczy Gy, Juhász P, Bakos J, Sinay H, László J	Effects of homogeneous and inhomogeneous static magnetic fields combined with gamma radiation on DNA and DNA repair	Bioelectromagnetics 31:488-494		175	
László J, Pivec N	Effect of inhomogeneous static magnetic field on dental pain in humans	Clinical Journal of Pain 26:49-55		205	Wolters Kluwer
Gyires K, Zádori ZS Rácz B László J	Analysis of inhomogeneous static magnetic field-induced antinociceptive activity in mice	Progress in Electromagnetics Research Symposium Online 6:307-313		79, 97	PIERS Online

Authors	Article title	External reference	Year	Reference page number in this book	Publisher
Antal M, László J	Exposure to inhomogeneous static magnetic field ceases mechanical allodynia in neuropathic pain in mice	Bioelectromagnetics 30:438-445	2009	125	Wiley
László J, Tímár J, Gyarmati Zs, Fürst Zs, Gyires K	Pain-inhibiting inhomogeneous static magnetic field fails to influence locomotor activity and anxiety behavior in mice: No interference between magnetic field- and morphine-treatment	Brain Research Bulletin 79:316-321		63, 79	Elsevier
Gyires K László JF	3 T homogeneous static magnetic field of a clinical MR significantly inhibits pain in mice	Life Sciences 84:12-17		91	
Gyires K, Zádori ZS, Rácz B, László J	Pharmacological analysis of inhomogeneous static magnetic field-induced antinociceptive action in the mouse	Bioelectromagnetics 29:456-462	2008	117	Wiley
László J, Reiczigel J, Székely L, Gasparics A, Bogár I, Bors L, Rácz B, Gyires K	Optimization of static magnetic field parameters improves analgesic effect in mice	Bioelectromagnetics 28:615-627	2007	79	
Sándor K, Helyes Zs, Gyires K, Szolcsányi J, László J	Static magnetic field-induced anti-nociceptive effect and the involvement of capsaicin-sensitive sensory nerves in this mechanism	Life Sciences 81:97-102		71	Elsevier

The Reader must be warned though that this book does not aim to summarize the complete craftsmanship accumulated about the medical applications of SMF-exposure, neither can it reveal all the gaps in knowledge. It certainly tries to untangle some areas that seem to be important from the clinical viewpoint. This book is not intended to be a review even if it contains a large enough amount of references to start a research in this field for a newcomer. It basically accounts for the author's own experience in life sciences during the past 7 years. Having a background in electric engineering and a history of almost 2 decades of university physics lecturing, the biology-related topics collected in this book come from the fresh aspect of a particular and positively skeptic "outsider". By definition, a person is positively skeptic if he does not believe his own eyes, but is ready to learn, "to strive, to seek, to find, and not to yield" (from Alfred Lord Tennyson, English poet, 1809-1892). I personally take responsibility that every single statement I formulated in this book reflects evidence provided by our own experimental data, measured in the best possible way. Although double blinding could not always be carried out, we always strived after reproducibility.

In good faith,

János F. László,*
Budapest, Hungary, 2014
Email: anna.laszlo@connect.polyu.hk

*Dr. János F. László passed away after writing the manuscript. The book has been published posthumously. It is the manifestation of the author's deep dedication to science and it represents the helping hand that researchers can grab to further their research in this field.

Acknowledgement

I would never have been able to focus on the research enclosed in the present book without my family: My late parents, György and Éva László, my daughters, Anna and Júlia, and first of all my wife, Éva who has been a constant encouragement. Anna was an indispensable language corrector to this book.**

I am deeply grateful to my co-authors, I had the possibility to learn from and work with (in alphabetic order, **boldface** means multiple co-authorship):

Antal, Miklós	Bácsi, Attila	Bakos, József
Barnea, Eytan R.	Bogár, István	Boldogh, István
Bors, László	Carata, Elisabetta	Csathó, Árpád
Csillag, Anikó	Dini, Luciana	Domokos, Csaba
Ertl-Wagner Birgit	Farkas, Péter	Fényi, Anett
Fülöp, Vilmos	Fürst, Zsuzsanna	Gasparics, Antal
Gődény, Mária	Gyarmati, Zsuzsa	**Gyires, Klára**
Hajagos, Imre	Helyes, Zsuzsanna	Hernádi, István
Hernádi, László	Horváth, Csaba	Juhász, Márk
Juhász, Péter	Kamm, Katharina	Kásler, Miklós
Kellermayer, Miklós, Jr.	**Kiss, Balázs**	Kocsis, Dorottya
Kónya, Attila	Kotlán, Beatrix	Kovács-Bálint, Zsófia
Kuba, Attila	Kubinyi-Kaszás, Györgyi	Kumar, V. Brahma
Kutasi, József	Laubender, P. Rüdiger	Mészáros, Szilvia
Nagy, Viktor	Naszádos, György	Németh, József
Panzarini, Elisa	Papp, Zsuzsa	Pázmándi, Kitti
Pivec, Natalia	Pomschar, Andreas	**Pórszász, Róbert**
Rácz, Bernadette	Rajnavölgyi, Éva	**Reiczigel, Jenő**
Reiser, Maximilian	Ruscheweyh, Ruth	Sándor, Katalin
Sinay, Hanna	Solténszky, Judit	Straube, Andreas
Szabó, Krisztina	**Szalai, Andrea**	Szamosvölgyi, Zsuzsa
Szathmári, Miklós	Székely, Hajnal	Székely, László
Szilasi, Magdolna	Szilasi, Mária	Szilvási, Judit
Szolcsányi, János	Tabák, Ádám	Tenuzzo, Bernadetta Anna
Thuróczy, György	Tímár, Júlia	Tóvári, József

**After the passing away of the author, his wife, Éva and his daughter, Anna provided inmense help with the final editing of the manuscript.

Tulassay, Zsolt	Újhelyi, Judit	Újhelyi, Zoltán
Vágó, Péter	Vecsernyés, Miklós	Vergallo, Cristian
Zádori, Zoltán	Zeitler, Zsuzsa	

Those below contributed to my work as well to various extents. Something they did or said was important for me. I wish they were still all among us!

Ádám, Ágnes	Ádám, György	Ádám, Veronika	Alfano, Alan P.
Allan, Basbaum	Anand, Anjali	Andócs, Gábor	Antoniouk, Alexandra
Antonyák, Dóra	Antos, László	Antus, Balázs	Arányi, Péter
Arz, Gusztáv	Aszódi, Attila	Aszódi, József	Bábás, Géza
Bak, Erzsébet	Balassa, Tímea	Balázs, András	Bálint, Géza
Balogh, Tamás	Bancu, Ligia	Bánfalvi, Gáspár	Baranyi, Attila
Baráth, Zita	Bárdos, György	Barnea, Jacqueline	Bársony, István
Bartha, Viktória	Barthó, Lóránd	Basbaum, Allan	Battistig, Gábor
Bazyka, Dimitrij	Beck, Mihály	Bedőcs, József	Békeffy, Magdolna
Bencsik, Attila	Bencze, Pál	Benczúr, András, Jr.	Bender, Tamás
Benkó, Rita	Benyó, Zoltán, Jr.	Benyó, Zoltán, Sr.	Berkes, István
Berta, István	Bertha, Prieto	Beu, Titus	Bíró, Oszkár
Bíró, Péter	Boda, Miklós	Bognár, Gábor	Böhm, Gabriella
Bojtár, Imre	Bokotey, Sándor	Bozó, László	Brooks, William M.
Brückner, Huba	Buka, Ágnes	Bunyitai, Péter	Bushnell, Catherine M.
Búzás, Norbert	Capretti, Eleonora	Carmela, Marino	Carter, Amy
Ceruti, Stefania	Chass, Gregory	Chen, Jane	Chira, Kornél
Chit, Allan W	Colbert, P. Agatha	Csajági, Dezső	Csajági, Eszter
Csányi, Vilmos	Csendes, Tibor	Csépe, Valéria	Cser, Lajos
Csermely, Péter	Csikász, Tamás	Csillag, András	Csirik, János
Csirmaz, László	Csizmadia, Imre	Dagny, Sandnes	Damjanovich, Sándor
Daniela, Giuliani	De Chatel, Rudolf	De Vocht, Frank	Del Carmen L.L., Maria
Demcsik, Tamás	Demeter, Ildikó	Demeter, Kornél	Derka, István
Dixon, Dianne	Dóczi, Tamás	Dona, Maria Gabriella	Drochon, Agnès
Ducza, Eszter	Duda, Ernő, Jr.	Duncan, Lindsay	Dux, Mária
Eccles, Nyjon	Ecsery-Puskás, Mariann	Edison, S. Arthur	Elekes, Károly
Erkel, András	F. Tóth, Katalin	Fábián, Csaba	Faigel, Gyula
Falkay, György	Falus, András	Farkas, Norbert	Fazekas, István

Fehér, Andor
Fehér, János
Ferenc, Mária
Ferenczi, János
Ferenczy, Ira
Fésűs, László
Feuer, Éva
Fidy, Judit
Finberg, John
Finet, Michel
Fleming, Braden
Földesi, István
Fórizs, Szabolcs
Frank, Tibor
Friedman, Merle
Fritz, József
Fülesdi, Béla
Füstöss, László
Gál, András Levente
Gál, Dezső
Galloni, Paolo
Garab, Kinga
Garami, Miklós
Garami, Péter
Gáspár, Rezső
Gáspár, Róbert
Georgescu, Lia
Gera, István
Gerasimova, Elena
Gerber, Gábor
Gergely, János
Ghavanini, Ali
Giamberardino, M. Adele
Glassy, Mark
Gmitrov, Juraj
Gödény-Polónyi, Mária
Goldstein, E. Lee
Golik, Ahuva
Gornto, Deborah
Goubert, Dorien
Grosz, Ferenc
Gundy, Sarolta
Gupta, Aditya
Gürgen, Gülşen
Gyarmati, Gábor
Gyires, Béla
Győri, János
Gyulai, József
Hagymási, Miklós
Haney, Theresa
Haris, Ágnes
Hárs, Titanilla
Harta, Gyöngyi
Härtlein, Károly
Hartyánszky, István
Hatvani, László
Hauser, Péter
Hável Szatmári, Katalin
Hay, Diana
Hegedűs, Krisztina
Hegedűs, Lajos
Hegyi, Gabriella
Heinen, Florian
Hermans, James
Hermecz, István
Hofstetter, Harald
Holden, Arun V.
Hollósy, Ferenc
Horkay, Ferenc
Horváth, Ildikó
Horváth, Ilona
Horváth, Katalin
Horváth, Teréz
Hristov, Jordan
Huang, Haw-Ming
Hunyadi, László
Hunyadi-Gulyás, Éva
Ilijin, Larisa
Imre, Enikö
Imre, Mihály
Indig, Fred E.
Ivanics, Tamás
Iványi, Amália
Jagasics, Zoltán
Jancsó, Gábor
Jandó, Gábor
Jokela, Kari
Juhász, Béla
Juhász, Gábor
Kálmánchey, Rozália
Kapitány, Erika
Kapusi, Katalin
Kardon, Béla
Kardon, Tamás
Kardos, Júlia
Kaszuba, Jolanta
Kató, Erzsébet
Kékesi, Katalin
Kele, Krisztina
Kellényi, Lóránd
Kempler, Péter
Kereszty, Marcell
Kern, András
Keszthelyi, Gabriella
Keviczky, László
Kieffer, Brigitte
Kígyós, Attila
Kincses, Anna
Kindert, Judit
Kiss, Anikó
Kiss, Szilvia
Klein, Rebecca C.
Klukovits, Anna
Kóbor, István
Koczkás, Andrea
Kökény, Gábor
Koltai, Gábor
Komoly, Sámuel
Korcsmáros, Tamás
Körmendi, Sándor
Kovács, Adrienn
Kovács, Gábor
Kovács, Ilona
Kovats, R. Sari
Kozsurek, Márk
Krajcsi, Péter
Krisbai, István
Kriszbacher, Ildikó
Kroó, Norbert
Kun, Chim
Kürti, Jánosné
Kurutz-Kovács, Márta
Labancz, Anita
Laczkó, József
Lafrenie, Robert
Láng, István
László, Ádám
Le Chapellier, Pierre
Lénárd, László
Lerchner, Szilvia

Lévai Horváth, Éva	Lin, James C.	Liu, John	Long, Fanxin
Lörincz, Sándor	Lovász, László	Lovász, Sándor	Lovisolo, Giorgo
Lukowiak, Ken	Lusik, Uljana	Macsi, Magdolna	Madarász, Emília
Magyar, Éva	Magyar, János	Magyar, László	Makara, B. Gábor
Marino, Carmela	Markó, Katalin	Markov, S. Marko	Marku, István
Márta, Ildikó	Marton, Sylvia	McGhee, Kamilla	McLean, Michael
Medzihradszky, Katalin	Méreg, Zsuzsa	Meskó, Attila	Miheller, Pál
Mihók, Ildikó	Miklós, Zsuzsanna	Miklósi, József	Mikus, Endre
Milne, Ruth	Mischorr, Margret	Mituszova, Ludmilla	Möbius, Anja
Mojzes, Imre	Möller, Harald E.	Molnár, Csilla	Molnár, Imre
Molnár, Lajos	Molnár, Tünde	Mónos, Emil	Murthy, Narasimha
Nagy, Csilla	Nagy, Pál	Nemes, Réka	Német, Jánosné
Németh, Tamás	Németh, Vilmos	Nguyen, Xuan Trang	Niedeczky, Csaba
Nyerki, Emil	Oláh, Zoltán	Oláh, Zsuzsa	Orbán, György
Ormos, Pál	Orosz, Jenő	Orosz, László	Osváth, Szabolcs
Pach, János	Pachner, Orsolya	Pajor, Attila	Pakucs, János
Pál, László	Pálinkás, József	Palkovits, Miklós	Pandalai, Shankar
Pannonhalmi, Kálmán	Papp, László	Papp, Zoltán	Párducz, Árpád
Patkós, Ildikó	Pázmány, Tamás	Peng, Shang	Penke, Botond
Perczel, András	Perjésné, Judit	Pethö, Attila	Petrányi, Győző
Pfützner, Helmut	Pintér, Erika	Pintz, János	Pioli, Claudio
Pizzorno, Joseph	Pléh, Csaba	Pocsai, Enikő	Polgár Májer, Ildikó
Pollack, Gerald	Pomogaibog, Olga	Pongorné, Cs. Mariann	Poniedziaek, Barbara
Poór, Gyula	Powers, Tamara	Prékopa, András	Prieto, Bertha
Pucsok, József	Pungor, Ernő	Puskás, Zsolt	Rácz, Károly
Rácz, Sándor	Rajkovits, Zsuzsa	Rapcsák, Tamás	Rauer, Heiko
Rauth, Michael	Ravazzani, Paolo	Regös, Ágnes	Reisz, Judit
Reith, János	Reményi, Edit	Remenyik, Bence	Réthelyi, Miklós
Révész, Mónika	Rigó, János	Ristic, Goran	Romics, Imre
Rónyai, Lajos	Rosen, Arthur	Rosivall, László	Roska, Tamás
Rothermich, Wayne	Rudas, Gábor	Rudy, Yoram	Salamon, Gábor
Salczer, Rita	San, Naty	Sandell, Linda	Sántha, Péter
Schmaus, János	Schuler, Ágnes	Schuler, Dezső	Schulteisz-Takács, Mária
Seaman, Ronald	Sebestyén, Imre	Segars, Paul	Sert, Cemil
Shi, Jiong	Shultz, Lenny	Siklós, László	Simkó, Myrtill

Simon, Jürgen	Simonovits, Emília	Sindrup, H. Søren	Sípos, Alíz
Smith, J. C.	Soltész, Pál	Somogyi, Miklós	Sós, Péter János
Sperlágh, Beáta	Stépán, Gábor	Stoyan, Gisbert	Strausz, János
Summerfield, Claire	Süth, Zsuzsa	Szabó, Emese	Szabó, Erika
Szabó, Izabella	Szabó, Sándor	Szabó, Szilvia	Szabó, Zsolt
Szakács-Nemere, Györgyi	Szalai, Istvánné	Szalai, László	Szalkó, Márta
Szamkó, Gabriella	Szántó, András	Szász, András	Szász, G. Krisztián
Szász, Máté	Szatmári, István	Szegö, Károly	Szeidl, László
Szekeres, Béla	Szél, Ágoston	Szemerszky, Renáta	Szemes, Imre
Szendrői, Miklós	Szieb, Katalin	Szigeti, Gyula	Szigetlaki, Zsolt
Szivi, Orsolya	Szőllősi, János	Szombathy, István	Szondy, Zsuzsanna
Szűcs, Attila	Takács, Gyula	Teodori, Laura	Tholkes, Katie
Thownsend, John	Tigyi, Attila	Tókos, Edit	Tolnai, Márton
Tompa, Kálmán	Torgyán, Sándor	Tóth, András	Tóth, Andrea
Tóth, Ferenc	Tóth, G. László	Tóth, Veronika	Traikov, Lubomir
Tretter, László	Tuba, István	Turi, Gabriella	Tusnády, Gábor
Ulbert, István	Urbán-Szabó, Katalin	Van Rongen, Eric	Varga, Mária
Várkonyi, László	Vas, Ádám	Vécsei, László	Vecsernyés, Miklós
Végh, János	Vehovszky, Ágnes	Vékás, Gusztáv	Vellai, Tibor
Vértessy, Gábor	Veszely, Gyula	Vidnyánszky, Zoltán	Vígh, Béla
Vizi, E. Szilveszter	Walsh, Linda	Wikonkál, Éva	Wisnovszky, Ágnes
Wittner, Lucia	Wöhrle, Natalie	Wolf, János	Wood, Andrew W.
Worthington, Brad	Yokuş, Beran	Yu, Shuguang	Zempléni, András
Zhan, Wei	Zilahy, Péter	Zoller, Vilmos	Zombory, László
Zsidó, László	Zupkó, István		

Professor Vizi, then President of the Hungarian Academy of Sciences was the open-minded researcher, who directed me to the Department of Pharmacology and Pharmacotherapy at Semmelweis University in the very beginning of my interest. Here Professor Klára Gyires took me under her wings. The cooperation and later friendship with her holds ever since.

Special thanks are due to my young colleagues (beyond co-authors, in alphabetic order):

Balaton, Attila, Loránd Eötvös University (student)
Keszthelyi, Gabriella, Loránd Eötvös University (student)
Kóbor, István, Péter Pázmány Catholic University (Ph.D. student)
Lerchner, Szilvia, Loránd Eötvös University (student)
Sándor, András, Kaposvár University (Ph.D. student)
Szabó Emerencia, Loránd Eötvös University (student)
Wittner, Lucia, Hungarian Academy of Sciences (Bolyai grant awardee)
Horváth, Katalin, Loránd Eötvös University (student)
Kézér, Tamás, Loránd Eötvös University (student)
Kozsurek, Márk, Semmelweis University (Ph.D. student)
Molnár, Tünde, Hungarian Academy of Sciences (Ph.D. student)
Slozár, Zsófia, Loránd Eötvös University (student)
Szekeres, Béla, Loránd Eötvös University (student)

It was an honor to have the opportunity of cooperating with the following institutions (in alphabetic order, **boldface** means multiple occasions):

• Budapest University of Technology and Economics, Budapest, Hungary: Broadband Infocommunicatons and Electromagnetic Theory Department
• Central Institute of Stomatology, Budapest, Hungary:
• L'Energia e l'Ambiente: Section of Toxicology and Biomedical Sciences, Ente per le Nuove Tecnologie, Casaccia, Italy
• **"Frédéric Joliot-Curie" National Research Institute for Radiobiology and Radiohygiene, Budapest, Hungary: Department of Non-Ionizing Radiation**
• Hungarian Academy of Sciences, Hungary:
  ○ Biological Research Centre, Szeged, Institute of Biophysics
  ○ **Centre for Ecological Research, Balaton Limnological Institute, Department of Experimental Zoology**
  ○ Chemical Research Center, Department of Neurochemistry
  ○ Computer and Automation Research Institute, Cellular Sensory and Optical Wave Computing Laboratory
  ○ Institute for Technical Physics and Materials Science
  ○ Institute of Cognitive Neuroscience and Psychology, Research Group of Comparative Psychophysiology
  ○ Institute of Experimental Medicine, Department of Gene Technology and Developmental Neurobiology
• Loránd Eötvös University, Budapest, Hungary:
  ○ Institute of Biology, Department of Genetics
  ○ **Institute of Mathematics, Department of Applied Analysis and Computational Mathematics**
• Ludwig-Maximilians-Universität München: Institut für Klinische Radiologie, Grosshadern, Germany

- Medical University of Sofia: Department of Medical Physics and Biophysics, Sofia, Bulgaria
- National Institute of Oncology, Budapest, Hungary:
  - Department of Experimental Pharmacology
  - Department of Radiological Diagnostics
  - **Surgical and Molecular Tumor Pathology Centre**
- National Research Council: Istituto di Ingegneria Biomedica, Milano, Italy
- Péter Pázmány Catholic University, Budapest, Hungary: Ányos Jedlik Research and Development Laboratory
- Politecnico di Milano: Dipartimento di Bioingegneria, Milano, Italy
- Pro Vitae Hospital: 1st Department of Internal Medicine, Gelnica, Slovak Republic
- Semmelweis University, Budapest, Hungary:
  - 1st Department of Internal Medicine
  - 2nd Department of Internal Medicine
  - 2nd Department of Obstetrics and Gynaecology
  - 2nd Department of Paediatrics
  - Department of Anatomy, Histology and Embryology
  - Department of Biophysics and Radiation Biology
  - Department of Human Morphology and Developmental Biology
  - Department of Medical Biochemistry
  - Department of Neurology
  - Department of Orthopaedics
  - Department of Pathophysiology
  - **Department of Pharmacology and Pharmacotherapy**
  - **Institute of Human Physiology and Clinical Experimental Research**
  - Szentágothai János Knowledge Centre
  - University Pharmacy Department of Pharmacy Administration
- Universidad Nacional Autónoma de Mexico: Departamento de Fisiología, Facultad de Medicina, Mexico City, Mexico
- University of Debrecen, Debrecen, Hungary:
  - Department of Anatomy, Histology and Embryology
  - Department of Pharmaceutical Technology
  - Institute of Immunology
  - **Institute of Pharmacology and Pharmacotherapy**
- University of Medicine and Pharmacy, Tirgu Mures, Romania:
  - 2nd Department of Internal Medicine
  - Department of Rheumatology

• University of Pécs, Pécs, Hungary:
  Department of Pharmacology and Pharmacotherapy
  ○ Institute of Behavioral Sciences
  ○ Institute of Biology, Department of Experimental Animals and Neurobiology
• University of Strasburg: Institute of Genetics and Molecular and Cellular Biology, Strasburg, France
• University of Szeged, Szeged, Hungary:
  ○ Institute of Informatics, Department of Image Processing and Computer Graphics
  ○ Institute of Mathematics, Department of Analysis
  ○ Institute of Pharmacotherapy and Biopharmacy
  ○ Institute of Physiology
• Universitá del Salento: Laboratory of Comparative Anatomy and Cytology, Department of biological, environmental science and technology, Lecce, Italy

Companies that helped my work (in alphabetic order, boldface means multiple occasions):

• Albitech Ltd., Hungary
• **Borsmagnet Ltd., Hungary**
• **ChenYang Technologies, Germany**
• Dentsana-TA Ltd., Hungary
• **e-Comers LLC., Hungary**
• Exasol Ltd., Hungary
• Gradient Technologies LLC, USA
• Innovo Ltd., Hungary
• Neuromagnetics Australia Pty Ltd., Australia
• **Optometal Ltd., Hungary**
• Procura Ltd., Hungary
• Saniplant Ltd., Hungary
• Supertech Ltd., Hungary
• Tenerum Ltd., Hungary
• **Toxi-coop Ltd., Hungary**

The following grants were used in the research projects included in this book (in alphabetic order):

• Alexander von Humboldt research grant
• Bridging Fund 2012 from Faculty of Medicine Research Fund from the University of Debrecen

• Egészségügyi Tudományos Tanács (ETT 079/2006, 284/2006, and 529/2006)
• Natural Rural Development Plan (NRDP1A/005/2004)
• Nemzeti Kutatási és Technológiai Hivatal (NKTH: INNO 2006-0249 and 2009-0248)
• Országos Tudományos Kutatási Alap (OTKA F-046635, NK-101538, K-73347, K-109595, K-72120, and T-046589)
• Társadalmi Megújulás Operatív Program (TÁMOP 4.2.2/B-10/1-2010-0024, TÁMOP 4.2.4.A/2-11-1-2012-0001, TÁMOP-4.2.2.C-11/1/KONV-2012-0001, TÁMOP-4.2.2.--11/1/KONV-2012-0023)
• US National Institute of Health (RET-008/2005)

Last but not least, a big thank you is due to the publisher, specifically Ms. Humaira Hashmi and Ms. Hira Aftab, for her continuous help, support, and encouragement with regard to the finishing touches of this manuscript. Thank you!

CONFLICT OF INTEREST

The author confirms that author has no conflict of interest to declare for this publication.

Dedication

To my daughters, Anna and Júlia,
the greatest motivators

2

CHAPTER 1

Introduction

A special tribute is due here to those Hungarian researchers who substantiated the area of biophysics dealing with how different living tissues respond to SMF-exposure. Júlia Lengyel, a Hungarian physicist, was probably the first scientist, to have "scientifically conducted investigations" on SMF-exposure-related issues specifically on cancer more than 80 years ago [1] as referred to in the 2nd chapter: "Rejection of transplanted tumors in mice" by J. Barnóthy in the book Biological Effects of Magnetic Fields first published in 1964 [2]. The Barnóthy family, Jenő (who died 20 years ago) and Madeleine (born Magda Forró 110 years ago) primarily deserve the Reader's attention since they worked and published extensively in the area.

The present book does not need to prove that natural SMF like that of the Earth otherwise known as geomagnetic field influences living objects in multiple modalities. This fact has been evidenced and can be regarded as notorious. In the course of the 100 million years of phylogenesis, living organisms have gotten used to the geomagnetic field which has a vertical component of 43.6814 μT, a North-South component of 21.1571 μT, and an East-West component of 1.5483 μT at the place and in the time of my writing this text, 150 m above sea level [3]. Some animals developed special receptors that assist them in navigation. Magnetotactic bacteria [4], migratory fish, and bird species [5] have such animal "GPS". A receptor sensitivity level of 2 orders of magnitude below geomagnetic field induction of the Lorenzini ampoules help cartilaginous fish (rays and sharks) detect the hidden prey [6]. It has recently been revealed that even a type of mammal (a bat species) uses the geomagnetic field for navigation [7].

Human habitat on Earth creates a very complex system. Concentrating on merely natural magnetic phenomena, we can create a triangle with the vertices magnetism, climate, and biosphere, see Fig. (**1.1**). It has not yet been decided whether the geomagnetic field has a direct measurable effect on mammals, but little doubt occurs as to whether its changes in time cause measurable responses [8, 9].

János F. László

Alterations in the geomagnetic fields, on the other hand undoubtedly lead to climate changes. Needless to say that this indirect effect of the magnetic field determines the health of a human, *i.e.* his homeostasis [10].

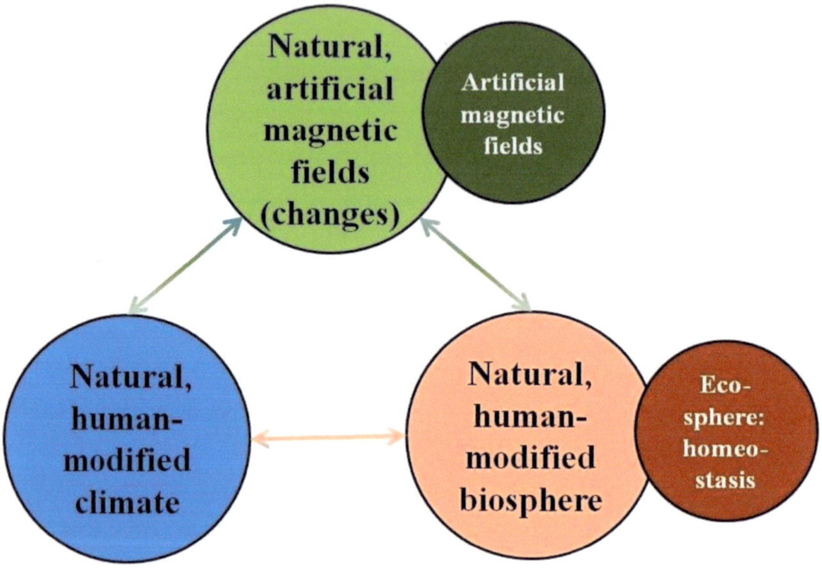

Fig. (1.1). Model of human habitat concerning magnetism, the essence of which is that the effects are introduced through time-dependence.

All 3 above mentioned components are interrelated directly as well as indirectly. The present book will allow me to focus only on a small but singular part of this complex system: The relationship between artificial SMF and human homeostasis within the global ecological biosphere.

We can suppose that the effect of artificial SMF-exposure on humans is also widely known. Nuclear magnetic resonance spectroscopy (NMR) was invented in 1945. Later, in the seventies it was completed with scanning and computer image processing, and was called magnetic resonance imaging (MRI). MRI has since become an important tool as a non-invasive method in modern medical diagnostics primarily useful for soft tissues. The importance of NMR (and MRI) has been punctuated 7 times so far, when 9 excellent scientists were rewarded with the Nobel Prize: Otto Stern in 1943, Isidor I. Rabi in 1944, Felix Bloch and Edward Purcell in 1952, Richard Ernst in 1966, Nicolaas Bloembergen in 1981,

Kurt Wüthrich in 2002, Paul C. Lauterbur and Sir Peter Mansfield in 2003. Raymond V. Damadian was the first in 1971 who initiated the “MRI industry” with his publication in Science as well as with the first whole-body diagnosis [11]. Magnetic fields were in the focus of research of Hendrik A. Lorentz and Pieter Zeeman, who won a Nobel Prize in 1902, Willis E. Lamb and Polykarp Kusch were awarded in 1955, while Robert B. Laughlin, Horst L. Störmer, and Daniel C. Tsui received one in 1998.

One current concern of MRI designers is how to improve visual resolution. One method is relatively straightforward; the SMF component of the MRI, B_0 should be increased. One of the first commercial MRI devices had a B_0 of 50 mT; companies today offer a wide range of machines in the 3-14 T range. Such high fields can be sustained exclusively by superconductive magnets, the cooling of which requires significant technical background, maintenance, and huge overhead costs.

Since the European Union (EU) banned the trade restrictions regarding the sale of medical devices with permanent magnets in 2002, the market was swarmed with “magic” and “enchanting” devices for practically all purposes: The same apparatus would increase low blood pressure (BP), while decreasing high BP at the same time. The question obviously arose: Do these devices have any influence on the human organism beyond psychosomatics?

SMF-exposure (MRI included) has progressed step by step to become a broadly examined physical agent; the database of NCBI (National Center for Biotechnology Information, in short PubMed) produces the following time development (Table **1.1**) if searched for “static magnetic”:

Table 1.1. Number of publications in PubMed database, which contain “static magnetic” in the decades after 1960.

	before 1960	sixties	seventies	eighties	nineties
number of publications	1	10	31	258	1136

Similar data for this century until February 14, 2014 (Table **1.2**):

Table 1.2. Similarly to Table 1.1 detailed for years starting with year 2000.

	2000	**1**	**2**	**3**	**4**	**5**	**6**	**7**	**8**	**9**	**10**	**11**	**12**	**13**	**14**
number of publications	259	259	233	282	312	380	412	405	436	469	503	522	527	498	53+?
5 year sum	1345					2102					2103+?				
10 year sum	3447														

The numbers are probably not exact. They are partly low estimates because PubMed does not have a track record for the far past (most publications before 1960 have never made it into the database); they are partly high estimates because publications may have been included that have nothing to do with life sciences. All in all, the trend is probably true that the number of publication shows an almost monotonic rise in time. Both World Health Organization (WHO) and the EU require such research. The importance of the therapeutic applications of SMF and the knowledge we lack in this field of science is reflected in the report of WHO from 2006 [12] in the Research Agenda for Static Fields: Introduction): "For static magnetic fields, research carried out to date has not been systematic and has often been performed without appropriate methodology and exposure information. Coordinated research programs are recommended as an aid to a more systematic approach. There is a need to investigate the importance of physical parameters such as field intensity, exposure duration and field gradient on biological outcome."

Here is another citation issued by Scientific Committee on Emerging and Newly Identified Health Risks of the EU from 2009 [13], in the Health Effects of EMF Exposure, Abstract): "Although a fair number of studies have been published since the last opinion, the conclusion drawn there stands: There is still a lack of adequate data for a proper risk assessment of static magnetic fields. More research is necessary, especially to clarify the many mixed and sometimes contradictory results. Short term effects have been observed primarily on sensory functions for acute exposure. However, there is no consistent evidence for sustained adverse health effects from short term exposure up to several teslas."

The official statement of WHO and the EU in effect says that up to a magnetic induction of 8 T, the human body will not be jeopardized by an external SMF. A fresh statement was due in 2008 about devices with higher fields but due to the lack of experimental research data, the EU postponed the issuance [14]. Instead, SCENIHR published the report mentioned above [13] about the potential hazards of SMF-exposure in January 2009.

The secret to the beauty of this research field lies in its complexity, its interdisciplinary or rather transdisciplinary nature. Without being exhaustive, Fig. (**1.2**) shows some of the inter- and trans-connected areas.

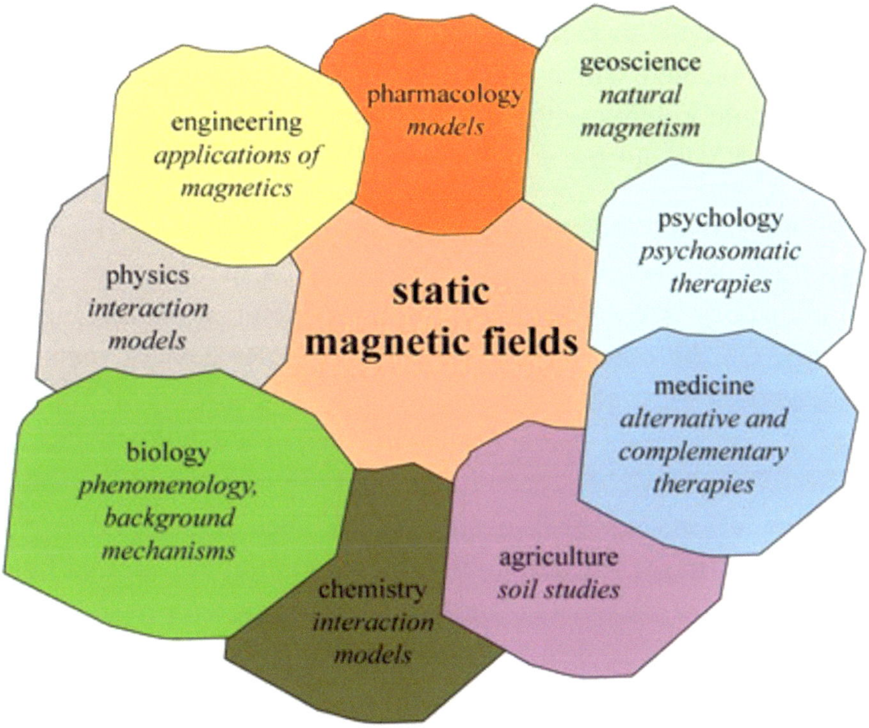

Fig. (1.2). Inter- and transdisciplinarity among different research areas dealing with static magnetic fields.

The description of SMF and the circles of application belong to physics. The generation of SMF is typically a task for technical and material sciences. The effects caused concern the field of biology and medicine affecting geosciences (natural SMF), psychology (psychosomatic therapies), agriculture (plant, soil bacteria), and chemistry (interaction models). Last but not least, we have mathematics providing the basis of all models including science supplying statistical models. The research detailed in this book is therefore, a field to be regarded as not only multi- and interdisciplinary, but also transdisciplinary since there is not only an overlap between fields, but in some cases these areas are inseparable.

Here are some world record holder SMF, just for the Reader's information. A fully functional SMF generator in the USA at Los Alamos National Lab produced 100.73 T magnetic induction in pulse mode. The maximum achievable magnetic induction today in continuous mode is 45 T. This device can be found at the National High Magnetic Field Laboratory in Tallahassee (Florida, USA) belonging to Florida State University. The exposure chamber for experimental use contains 15 sample holders with a diameter of 32 mm each. The generator is powered by a 29.3 MW electric supply.

In spite of the amount of publications providing medical evidence for the beneficial effects SMF-exposure can exert on living matter, a researcher must keep his obligatory skepticism due to the difficulties comparing different measurements. On the other hand, the spread of MRI devices (many hundred thousand diagnoses were going on around the world already in 2009) and the increase of B_0 components make it not only important but also necessary to conduct research in this field. Accordingly, a large part of physiological research concerning the effects of SMF-exposure has been started on a pure epidemiological basis. In these studies, those persons who work around functioning MRI devices are under examination since they are exposed for longer time periods and/or more frequently to fringe fields around MRI devices. Similarly, an increased risk may be attributed to particle accelerators in high energy labs, affecting research personnel. There is an increased duration of SMF-exposure to some workers in special areas of industry, such as aluminum processing or accumulator production. At these locations regular medical surveillance and check-up are compulsory.

If electrically charged particles (objects) move in an external SMF with non-relativistic velocities with a component non-parallel to the SMF, the SMF diverts the particles from their original path as described by the Lorentz force. Living tissues consist of electrically charged particles most of which are in motion even if the object itself is stationary. There is no wonder that SMF-exposure becomes a crucial factor. The question, therefore, is whether such effects remain observable even if the *ab ovo* magnetic disorder in the mostly diamagnetic matter (of water) and the induced elevated heat transfer show a trend of reducing the effect below measurable thresholds.

Some suggest that the magnetic interaction is only indirectly responsible for the physiological effects induced by electromagnetic fields (including zero frequency, SMF). Time-dependent magnetic fields generate a magnetic flux on a certain surface (transformer induction) that causes an electric potential difference, and this can lead to the production of electric currents. The other possible source of induction can be if a conductor moves within a homogeneous or inhomogeneous SMF (motion induction). When a patient is moved into the bore of a 3 T MRI from a magnetic background of some mT in a path of 1 m within a time period of 20 s, his body is exerted to a sudden gradient in the SMF in the 3 T/m range. This is an extreme magnetic and, thus, electric load for the body. It is widely accepted that the human body is rather sensitive to changes in electric current densities. Magnetic induction concerns neuroscience since the peripheral nerves are the most sensitive parts in our body to get stimulated by external magnetic fields. These peripheral nerves are our primary SMF receptors specialized to sense electric currents as well. For their stimulus, 480 mA/m^2 electric current density [15] or 40 T/s magnetic induction change [16] seem to be satisfactory.

As mentioned before, even a human body at rest is subject to changes in the magnetic flux in a perfectly homogeneous SMF. Without self-motion there are numerous currents in the body carrying electric charges, electrons, ions, and charged molecules. Before being examined, the patient's head will be fixed on the table of the MRI. Even so, patients often complain about unusual sensations at one or multiple modalities of perception: Sparkling stars (phosphenes, visual leve l), nausea or vomiting (proprioceptive level), vertigo (vestibular level), metal taste (gustatory level), and/or headache (multimodal level). These symptoms are probably primarily due to magneto-hydrodynamic interactions [17] and as a consequence, simultaneous inputs in the brain get into conflict [18].

Taking into account the scanning function of a clinical MRI, the complicated picture becomes even more implied. The B_1 component of the MRI is a gradient SMF, which is not only a varying SMF in all 3 dimensions in space, but is a time-switching SMF as well. The research exploring the effects of such SMF is a separate area of research [19] and will not be discussed in the present book.

What role can SMF-exposure have in therapy? As an example let us look at neuropathic pain... Neuropathic pain affects 44-98 million people worldwide. The lower estimate does not include patients with low-back pain associated with neuropathy. Neuropathic pain has long-term consequences regarding the quality of life of the patient as well as his insurance costs. Neuropathy is a disease of the nervous system. The 3 major forms of nerve damage are: Peripheral neuropathy, autonomic neuropathy, and mononeuropathy. Neuropathy is classified according to its cause: Diabetic peripheral neuropathy 0.6%, postherpetic neuralgia 0.5%, cancer-associated 0.2%, spinal cord injury 0.12%, causalgia and reflex sympathetic dystrophy 0.1%, multiple sclerosis 0.05%, phantom pain 0.05%, post stroke 0.03%, human immuno-deficiency virus (HIV)-associated 0.015%, trigeminal neuralgia (tic douloureux) 0.015%, low-back pain-associated 2.1% in % in 100,000 cases [20]. Nerve damage is likely due to a combination of factors: Metabolic factors (high blood glucose, long duration of diabetes, possibly low levels of insulin, and abnormal blood fat levels), neurovascular factors leading to damage to the blood vessels that carry oxygen and nutrients to the nerves, autoimmune factors that cause inflammation in nerves, mechanical injury to nerves (carpal tunnel syndrome), inherited traits that increase susceptibility to nerve disease, lifestyle factors such as smoking or alcohol consumption. Its symptoms are: Allodynia, anesthesia, dysesthesia, hyperalgesia, hyperpathia, hypoesthesia, paresthesia, phantom pain, referred pain including numbness, tingling, or pain in the toes, feet, legs, hands, arms, and fingers, wasting of the muscles of the feet or hands, indigestion, nausea, or vomiting, diarrhea or constipation, dizziness or faintness due to a drop in postural BP, problems with urination, erectile dysfunction (impotence) or vaginal dryness and weakness.

Pain attached to neuropathy (diabetic peripheral neuropathy, post herpes neuralgia, tumoral disease, injury of the spinal marrow or multiple sclerosis, phantom pain, pain following stroke and trigeminus neuralgia, lower back pain) causes long-lasting decrease in life quality of 44-98 million people worldwide. (The higher value contains those who have lower back pain, possibly due to neuropathic pain, such as sciatica or lumbago.) At least one third of the world's population is affected by this kind of pain throughout their life. This pain must be released. Current therapy options are rather restricted. Conventional therapy includes steroids (*e.g.* betametazon, prednisolon, and hydrocortisone) and non-steroidal anti-inflammatory drugs (NSAID, *e.g.* ketoprofen, metamizol, diclo-fenac, naproxen, piroxicam, cloxinin, ibuprofen, nimesulid, paracetamol, and meloxica m), anti-inflammatory drugs, antiepileptics, local anesthetics, anti-depressants, antiarrythmics, opioid analgesics, NMDA-receptor antagonists, as well as all of these combined.

These methods work on different background mechanisms, with different effectiveness, but their common advantage is that they contribute to the lowering of inflammation. Although these drugs are effective, their application warrants extra prudence. Their use often triggers undesired side effects and almost always unperspicuous interactions. These therapy options involve real hazards (*e.g.* allergy, ulcers in the gastric tracts, *etc.*). Iatrogenesis (health degradation following medical treatment or advice) is number 5-9 leading death cause in the USA [21, 22].

Is there anything wrong with medicines in general? Well, the different phases of research and the marketing authorization take about 10-12 years; meanwhile, the legal protection of the patent lasts for 20 years. Is 8 years enough to realize profit for the shareholders? Will patients not die before even commencing treatment? Molecules are not selective enough to exclusively get to the target receptor and receptors are not selective enough to exclusively get to the donor molecule.

Does the Reader agree that everyone would be interested in a therapy option that is able to kill pain, inhibit inflammation, reduce edema and handicap with a method that is non-drug, non-invasive, non-contact, non-psychoactive, not painful, has a prompt and local effect, can be used comfortably at home, uses the endogenous sources of the human body, is evidence-based with a device that does not need care or even maintenance, has a lifespan over that of humans, does not contain moving parts, is inexpensive, does not need external power, and its use does not require expertise? Many researchers and clinicians would, indeed, be interested in such a therapy option, and, in fact, hope to have found one in SMF-exposure devices.

Human ingenuity has supplied everyday life with apparatuses in a wide range of the electromagnetic spectrum. Why did I choose the zero frequency limit for the subject of this book? I decided long ago that I wanted to contribute to the understanding of the background mechanism of how magnetic fields act on living matter. The zero frequency limit seemed to be the only choice providing the possibility of studying an electricity-free action of SMF even if, in practice, this electricity-free action can rarely be realizable.

The critics may ask why I chose to investigate many different fields of life sciences rather than digging deeper in one single field. I have a theoretical and a practical answer to this. The theoretical reason is that we are still lacking systematic phenomenological knowledge in many areas of medicine. Systematic research is typically carried out by several research groups cooperating and exploring a certain area. This is how we have been working. The practical reason is even simpler; the lower the well in a fundamental field of science, the higher the costs.

The structure of the life sciences chapters in this book follows basically phylogenesis (chronology). It starts with experiments on microorganisms (***In Vitro* Experiments on Microorganisms**) and through inver-tebrates and mammals (***In Vivo* Animal Experiments**), consolidates in human trials (**Human Investigations**). At the beginning of coherent sections, preliminaries inform the Reader about the antecedents. Tables, summarizing Chapter 5 and 6, help further orientation. In case of analgesia, I introduced a special summary, partly because of the complexity of the topic and partly because of the depth of the discussions. Chapters 2 (**Physical Properties of Static Magnetic Fields**) and 3 (**Sources of Static Magnetic Fields**) only serve the purpose of assisting the Reader in getting acquainted with the physics background and the problems arising from mixing natural and life sciences.

CHAPTER 2

Physical Properties of Static Magnetic Fields

Keywords: Hall-effect, Magnetic induction, Magnet therapy, Physical properties, Vector.

An SMF is conventionally described by the 3 dimensional magnetic induction ($\vec{B}$) or magnetic field strength ($\vec{H}$) vector. Since most applications in this book use SMF perpendicular to the surfaces of the living matter (except the 3 T clinical MRI), we choose to use magnetic induction whose component perpendicular to the interface between materials with different susceptibilities remains unchanged. I shall sometime abbreviate magnetic induction vector to induction bearing in mind that magnetic induction is a quantity, not a phenomenon. SMF is a special type of magnetic field in which induction does not change in time. In other words, it is time-independent, its time derivative is zero, or the field is simply static. However, even an SMF can and, as a matter of fact, always does change is space. We refer to SMF as inhomogeneous if at least one of its components has a non-zero induction derivative (gradient) in space. In the hypothetical situation when a magnetic field does change neither in time, nor in space, we call it homogeneous SMF. This is a mathematical model, an abstraction, since there are no infinite sources of magnetic fields, not to mention that along the edges the SMF will necessarily be inhomogeneous. The sources of SMF are electric currents or atomic particles (molecules) that have a net magnetic spin. We shall speak about the sources a little more in a little more detail in Chapter 3 (**Sources of Static Magnetic Fields**). Earth itself is a complex natural source of SMF due to the huge amount of minerals that are either magnetically anisotropic or in motion. Anisotropy is a term for being directionally dependent. Artificial magnetic fields generated by man are usually produced by electric currents. If the current is direct (DC) the resultant field is SMF; otherwise it becomes an electromagnetic field in the broader sense (AC, non-zero frequency). Nowadays, due to the development of materials science, permanent magnets that generate SMF easily 5-6 orders of

János F. László

magnitude beyond that of Earth and 2-4 orders of magnitude beyond that of natural magnetic ores can be manufactured. In some of the experiments reported in this book, we used magnetized cubes of size 10×10×10 mm that have a remanent magnetic induction (induction remaining even if the source magnetic field strength gets back to zero) of 1.47 T!

We stick to SI units in this book; accordingly, magnetic induction (or magnetic flux density or intensity in the English literature) has a unit named after Nikola Tesla (1856-1943), Serbian inventor. T (=Vs/m^2=Wb/m^2=N/A/m). magnetic flux is measured in Wb (=J/A=Tm^2) named after Wilhelm Eduard Weber (1804-1891), German physicist (the surface density of 1 Wb magnetic flux is 1 T, this is where the English nomenclature for magnetic induction originates from). magnetic field strength is in A/m (named after André-Marie Ampère, French physicist, 1775-1836). A particle carrying a charge of 1 C (after Charles Augustin de Coulomb, French physicist, 1736-1806) and passing through a magnetic field of 1 T at a speed of 1 m/s perpendicular to SMF experiences a force with magnitude 1 N (after Sir Isaac Newton, English physicist, 1642-1727). The unit V was named after Alessandro Giuseppe Antonio Anastasio Volta (Italian physicist, 1745-1827).

The grade of a permanent magnet relies on the maximum energy product of the materials the magnet is made of ($B \times H$), frequently provided by the manufacturers in English units. A grade N50 magnet, for example, is made of a material with a maximum magnetic load of 50 MGOe (megaGauss Oersted named after Carl Friedrich Gauss, German mathematician, 1777-1855 and Hans Christian Ørsted, Danish physicist, 1777-1851), *i.e.* about 4×10^5 TA/m.

MEASUREMENTS

In principle, the $\vec{B}(\vec{r})$ vector-vector function must be known (measured or calculated) at all $\vec{r}$ positions within the finite volume of the exposure chamber to fully describe the SMF. We actually measured all 3 components of the specific magnetic induction vector in our studies. Usually 2 of them were ignorable for their absolute values were orders of magnitude below the so-called dominant component as well as they decayed in the magnetic background. Such negligible components were regarded as fringe field components.

TOOLS, SAMPLING

Magnetometers are used to determine the direction or magnitude of an SMF. Basically a magnetometer can be either "fluxgate" or based on the Hall-effect (named after Edwin Herbert Hall, American physicist, 1855-1938). Either way, one vector component can be measured at a time. The fluxgate magnetometer is a sensitive device; the mechanism is based on the different magnetic saturation of ferromagnetic materials. The probe consists of 2 parallel ferromagnetic cores, close to each other. A coil is wound around the cores, and thus the secondary AC current generated in the coil is detected. The signal of the coil is proportional to the induction of the external SMF, depending on the orientation of the SMF and the cores relative to each other. Fluxgate magnetometers have a measurement range between 1 nT to 10 mT. A special application of such magnetometers is using the corresponding component of the geomagnetic field as a basically constant bias allowing for the detection of SMF below that of Earth.

A probe based on the Hall-effect consists of a thin square pad or foil made of gallium- or indium arsenide semiconductor furnished with 4 electric terminals. DC is lead through the pad or foil between 2 opposing main terminals, and the potential difference between the other 2 cross terminals gets measured. The so-called Hall-potential is proportional to the magnetic flux through the pad or foil, to the cosine of the angle formed by the magnetic induction, to the main direction of the pad or foil (polarization dependence!), and to the DC current between the main terminals. Hall-probes can measure between 100 μT up to 100 T, in principle.

I wish to mention the superconducting quantum interference device (SQUID) here that is capable of measuring very small magnetic inductions (down to 5×10^{-18} T) based on superconducting loops containing Josephson junctions (after Brian David Josephson, Welsh physicist, 1940).

We used Hall-probes exclusively. In order to scan SMF along lines in a generator, the generator was set up on its side on a stable, solid surface, and its position was marked for repeated measurements. The active part of the Hall-probe (Model 420

Gaussmeter; Lake Shore Cryotronics, Westerville, OH, USA) was at the end of a rigid and long shaft. The passive part of the probe, including the electronics, was fixed to the arm of the robot so that the active part would penetrate into the interior of the exposure chamber. The arm, holding the probe, was controlled by a computer equipped with dosimetric scanning software. The probe was moved parallel to the magnetic matrices of the chamber. Line scans were executed at 5 different planes between the matrices. Since a transverse probe can measure only one component of the induction at a time, the measurement was repeated after rotating the plane of the shaft (including the active part) by 90°. The third component was measured by a different probe with a flexible shaft. The active part of the probe was fixed perpendicular to both previous directions. These measurements were performed separately from the life sciences studies.

Whenever something is asserted about the magnetic induction of a certain SMF, it is based on a sequence of dosimetric experiments as well as on multiple measurements at the same point. The number of sampling points was between several tens to hundreds depending on the inhomogeneity of the SMF. These values were averaged provided that averaging was not counter-indicated. Counter-indication occurred when the sampling points were different. For example, sampling SMF along the symmetry axes of cylindrical magnets with identical pole directions in the isocenter of an arrangement, the search for local maxima was definitely not counter-indicated. When determining the gradient components of the magnetic induction in a given distance from magnets, the local extremes of the induction of all neighbors were collected in a given distance from the surface. These values were then divided by the distance of neighboring extremes, and the ratios were averaged. The lateral distance between nearest neighbors was always held constant because the lateral periodicity of the magnet lattices (lattice constants) was fixed. If the number of individual magnets permitted, the SMF of magnets close to the edges were disregarded due to counter-indication; they had fewer neighbors than the ones in the bulk. In most experiments, we succeeded in leaving the edges of the SMF outside the exposure chamber excluding special SMF ranges from the experiment. Thus, such non-special induction and gradient values characterized the SMF of a specific magnet arrangement. These values will be summarized in Chapter 3 (**Sources of Static Magnetic Fields**).

CONSTRAINTS, SOLUTIONS

Physical perception has its obvious limits. Whether we look at the direct effects SMF-exposure can exert on biological systems or the indirect effects of SMF-exposure through induced electric fields, we need signals that are measurable and large enough compared to the physiological signals produced by the background of thermal motion. This background exhibits constraints in the measurability of signals in biological systems [23, 24]. Energy approximations are used for the lower limit of detection taking into account the average thermal energy of the environment as a background and the energy of the occurring biological phenomenon. SMF-induced effects, probably due to radical pair interactions, are weak interactions compared to thermal motion [25].

A typical surface scan of the component perpendicular to the surface at a distance of 10 mm can be seen in Fig. (**2.1**). Individual neodymium-iron-boron (NdFeB) grade N50 cylindrical magnets were positioned with alternating poles by one another in a checkerboard-like configuration. This configuration is called "bidirectional", as opposed to "unidirectional" when magnets are oriented with their identical poles in one direction. The line-scanned area within the isocenter of the arrangement was 41×41 mm in size. The contribution of the asymmetric magnetic induction near the edges can be disregarded within this area since the arrangement has a lateral extension of at least twice the 41 mm distance.

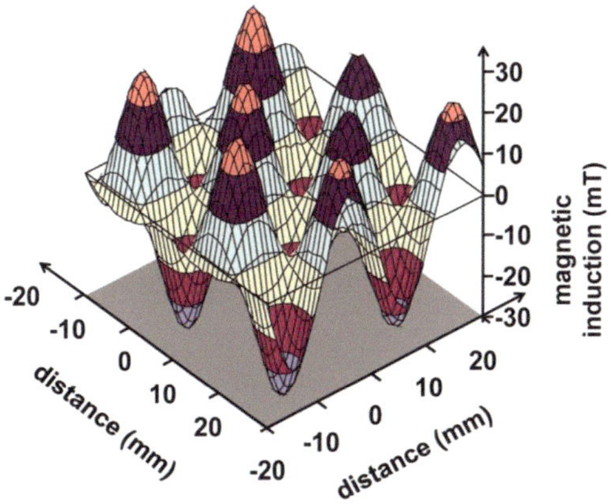

Fig. (2.1). A typical field scan of SMF at a distance of 10 mm from the magnets' surface for the case of NdFeB N50 cylindrical magnets sitting one next to another with alternating polarity.

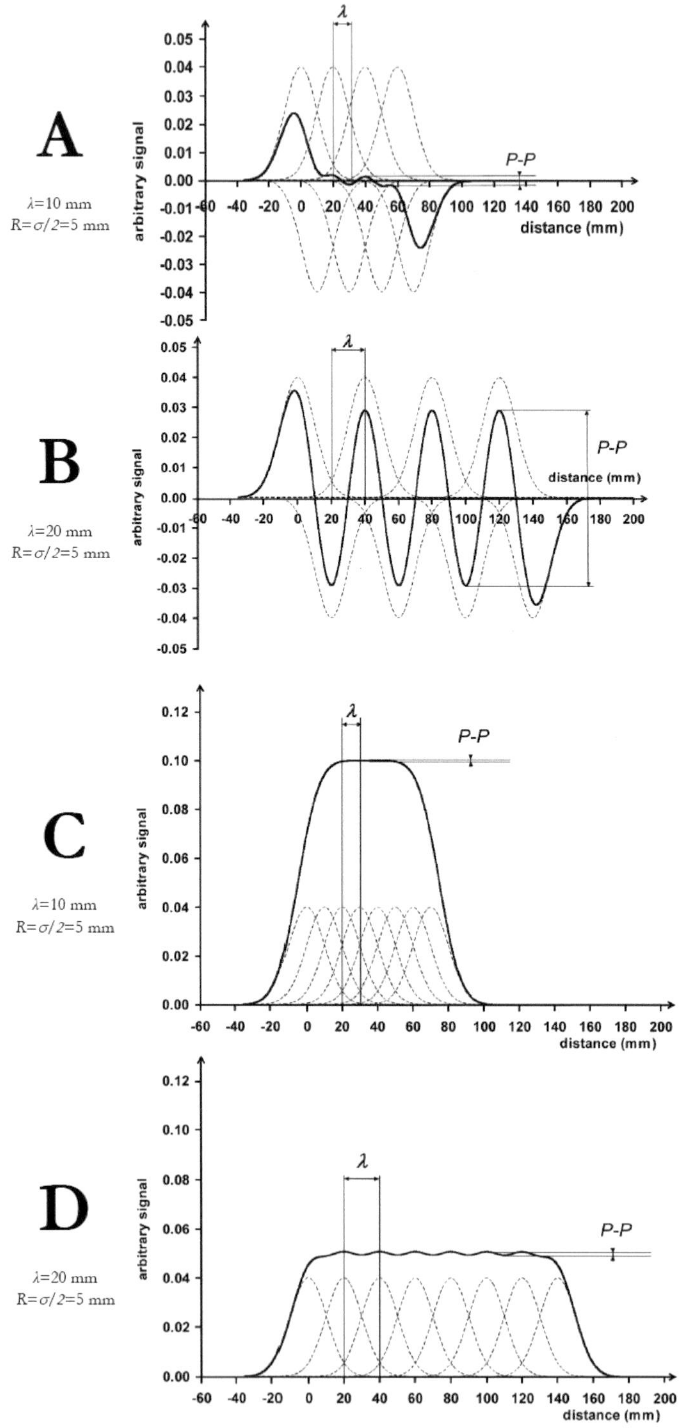
A
λ=10 mm
R=σ/2=5 mm
B
λ=20 mm
R=σ/2=5 mm
C
λ=10 mm
R=σ/2=5 mm
D
λ=20 mm
R=σ/2=5 mm
λ
P-P
arbitrary signal
distance (mm)

Fig. (2.2). Schematic figure of a resultant arbitrary signal (*e.g.* magnetic induction) distribution of a bidirectional magnet arrangement. The resultant signal can be drastically different from the individual signals depending on the arrangement of the individual magnets. Dashed and solid lines denote the individual and the resultant signals, respectively. **A)** Cylindrical magnets of 5 mm radius are arranged with alternating polarity along a line 10 mm away from each other. **B)** Same as in (A), but the magnets are 20 mm away from each other. **C)** Same as in (A), but the magnets are arranged with identical polarity along a line 10 mm away from each other. **D)** Same as in (C), but the magnets are 20 mm away from each other.

Approximating the scanned values of the SMF distribution along the x axis, we fitted normal distribution functions to the individual peaks, where the contribution of the kth peak to the distribution was $\pm\frac{1}{\sigma\sqrt{2\pi}}e^{-\frac{[x-(k-1)\lambda]^2}{2\sigma^2}}$, with k=1,2,…,n (σ was considered equal for the peaks), and λ the distance between the means (the lattice constant). In this simple approach, widely used for finding the spatial resolution in laterally or vertically periodic systems (see *e.g.* in the review of Hofmann [26]), the magnets were bidirectionally arranged and the R radius of each individual magnet was 5 mm (equals to one half of σ), See Fig. (**2.2A**) and Fig. (**2.2B**). Dashed lines represent arbitrary signals (*e.g.* magnetic induction values) belonging to each contributing magnet, whereas the solid line shows the resultant signal due to the interaction between the magnets. If λ is small and we neglect the non-symmetrical side peaks, the peak-to-peak (*P-P*) value of the resultant signal can be significantly smaller than what the individual peaks would suggest. *E.g.* if $\sigma/2=R=5$ mm and $\lambda=10$ mm, the signal is reduced to 15% of the *P-P* value (Fig. **2.2A**). For $\sigma/2=R=5$ mm and $\lambda=20$ mm, the signal is reduced to only 73% (Fig. **2.2B**). For a similar situation when $\sigma/2=R=2.5$ mm, $\lambda=5$ and 10 mm, the corresponding values are 32% and 73%, respectively. The spatial resolution gets better with decreasing λ.

Similarly to Fig. (**2.2A**) and Fig. (**2.2B**), Fig. (**2.2C**) and Fig. (**2.2D**) show the situation when the magnets are placed one next to another unidirectionally. If $\sigma/2=R=5$ mm and $\lambda=10$ mm, the magnitude of the resultant magnetic field becomes 2.5 times bigger than the individual signal. At the same time, the distribution in the center can be considered homogeneous since since the *P-P* value is almost zero. However, the *P-P* value becomes measurable if $\sigma/2=R=5$ mm and $\lambda=20$ mm, as shown in Fig. (**2.2D**).

In order to be able to take this effect into account, we defined "surface roughness" as $a=\Delta B/\lambda$ in T/m. Here, the induction difference (ΔB) was considered equal to the *P-P* value over the distance between the adjacent positive and negative peaks in both directions (because of symmetry reasons λ was equal in both x and y directions). The Reader will see how surface roughness affected the measured induction values in case of concrete applications of generators in the Section **Generators 1-16**. The average values for all peaks, *P-P*, and $\bar{\alpha}$ are collected in Table **3.4**. In this sense, a homogeneous field has $\bar{\alpha}=0$ (see *e.g.* Fig. **2.2C**).

No special efforts were made during the biology experiments to shield the experimental setup from the geomagnetic field of Earth since the shielding itself could generate unwanted side effects [27]. Horizontal components of the SMF in the exposure chambers and all components of Earth's magnetic field were regarded as stray field components. Control samples were always exposed to at least the horizontal component of the geomagnetic field, magnetic induction values of which were a minimum of 4 orders of magnitude lower than those at the target position in the exposure chamber.

RELEVANT INTERACTIONS IN BIOLOGY

According to the classification of WHO [12], the interaction between SMF-exposure and a living tissue can be of the following nature:

- Electrodynamic interactions
  - Magnetic induction of electric fields and currents
  - Lorentz force
    - Flow potentials
    - A theoretical study of the possible effects of flow potentials on the heart
  - Magnetohydrodynamic model
- Magnetomechanical interactions
  - Magnetomechanics (torque on magnetic dipole moment)
  - Magnetophoresis (force on magnetic dipole moment)
  - Anisotropic diamagnetism
- Radical recombination rates
- Biogenic magnetite

  - Single-domain crystals
  - Superparamagnetic magnetite
  - Other ferromagnetic inclusions
  - Local amplification due to ferromagnetic material
- Mechanistic co-factors and other mechanisms
  - Light as a co-factor
  - State dependence

Although some discussion will follow in Section **Clinical MRI**, an overview of all possible interactions and related studies would well exceed the volume limitations of this book. The Reader is, therefore, referred to the most comprehensive review papers available: From a physicist [17] and from a physician [28]. Meanwhile, some specific topics were reviewed by Colbert *et al.* [29], Kangarlu [30], Heinrich *et al.* [31], Yamaguchi-Sekino *et al.* [32], and Ueno [33].

MAGNET THERAPY, DEFINITION OF DOSE

Magnet therapy (magnetic therapy, biomagnetic therapy, or magnetotherapy) is a complementary or alternative medical practice part of which is SMF-exposure. Clinicians claim that SMF-exposure can have a beneficial effect on the body part exposed. Such effects include anesthesia, analgesia, increased speed of blood flow, more effective and faster wound healing with fewer scars. Beyond the occurrences of "magnetic therapy" in publications (presented in the **Introduction**), "magnetic therapy" appears in 237 titles of patents in the USA (USA Patent Database at http://www.uspto.gov) and 2239 titles among European patents (European Patent Database at http://ep.espacenet.com) as of February, 2014. These numbers show an undeniable trend of favoring this type of therapy. The reason for this interest in SMF-based medical devices especially SMF-based medical devices is obvious: Patients like it that such devices offer a simple solution for analgesia, for example. Also, they are safe and long-lasting, and the method is drug-free and non-invasive. Most of such devices are relatively inexpensive too. SMF-therapy can be classified as a self-healing therapy option due to it being comfortably applicable at home.

The direct or assisted effects of SMF-exposure on acute or chronic diseases are an intriguing although little "exotic" and somewhat "miraculous" territory of science for those in clinical practice. Experimentalists, on the other hand, simply accept it as a valid option once the method can be supported by evidence. Most of us, fundamental scientists and practitioners, are waiting for an éclat, for the unambiguous background mechanism(s) to be revealed. This mechanism should be describable by physical interactions, should have a range of side effects and interactions with drugs, and a wide spectrum. These are the characteristics that make an evidence-based method practical. Needless to say that so-called conservative medicine lacks such comprehensive characteristics in almost all methods in everyday practice. As mentioned in the Introduction, the development of a new drug is far too expensive and takes too much time, and even if it gets to the market, the agent substance may still not reach the targeted receptor or may reach other receptors. Human studies related to SMF-induced analgesia, for instance, make the decision difficult, whether the effect experienced by healthy volunteers or even patients would go beyond placebo [34 - 38], since the effect gets mediated partly through the same set of endogenous opioid receptors. As mentioned in the Preface, placebo effect was shown to produce side effects already in 1974 [39].

Several reports were dedicated to the comparing of existing results, and almost all of them concluded that the studies were difficult to compare [40 - 42]. Colbert *et al.* [43] however, made serious progress by suggesting a standard to describe the devices and exposure conditions in human trials. They proposed to include the material magnets are made of, magnet shapes and sizes, pole configuration in case of multiple magnets, measured magnetic induction or field strength map (especially those at the target site), exposure frequency, duration, target tissue location, quality and distance from the magnets' surface, as well as the structure holding the magnets. Such tables will be presented with regard to all human studies in this book (Sections **On healthy volunteers**, **On visitors of a dental clinic**, **Stomatological pain**, **Erosive gastritis**, **Allergy**, **Pain perception and bone turnover**).

Since SMF-exposure is not attached to radiation, we cannot expect results we are used to in radiation biology. In radiology terms, "dose" is an amount of energy absorbed in the target tissue. In case of SMF-exposure this definition cannot be used. Radiation biologists use the dimensionless *N* number for dose-equivalence, but this is useless for us as well since the quantities *N* depends on are not at all, or if they are, they are not well -defined (for example the duration of dose transfer, the volume in which it is absorbed, and also the subject of exposure). The routine use of *N* for magnetic induction as a routine in the MR literature for the homogeneous SMF component of the MR (B_0) seems to be an oversimplification.

When trying to define dose for SMF-exposure, we need to tackle the following questions:

Biological effect: Type of model, definition of effect and/or response.
Subject exposed: Type (strain), gender, age, mass, character of the subject (static like during anesthesia or dynamic when freely moving), area of exposed surface, individual subject, period of examination, average (median) of measured values.
Location: Circumstances preceding and during the experiment (temperature, air pressure, nutrition and water quality and quantity, sample size per group and overall, lighting, circadian cycle, background noise and vibrations, magnetic background, *etc.*).
Magnetic field in air: Time dependence (static, dynamic), induction (absolute value and direction), homogeneity (induction gradients' absolute value and direction), *P-P* induction at different distances from the magnetic surface, surface roughness.
Magnetic field in subject tissue: The same as in air, plus subject tissue quality, penetration depth of SMF-exposure into tissue (crossing and distracted lines).
Source of magnetic field: Material (its grade if applicable), remanent induction, shape, height, radius or side lengths, lattice constant, number of neighbors, induction on the magnets' surface, magnetic coupling, polarities.
Timing: Durations attributed to different biological responses following or during SMF-exposure (especially if response times are short or if the field is time-dependent), multiple (repeated) exposures, and time points of measurement (s) relative to exposure(s).

Let us now inspect a concrete situation in life when we want to perform a specific animal *in vivo* experiment where the aim is to illuminate the effect SMF-exposure might have. We assume that the subjects are individuals of an ordinary mouse strain of identical age and similar body mass. The subjects are free to move within geometric constraint during whole-body SMF-exposure. We have enough sources and time to include a sample size to realize a statistical power of 80%. The model in question is a well-known and widespread acute pain assay with well-characterized responses in case of a complete family of pharmacological treatment options. We know all production specifications of the magnets used for generating the SMF; we measured the magnetic induction and gradients vectors of the SMF in 3 dimensions in advance with a certified magnetometer. We have a picture of SMF inhomogeneities, including the spatial edges of SMF. We can now establish that our SMF is as homogeneous within a good approximation, and the direction of the dominant component of the SMF is perpendicular to the cage. With the help of MRI measurements we clarified earlier what type of magnetically anisotropic materials occur in the body of a mouse and we also executed a computer simulation to find out the penetration depth of SMF into the subject's body. Now we can begin designing the experimental protocol. In order to verify dose-dependence, we need at least 4 different SMF and 4 different single exposure durations. The evaluation of data should be done after the same time period, excluding an undesired parameter in the model; namely, the spontaneous decay duration of the effect. We measure 4 time periods per SMF-exposure. We also need to carry out the experiment in preferably one, but definitely not more than 2 days, during the same hours. Since the minimum sample size is 10/group, we need to experiment on 50 animals per day, including daily control. We can achieve this by either chosing short exposure durations, or having many generators and human power to perform the experiments simultaneously. Both choices are risky: Decreasing exposure time may result in the lack of effects, and the simultaneous experimenting may result in differences compared to single animal-experiments because of the social behavior of mice [44]. Even if we can afford single-animal experiments, we would face difficulties: We would like to have the same (preferably blinded) person do the experiments in order to avoid the variability in judgment. The following day we use another SMF, then another, and again another. During the 4 days we accumulate data on 200 animals. A physiological response function (φ) develops which depends on at least 2 parameters: Absolute value of magnetic induction (B) and exposure duration (τ). We necessarily assume that all circumstances in the lab remain unchanged during the 4 days. On the basis of our experiment, we determine whether our function φ is really a classical dose function depending on ($B\tau$ or $B\tau^2$) only. This means that φ corresponding to unit induction and unit duration is equal to double induction and half (or quarter) duration. Is the biological response of our mice to SMF-exposure with a double magnetic induction for a halved time identical? This condition might seem too rigid for a life sciences experiment. However, if this assumption does not hold, our chances of a true extrapolation and, consequently a true prognosis from a low number of experiments degrade severely. There still remains a question: Even if we succeed in determining function $\varphi(B,\tau)$ reliably in a certain experiment, what can we conclude from this function regarding (i) another model under identical exposure conditions or (ii) the same model under different exposure conditions?

The Reader is now probably convinced that the effective dose problem has no simple solution. A third phase clinical trial, however, requires that an SMF-exposure device be optimized and validated through many series of *in vitro* and *in vivo* tests. It would be an amazing step towards comparable (maybe even reproducible) tests if scientists could be motivated to design and execute their tests according to how they are presented here, they did not mind the excess work, and described the applied technology and exposure conditions already in the preclinical phase. As long as this is only a hopeful perspective, we cannot draw reliable conclusions about the real efficiency and possible benefits of SMF-therapy.

FROM TRANSCUTANEOUS ELECTRIC NERVE STIMULATORS TO GRADIENT STATIC MAGNETIC FIELDS

In Chapters 4 (***In Vitro* experiments on microorganisms**), 5 (***In Vivo* Animal Experiments**), and 6 (**Human Investigations**) dealing with measurements, the Reader will face the fact that a moving object in an SMF is a similar physical phenomenon as a stationary object in a time-dependent magnetic field. I kindly refer the Reader to the Bioelectromagnetics book of Malmivuo and Plonsey, especially Chapters 21 and 22 *ibid.*

Nerves can be stimulated by electric currents. These currents may be the consequences of non-isopotentially charged external electrodes. By choosing the right parameters of the external electrodes, the electric current appearing in the living tissue may overcome the threshold of the nerves to the given stimulus requiring them to respond. Such action potential responses may eventually get to the brain to be processed there for further action. This phenomenon is widely known and accepted and is used in a wide range of biomedical devices from cardiac pacemakers to transcutaneous electric nerve stimulators (TENS).

Non-isopotentially charged external electrodes are not the exclusive source of electric currents in the tissues, though. A time-dependent external magnetic field can obviously achieve such currents on the basis of magnetic field induction. Due to the changes in the induction of the magnetic field, the magnetic flux over a surface varies in time; consequently, an electric potential, possibly an electric current can be generated. This phenomenon has also been known for 150 years or so.

Is it possible that an SMF (where the magnetic induction does not change significantly with time) induces an electric current? It is and this phenomenon is known as motion-induced (or Faraday) currents. If the (electrically charged) object exposed to the SMF moves with a finite (but not relativistic) velocity not parallel to the induction of the SMF, the SMF changes the trajectory of the object. Cyclotrons, Hall probes, and other magnetic devices operate today on the basis of this phenomenon.

Is it possible to create an electric current by an external SMF in the living tissue in a stationary object (without self-motion)? For example, if strong permanent magnets are attached (or moved closer) to the human tissue, charged particle flows within the tissue may react. Blood itself (microcirculation), currents of the endocrine system, and intercellular currents in a human are all representative of such a flow. The stimulation of nerves under such conditions is possible as evidenced by researchers in relatively recent examinations and trials in the past 20 years. Note that this phenomenon actually constitutes a handicap from the epidemiological point of view with regard to stationary working forces around magnetic resonance devices.

If the SMF is a so-called gradient field where the magnetic induction changes in space, the probability of nerve stimulation increases due to the fact that the action of electric charges between magnetically non-isopotential points is more expressed than between isopotential points.

Consistent with this is the idea that exposure to an external gradient SMF may, in practice, have the same induced response as a TENS. It is interesting to note here that while different TENS devices have been approved by the FDA, no gradient SMF generating device has ever been.

PERCEPTION OF STATIC MAGNETIC FIELDS

The perception of SMF is a frequent phenomenon in the fauna, used for orientation, hiding, and hunting. Do humans also have endogenous SMF detectors that they can use for self-motion perception in an external SMF? We have a body that contains magnetically anisotropic matter *ab ovo*; it employs flowing fluids for different material transport processes, and it maintains a nervous system based on electrically charged particle transfer. Thus, it is evident that many parts of our organism are subject to changes in an external SMF. Accordingly, patients often report on mild and temporary (patho)physiological effects while spending time in the bore of a high field MRI. This book is a step forward in the search for potential SMF sensors in humans.

During the past decades, interest has turned towards the scientific exploration of the way the human body creates and handles signals due to motion perception. However, beyond visual, vestibular, auditory, tactile, and proprioceptory modalities of sensing motion, little is known about magnetic detection in spite of the fact that the existence of geomagnetic biosensors in bacteria, bees, sharks, rays, migrating birds, and even in bats has been discovered [4 - 7]. The 100 million years of phylogenesis has not degraded magnetic sensory functions in these animals. Do humans have magnetic sensors that can be used for motion perception?

We perceive motion of objects around us and we perceive self-motion as well. Motion perception is most frequently attributed to the process of inferring speed and direction of an element based on visual (90%), vestibular (7%), and proprioceptive (2%) inputs. The visual system is influenced by external electromagnetic waves in the visible spectrum, ranging from 390 to 750 nm. The vestibular system responds to external mechanical inputs (*e.g.* pirouette), whereas the sensory organism for proprioception can be stimulated by mechanical, chemical, or electrical stimuli from the inside (*e.g.* life signs of a long distance runner, the feeling in a moving roller coaster or in an accelerating elevator). Other stimulus modalities contribute to motion perception as well. These are either auditory (*e.g.* hearing the apparent wind) or tactile perception (*e.g.* feeling the apparent wind). The way specific bat and dolphin species utilize an ultrasound generator and detector to assess their dynamic distance from objects is a representative example of auditory motion perception. The adaptation of gliding birds to winds is an example of tactile motion perception. The complicacy of our sensory system is well characterized by the fact that motion perception is not restricted to relative motion. We all have experienced the sensation of a rising stomach when watching a movie from the viewpoint of a person in a moving roller coaster while comfortably sitting in an immobile seat in a cinema. What is certain is that the stimulation of the motion perceptual system requires either dynamism (change in time) or inhomogeneity (change is space). If both the time derivative and the gradient of a potential perceptional input quantity are zero, motion perception does not occur. If a signal is periodical in time and/or in space, it increases the possibility of it causing a response in the perceptual system. Using an artificial periodicity in the gradient of an optical signal can trick our vision; this effect is referred to as an optical illusion.

Those who have ever entered or gotten close to a strong SMF do not deny that they could feel the SMF. The lower threshold value of the magnetic induction as a sensory input shows large variety among individuals, similarly to other sensory threshold values. A strong SMF interacts with those static particles in our body that are originally magnetized as ferro-, dia-, or paramagnets. Our body material has diamagnetic characteristics overall due to its high percentage of water, making the medical diagnosis method of MRI possible. The high concentration of hemoglobin makes the arterial blood ferromagnetic, while the venous flow remains paramagnetic. Due to the net magnetization of hemoglobin and oxygen molecules, an interaction with the external SMF would also occur even if blood was at rest.

SMF also influences the trajectory of electrically charged particles in our body that are in motion relative to the SMF even if these particles do not possess a non-zero net magnetization. The external SMF can be uniform (where the distribution of the magnetic induction is homogeneous) or non-uniform (where the magnetic induction is inhomogeneous).

It is the uniform SMF component of an MRI (with B_0 magnetic induction) that makes it possible for magnetized molecules to get arranged in our body. Still, complaints of patients show that exposure to this SMF induces biological responses as mentioned before. Vertigo, for example, is explained by a conflict in the brain occurring due to discordant sensory inputs [18]. On the other hand, the natural requirement for improving image resolution in MRI resulted in the application of ever stronger B_0 components up to a point where no more experimental evidence supported the use of such high fields any more [45].

Besides the gradient magnetic field (of induction B_1) that is an inherent part of the MRI, another non-uniform SMF manifests itself for MRI patients between the internal section of the MRI (*e.g.* bore) and its external part (MRI room). Nowadays, 3-4 orders of magnitude difference occurs between magnetic induction inside and outside the MRI. On the meter long way between the inside and the outside of the MRI, a patient experiences this gradient on the rolling table. Longer exposure to stray SMF gradients has raised epidemiological concerns in those who work close to an MRI (*e.g.* [46]).

Due to their high concentration of nociceptors, the part of our body that is the easiest to stimulate by electric fields or SMF is the system of peripheral nerves. Peripheral nerves as such, represent an SMF detector. Switching off all our other sensory inputs, SMF sensors can easily satisfy self-motion perception, *e.g.* lying on the table of an MRI, getting slowly rolled into the bore; the motion can at least be perceived in the form of a mild discomfort. For an equal response, viscera need stronger excitation/stimulus than peripheries.

CHAPTER 3

Sources of Static Magnetic Fields, Generators

Keywords: Generator description, Magnet arrangement, Magnet origin.

Several SMF types have been tested and are reported in this book. As mentioned in **Measurements**, from the viewpoint of a life sciences experiment an SMF must be considered a 6 dimensional vector space, given that every point of the SMF should be described by 3 components of the magnetic induction and 3 components of its gradient. It has been proven (and the Reader will see this shortly) that both induction and its gradient play an important role in the evocation of biological response independently of each other in certain ranges. If the sources of the SMF are permanent magnets, these 6 components depend on different parameters: Individual magnets (shape, size, and magnetization), and arrangement of the magnets (number, position, and polarity). The first step for us was to investigate 17 different arrangements and watch, which one induced the highest average response rate in a specific *in vivo* acute pain test, the writhing test in mice (see **Visceral action: The writhing test**). The optimal arrangement or its variations have then been used for a number of different measurements. We also developed more sophisticated SMF generator models in the hope that these will be more effective than the previously chosen ones regarded as optimal in selected tests. Such a special generator was used, for example, in section **On healthy volunteers**. The highest magnetic induction we used was the 3 T SMF provided in the bore of a clinical MRI in everyday use at Szentágothai János Knowledge Centre of Semmelweis University.

MAGNET MATERIALS

Since Hungary has never been famous of its magnet production, most individual magnets had to be imported. The question then raises, which country, which company would provide the highest quality for the most reasonable price. A company should be preferred, where production and trade is in one hand, so

János F. László

quality control is not autotelic. At the same time, reliability should be present not only in the quality of the product, but in shipping and payment as well. What exactly did we expect from a magnet? Table **3.1** and Table **3.2** gives the answer with respect to the materials we finally used.

Table 3.1. Manufacturing, magnetic, mechanical, and material features of the material individual magnets were made of.

NdFeB	Barium ferrite
History	
Neodymium-iron-boron ($Nd_2Fe_{14}B$) tetragonal crystalline structured magnets were developed in 1982 by General Motors and Sumitomo Special Metals. This is the newest and strongest (per mass) type of permanent magnets. The alloy they are made of, together with samarium-cobalt, belong to rare earth metals group of materials. Their production technology is very similar.	A ferrite is a chemical compound of ceramic materials mostly consisting of iron oxide (Fe_2O_3). They were invented in 1930 at Tokyo Institute of Technology. Due to the low price and inexhaustible source of ingredients, their price is the lowest. On the other hand, because of their beneficial magnetic features, they present a good price/value ratio. Especially one type of hard ferrites is barium ferrite with the composition of $BaFe_{12}O_{19}$ ($BaO \cdot 6Fe_2O_3$).
Manufacturing	
First raw material containing the necessary composition of ingredients are melted in a furnace, cast into a mold, and cooled to form ingots. Ingots are pulverized and milled to fine dust. This material undergoes a process of liquid-phase sintering which the powder is magnetically aligned into dense blocks. The blocks are then heat-treated, cut to shape, surface treated, and finally magnetized. Preventing corrosion, a galvanic coating with nickel or zinc is used. Better magnetic features and much lower price are the advantage of such magnets over samarium-cobalt ones.	Ferrites are produced by heating a mixture of finely-powdered precursors of 80% iron oxide and 20% barium carbonate ($BaCO_3$) pressed into a mold. The resulting mixture undergoes sintering (ferritization). Afterwards, the cooled product is milled to single crystals with particles small enough to consist of a single magnetic domain each. The powder is then dry- or wet-pressed into a shape, dried, and re-sintered. The shaping may be performed in an external magnetic field in order to achieve the preferred orientation of the particles (anisotropy). The volume of the material decreases by about 17% during the production, size tolerance is acceptable only after grinding.

(Table 3. 1) contd.....

NdFeB	Barium ferrite
Magnetic features	
The coercitive field strength of magnets made of neodymium-iron-boron is higher than for samarium-cobalt. Remanent induction is identical to that of AlNiCo magnets. Their maximal B×H product is 50% over that of samarium-cobalt. Disadvantages are the ability for corrosion and the limited range of allowed external temperature (T_{max}=80-180° C depending on material quality).	Isotropic magnets can be magnetized to any preferred direction and their features are basically independent of direction. Anisotropic magnets are produced in a strong external magnetic field during pressing, have therefore, a so-called easy direction of magnetization, in which direction the magnetic features are much better than in the other directions. Containing large crystal anisotropies, ceramic magnets have high coercitive field strength making them resistant toward external demagnetizing fields and provide them long-time stability. Due to the small remanent induction, higher pole surfaces must be designed. The maximum external temperature is 250° C.
Mechanical features	
Neodymium-iron-boron are very rigid and brittle, grounding needs diamond tools. Because of their rigidity and strong magnetic field they easily break or get damaged when clashed to other magnets. In case of bigger volumes this represents a high risk of accident. They corrode under standard circumstances; this is why they need galvanic coating.	Ceramic magnets are also hard and brittle, diamond tools are needed to grind them. They are excellently resistant to corrosion, acids, salts, oils, and gases.
Material features	
Made by powder metallurgy, chemical composition: $Nd_2Fe_{14}B$. High resistance against demagnetization. Magnetic field-characterizing values are high remanent induction (B_r), coercitivity of B (bH_c), intrinsic coercitivity (iH_c), and energy product (BH_{max}). Excellent ratio of price/power. The temperature coefficient of intrinsic field strength is high. Thermal stability is limited. Rigid and fragile. Susceptive to corrode, galvanic coating is needed. Not suitable for high operating temperatures.	Made by powder metallurgy, chemical composition: $BaO_6Fe_2O_3$. Highresistance against demagnetization. Intrinsic coercitivity (iH_c) is high. Has high electric resistance. Excellent ratio of price/power. The temperature coefficient of intrinsic field strength is high. Thermal stability is good. Rigid and fragile. Resistant to corrosion. Not suitable for high operating temperatures.

Table 3.2. Physical features and magnetization directions of the materials individual magnets were made of.

	NdFeB	Barium ferrite
Physical features		
Curie temperature (°C)	310-370	450
maximum operation temperature (°C)	80-240	250
resistivity (μΩm)	1.6	$>10^{10}$
hardness (HV)	560-580	480-580
density (g/cm^3)	7.40	4.8-4.9
relative permeability	1.05	1.05-1.20
saturation field strength (kA/m)	2400-3200	800
temperature coefficient of B_r (%/°C)	-0.12	-0.20
temperature coefficient of iH_c (%/°C)	-0.6	0.3
Directions of magnetization		
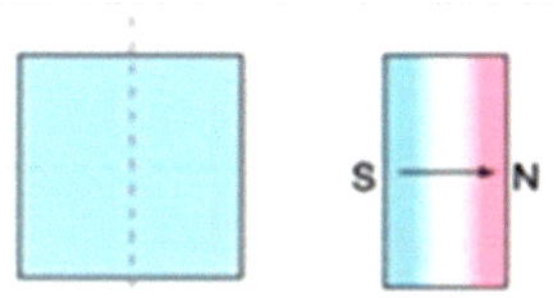 laterally magnetized	X	X
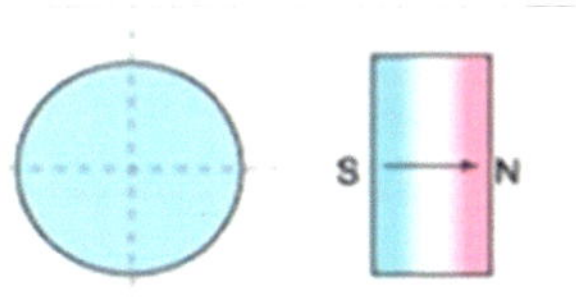 axially magnetized	X	X
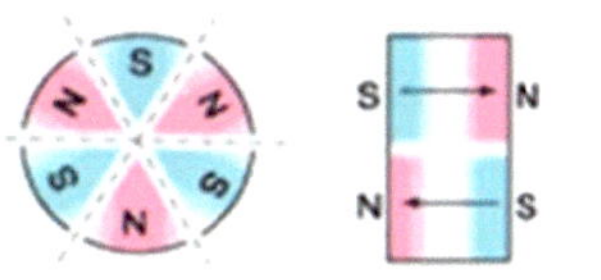 axially magnetized per segment*	X	X

(Table 3.2) contd.....

	NdFeB	Barium ferrite
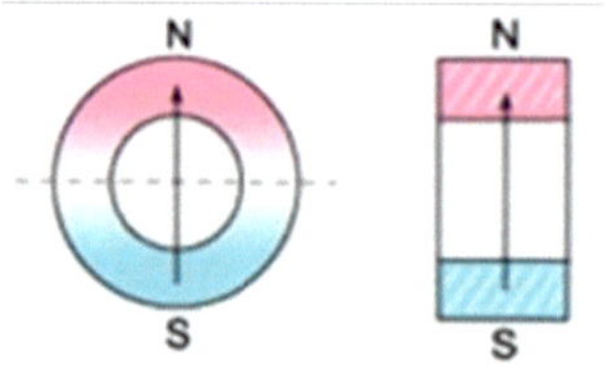 diagonally magnetized*	X	X
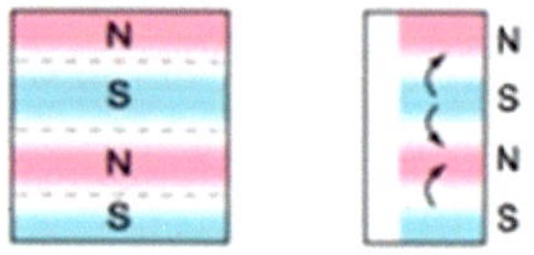 multipolarly magnetized on one side*	X	X
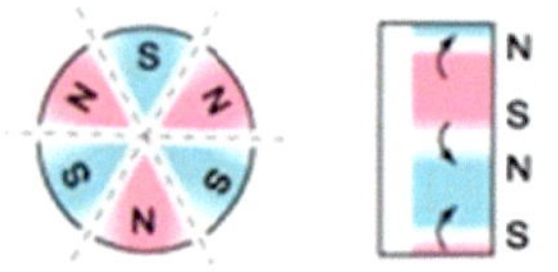 axially magnetized per segment on one side*	X	X
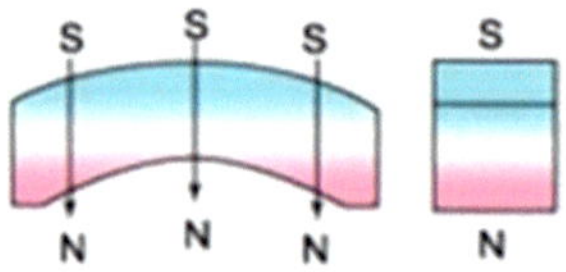 diagonally magnetized per layer segment	X	
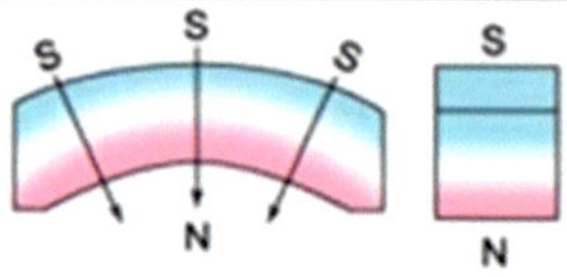 radially magnetized per layer segment		X
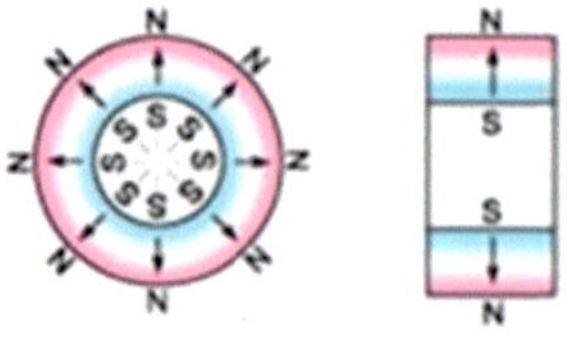 radially magnetized*		X

(Table 3.2) contd.....

	NdFeB	Barium ferrite
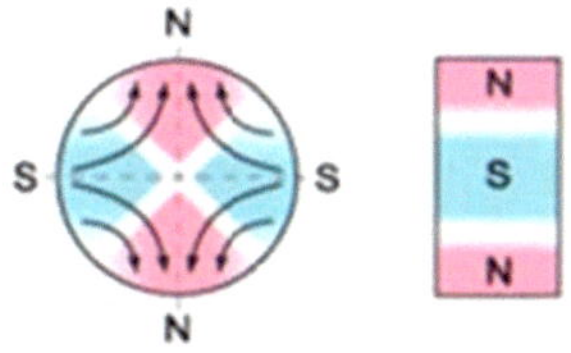 multipolarly magnetized on superficia*		X
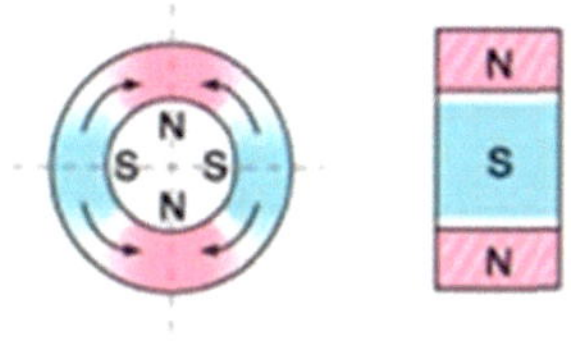 multipole ring, poles on the inner superficia*		X
* Special magnetizing coil is needed.		

After having investigated commercially available magnets (also beyond those mentioned before), the best choice for the biological investigations seemed to be axially magnetized cylindrical NdFeB magnets grade at least N35 with Ni-Cr coating. If budget allows higher grade (N38, N50) magnets would be more appropriate. The ratio of height to diameter of the cylindrical magnet may be important, 22×10, 6×6, 12×10, 20×10, 10×10, or 6×6.5 mm magnets seem applicable. If block magnets are needed, barium ferrite material is suggested first, if budget allows NdFeB magnets may be used.

GENERATORS 1-16

The animal experiments made it necessary to design SMF generators in which the magnets are held in matrices that can be easily and quickly exchanged. The SMF-exposure chamber was then the space between these replaceable matrices. We used ferrite or NdFeB magnets in block or cylindrical shape. The magnets were positioned in a way that they showed opposite poles to each other below and above the exposure chamber allowing, if possible, for an above background vertical component of the SMF. Table **3.3** shows data of these arrangements (generators). Table **3.4** presents the *P-P* magnetic induction values averaged, as described in **Tools, sampling**, surface roughness ($\overline{\alpha}$), and averages and standard deviations of magnetic inductions for the same generators. If $\bar{\alpha} \approx 0$ the SMF is homogeneous (see Fig. (**2.2C**)).

Table 3.3. Summarized technical data of the individual magnets and their arrangements used in the different experiments.

generator	individual magnet							magnet arrangement			
	material	grade	B_r remanent induction (T)	radius (mm)	height (mm)	side-length #1 (mm)	side-length #2 (mm)	polarity	number of matrices	magnetic coupling	matrix constant (mm)
1	NdFeB	N35	1.20	5	10	n/a	n/a	bidir.	2	no	10
2	n/a	n/a	n/a	n/a	n/a	n/a	n/a	n/a	n/a	n/a	n/a
3	NdFeB	N35	1.20	5	10	n/a	n/a	bidir.	1	no	10
4	ferrite	n/a	0.40	5	10	n/a	n/a	unidir.	2	no	10
5	NdFeB	N35	1.20	5	10	n/a	n/a	unidir.	2	no	10
6	NdFeB	N50	1.47	5	10	n/a	n/a	unidir.	2	no	10
7	ferrite	n/a	0.40	5	10	n/a	n/a	bidir.	2	no	10
8	NdFeB	N50	1.47	5	10	n/a	n/a	bidir.	2	no	10
9	NdFeB	N35	1.20	2.5	10	n/a	n/a	bidir.	2	no	5
10	NdFeB	N35	1.20	2.5	10	n/a	n/a	bidir.	2	no	10
11	NdFeB	N50	1.47	5	10	n/a	n/a	bidir.	2	yes	10
12	NdFeB	N50	1.47	5	10	n/a	n/a	bidir.	2	yes	20
13	NdFeB	N50	1.47	5	20	n/a	n/a	bidir.	2	yes	10
14	NdFeB	N50	1.47	5	20	n/a	n/a	bidir.	2	yes	20
15	ferrite	n/a	0.40	n/a	25	70	50	bidir.	2	yes	n/a
16	ferrite	n/a	0.40	n/a	25	70	50	unidir.	2	yes	n/a

In some cases the produced SMF was modified by magnetically coupling the lower side of the lower matrix with the upper side of the upper matrix in a horse-shoe like form (see column magnetic coupling of Table **3.3**). In order to demonstrate the effect of this coupling, I made use of a special arrangement of 5×5 pieces of NdFeB grade N50 cylindrical magnets of 5 mm radius and 10 mm height each (similarly to generator 17d). The effect is shown in Fig. (**3.1**). The absolute value of the magnetic induction perpendicular to the magnets' surface along the symmetry axis of the magnets in the isocenter is on the vertical axis, while the distance measured from the central magnet's surface is on the horizontal axis in the range of 10 mm $< z <$ 20 mm. In case of unidirectional arrangement, magnetic coupling (*mc*) increases the homogeneity of the SMF; consequently, the decay of the function is shifted towards higher distances. In case of bidirectional arrangement, *mc* also increases magnetic induction by exactly 59%, averaged in the given range, but it fails to change the shape of the function. Applying 3×3 pieces of magnets (generator 17c) the effects of *mc* were similar, whereas the induction enhancement was smaller (22%).

Table 3.4. Summarized measured and derived data of SMF as obtained with a calibrated Hall probe at a distance of 3, 10, and 15 mm from the magnet surface in the different experiments.

generator	*z*=3mm				*z*=10mm				*z*=15mm			
	average *P-P* value (mT)	$\bar{\alpha}$ average surface roughness (T/m)	average *B*(mT)	standard deviation of *B*B(mT)	average *P-P* value (mT)	$\bar{\alpha}$ average surface roughness (T/m)	average *B*(mT)	standard deviation of *B*(mT)	average *P-P* value (mT)	$\bar{\alpha}$ average surface roughness (T/m)	average *B*(mT)	standard deviation of *B*(mT)
1	389.46	39.25	200.88	108.79	17.94	1.78	202.28	4.17	2.97	0.22	202.47	0.66
2	0	0	0	0	0	0	0	0	0	0	0	0
3	192.28	18.89	198.11	47.16	10.16	1.01	197.67	2.12	3.19	0.31	198.23	0.64
4	25.30	2.82	159.33	5.08	7.21	0.80	160.32	1.89	4.83	0.58	160.84	1.51
5	10.59	1.15	88.94	2.60	4.38	0.43	82.60	1.24	6.90	0.78	81.56	0.87
6	6.39	0.62	87.72	1.16	4.38	0.69	83.72	1.80	2.21	0.50	81.36	1.46
7	110.65	11.14	196.08	28.54	7.64	0.69	83.72	1.80	2.21	0.50	82.61	1.46
8	513.69	51.37	208.82	137.00	57.20	5.72	201.67	13.33	5.74	0.69	201.40	1.44
9	62.83	19.59	201.56	21.80	1.09	0.31	199.51	0.33	0.74	0.22	199.31	0.20
10	120.38	8.63	197.88	19.78	2.26	0.46	202.96	1.01	0.77	0.13	203.03	0.27
11	783.22	74.16	212.90	191.62	108.68	10.69	200.62	25.01	1.46	0.15	201.08	0.29
12	337.43	16.55	196.60	76.67	65.54	3.22	197.18	15.67	30.62	1.58	200.96	7.73
13	259.36	25.82	206.01	72.87	17.28	1.47	203.61	3.29	4.52	0.44	202.86	0.92
14	321.82	16.55	196.60	76.67	72.85	3.64	201.97	17.90	30.77	1.67	202.07	8.39
15	258.39	5.16	200.01	101.78	220.80	4.34	197.57	67.07	169.90	3.40	199.26	46.02
16	16.18	0.78	83.75	6.99	4.98	0.9	81.57	1.03	1.55	0.03	81.86	0.37

The computer-aided design and the picture of generator 11 frequently used in the biology experiments can be seen in Fig. (**3.2A**) and Fig. (**3.2B**), respectively.

The development of magnetic induction in the exposure chamber was estimated in advance by a computer model (ANSYS, Canonsburg, PA, USA) as shown in Fig. (**3.4**).

Fig. (**3.5A-C**) demonstrate the results of line scans in the exposure chamber of generator 11 at 3, 10, and 15 mm from the magnets' surface, respectively. Scanning started at 0 mm and continued until 40 mm with an increment of 1 mm.

The other lateral direction remains hidden in the figure for symmetry reasons.

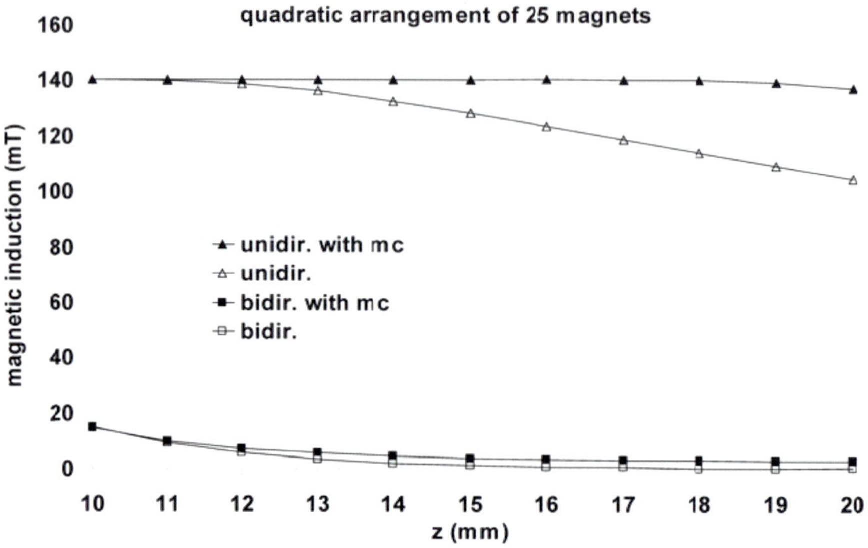

Fig. (3.1). The effect of magnetic coupling of the poles of the lower and upper magnets (mc) for a quadratic arrangement of 25 pieces of NdFeB cylindrical magnets of grade N50 with R=5 mm and L=10 mm. The magnetic induction perpendicular to the magnet surface is shown as a function of the distance from the surface of the axis of the central magnet (z coordinate between 10 and 20 mm).

A

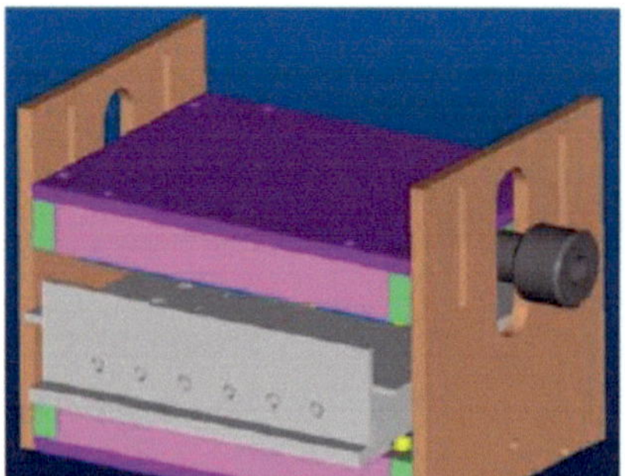

B

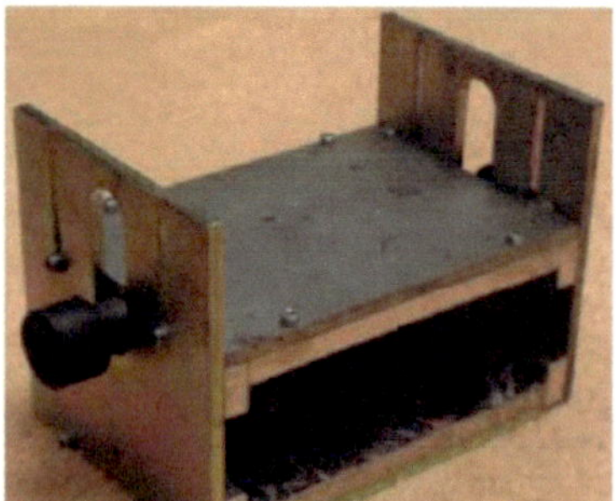

Fig. (3.2). A) Computer design of inhomogeneous SMF generator #11. The device consists of 2 ferrous matrices including 10×10 mm cylindrical N50 grade NdFeB magnets (remanent induction, B_r=1.47 T). The lateral periodicity of SMF is 10 mm. Individual magnets sit in a checkerboard configuration in the lower matrix and inversely in the upper one. In most of the experiments to be described, the distance between lower and upper magnets was fixed at 50 mm in order for comparison and to maximize the field induction through the cage. A Plexiglas animal cage is fitted into the exposure chamber. **B)** Photo of the device.

The optimum analgesic effect (*AE*) in the acute pain test was achieved with generator 11; therefore, it was used in most of the measurements where such detailed testing was not or would have hardly been executable.

Fig. (**3.3**) presents a conscious mouse in the Plexiglas cage in the exposure chamber of generator 11.

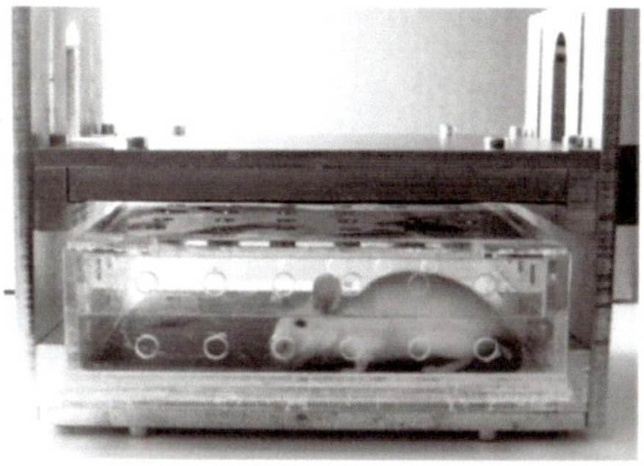

Fig. (3.3). Device for induction of static magnetic field (generator 11). The generator contains 2 magnet holding matrices, one below and another on top of the animal cage. The cage is made of Plexiglas, its size is L×W×H=140×140×46 mm. The poles below and above the cage facing each other are of opposite polarity allowing field lines to cross the cage; that is to say, SMF has vertical components.

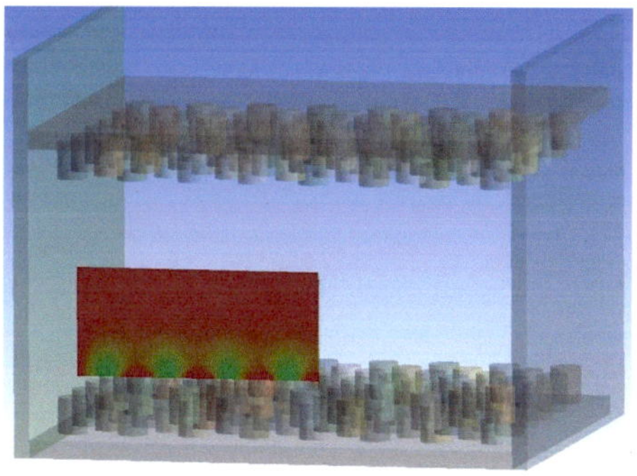

Fig. (3.4). Computer model of the SMF produced in the exposure chamber of generator 11.

GENERATORS 17a-e

Generator 11 was altered in a way that some magnets were unidirectional in a group of magnets, whereas the polarity of the neighboring magnet group was opposite. Such SMF was called *M*-SMF designating the number of magnets used per group. *M* was exactly the square root of the number of magnets. This "partitioned" arrangement was designed to test the effective lateral dimensions of a unidirectional arrangement on pain response in the writhing test (**Lateral**

gradients). *M* characterized a partition. The nomenclature of these partitions followed the rule: A group of 2×2 magnets was *M*=2 (Generator 17a), a group of 3×3 magnets was *M*=3 (Generator 17b), *etc.* up until 6×6 magnets, *M*=6 (Generator 17e). The upper matrix contained magnets with inverse pole structure. The original generator 11 in this system would have been 1×1 (*M*=1). Line scans of different partitions can be seen in Fig. (**3.6A**). Fig. (**3.6B**) presents a 3D view of the measured SMF created by generator 17d.

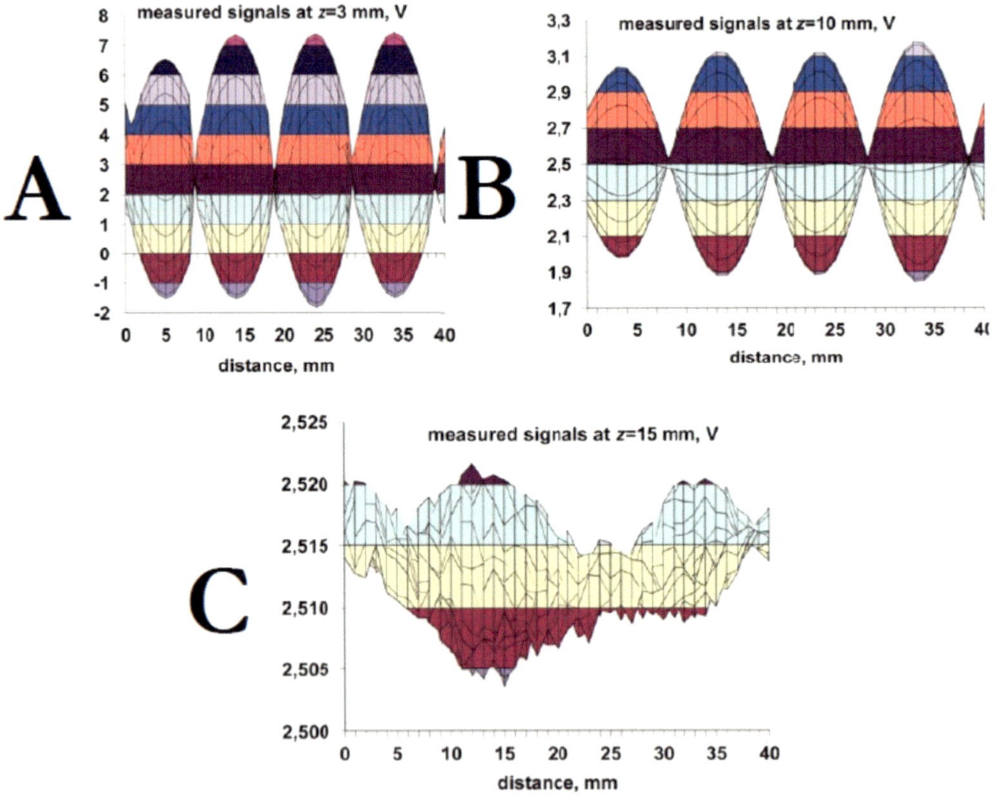

Fig. (3.5). Characteristic structures of the inhomogeneous static magnetic field (SMF) optimized for analgesia. Measured signals of a 5 V Hall probe with 12.3 mV/T sensitivity were taken at z=3 mm in panel **(A)**, 10 mm in panel **(B)**, and 15 mm in panel **(C)** from the surface of the top of the magnets. z is the coordinate perpendicular to the magnets' circular surface. Line scans were recorded from 0 to 40 mm in both directions (one of which remains hidden in the 2D figures) in steps of 1 mm.

GENERATOR 18

This generator was used in the human trial described in section **On healthy**

volunteers. The SMF-exposure system consisted of a metal frame that held 2 magnetically coupled ferrous matrices facing each other. The matrices contained cylindrical magnet blocks that were fixed onto a metal plate forming a square lattice with a lattice constant of 25 mm (for distance between block centers, see Fig. (**3.7B**). This layout generated an SMF that was strongly inhomogeneous in both lateral directions. Neighboring blocks were positioned with alternating poles. Magnets facing each other (in the matrices) were of opposite polarity. The distance between the 2 matrices was set constant at 50 mm. The exposure chamber of 140×100×50 mm^3 Fig. (**3.7A**) was big enough for a human palm and 4 fingers to fit in. The thumb remained outside the device.

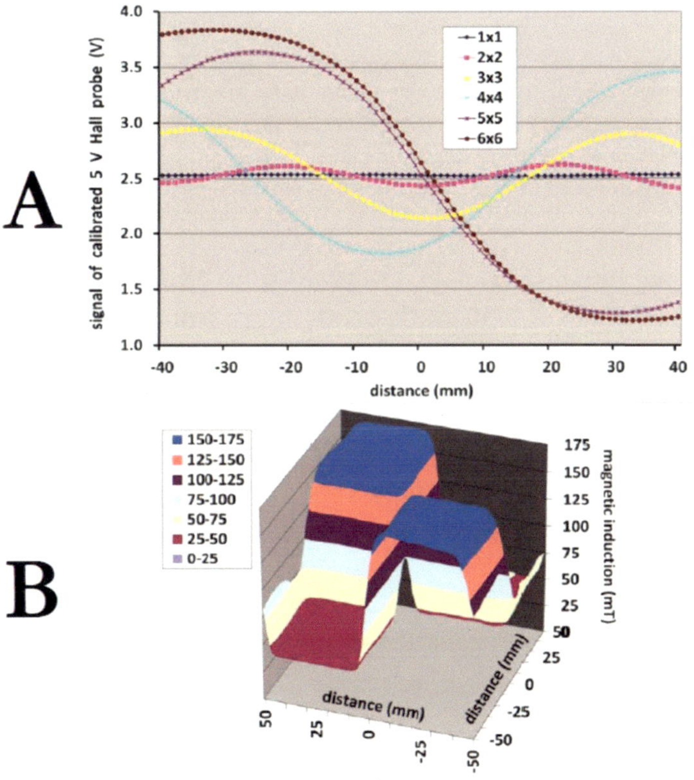

Fig. (3.6). Signals of the calibrated 5 V (12.3 mV/T sensitivity) Hall probe over generators 17a-e. The number of magnets sitting with identical poles in groups were different in the generators (2×2, 3×3, …, 6×6) in the lower matrix and inversely in the upper. **A)** Line scans were done at 3 mm above the upper surface of the magnets in the lower matrix between -40 and 40 mm. **B)** 3D view of the measured SMF created by generator 17d.

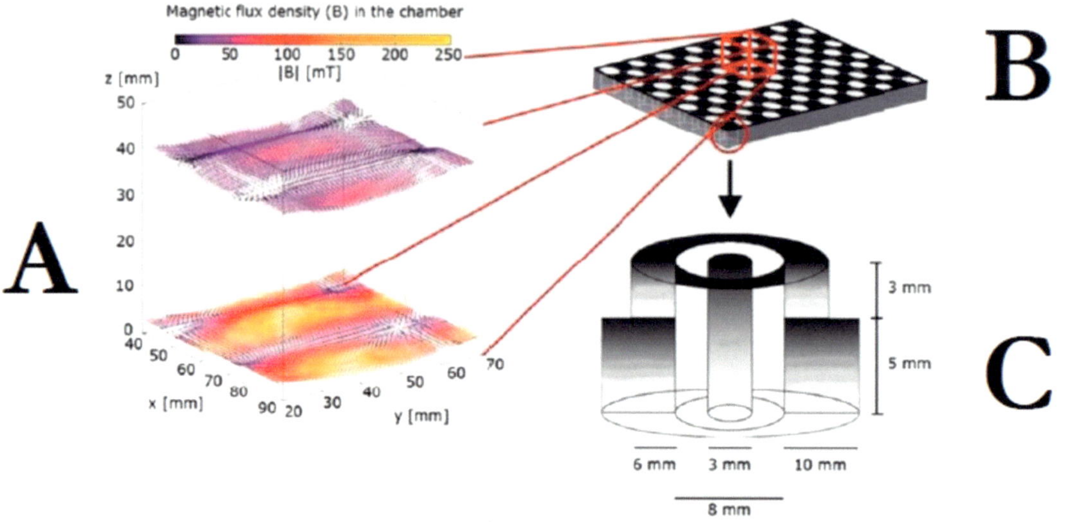

Fig. (3.7). Dimensions and polar configuration of the static magnetic field-exposure device used in the experiment. **A)** Magnetic induction components at 3 and 40 mm (distance measured from the lower matrix). **B)** Schematic presentation of the lower magnetic matrix. **C)** Single magnetic block containing an axially magnetized cylindrical permanent magnet. Magnetic poles are distinguished by black and white colors.

A single magnetic block (Fig. **3.7C**) contained an axially magnetized cylindrical permanent magnet made of N50 grade neodymium-iron-boron (NdFeB, B_r=1.47 T), coaxially surrounded by 2 ring-shaped magnets made of the same material with similar magnetization. The cylindrical magnets at the centre of a block were 8 mm high and had a diameter of 3 mm. The lower ring magnet was 5 mm in height, had 8 mm inner and 18 mm outer diameter, while the ring magnet on top had 3 mm height, 8 mm inner and 14 mm outer diameter. Magnetic poles pointed in the same direction within a block.

ANSYS computer model forecasted an optimally high number of magnetic field lines crossing the exposure chamber perpendicular to the surface of the magnets (Fig. **3.8**).

Typical *P-P* magnetic induction values were 330±0.1 mT at 3 mm, 103±0.1 mT at 10 mm, 19±0.1 mT at 20 mm, 22±0.1 mT at 30 mm, and 118±0.1 mT at 40 mm. These values of the vertical component of SMF were measured along the axis of a magnet block in the isocenter of the arrangement. The corresponding lateral gradient values were 13.2, 4.1, 0.8, 0.9, and 4.7 T/m, respectively. At z=10 and 40 mm within the chamber we expected identical magnetic inductions and gradients. The *P-P* values of the lateral components of the magnetic induction were about 70% below those of the perpendicular components. This arrangement was designed to maximize the flux of vertical magnetic field lines crossing the treatment chamber. The induction measurement followed the steps described in **Tools, sampling** for automation.

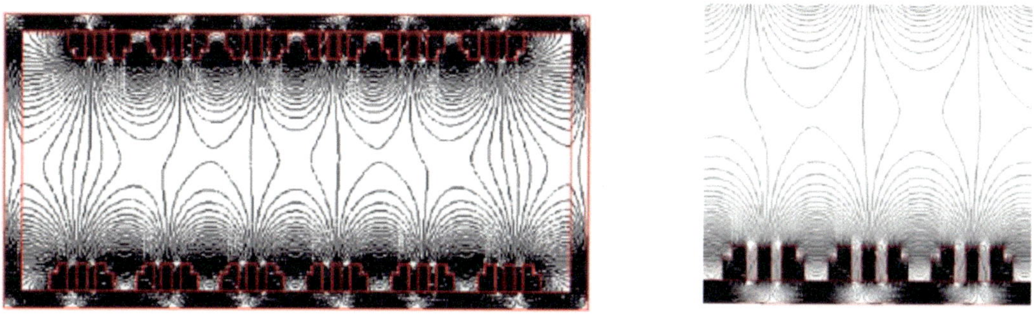

Fig. (3.8). Computer simulated magnetic lines of force (original and magnified for only 3 neighboring magnetic arrays) along a line in generator 18. In front and in back of those presented similar arrays are located with opposite poles (hidden in the 2D figure).

In this model, an analytic form of the magnetic induction ($B(z)$) along the axis of a pair of magnets can be found provided that R_1, R_2, R_3, L_1, L_2, D, B_{r1}, and B_{r2} are given (Fig. **3.9**).

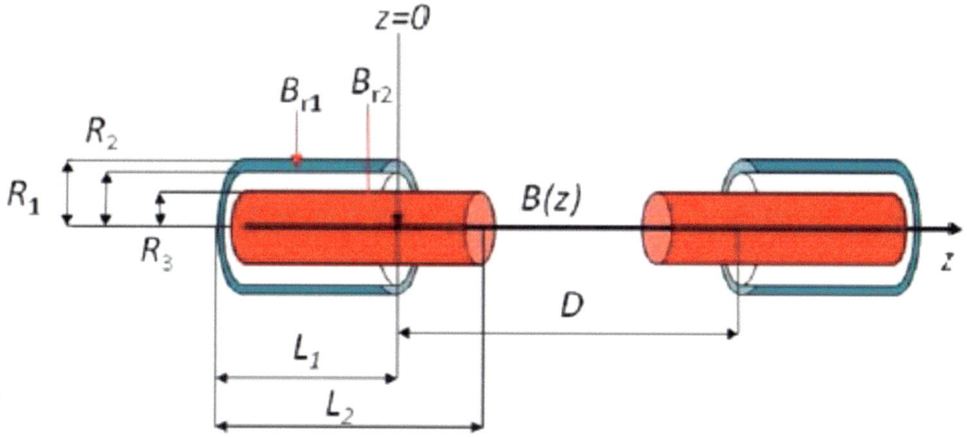

Fig. (3.9). Schematic arrangement of magnets of generator 18 and parameters of analytic form.

$$B(z)=\frac{B_{r1}}{2}\left[\frac{L_1+z}{\sqrt{R_1^2+(L_1+z)^2}}-\frac{z}{\sqrt{R_1^2+z^2}}\right]-\frac{B_{r1}}{2}\left[\frac{L_1+z}{\sqrt{R_2^2+(L_1+z)^2}}-\frac{z}{\sqrt{R_2^2+z^2}}\right]+$$

$$+\frac{\alpha B_{r2}}{2}\left[\frac{z+L_1}{\sqrt{R_3^2+(z+L_1)^2}}-\frac{z+L_1-L_2}{\sqrt{R_3^2+(z+L_1-L_2)^2}}\right]+\frac{B_{r1}}{2}\left[\frac{L_1+D-z}{\sqrt{R_1^2+(L_1+D-z)^2}}-\frac{D-z}{\sqrt{R_1^2+(D-z)^2}}\right]-$$

$$-\frac{B_{r1}}{2}\left[\frac{L_1+D-z}{\sqrt{R_2^2+(L_1+D-z)^2}}-\frac{D-z}{\sqrt{R_2^2+(D-z)^2}}\right]+\frac{\alpha B_{r2}}{2}\left[\frac{D+3L_1-2L_2-z}{\sqrt{R_3^2+(D+3L_1-2L_2-z)^2}}-\frac{D+3L_1-3L_2-z}{\sqrt{R_3^2+(D+3L_1-3L_2-z)^2}}\right]$$

Parameter a determines whether the magnets on one side have an identical (a=1) or opposite (a=-1) pole orientation.

GENERATOR 19

This exposure system originated in combining generator 3 with 17c. The SMF arrangement contained a single matrix of 3×3 individual cylindrical neodymium-iron-boron N35 magnets of size 10×10 mm (Borsmagnet, Budapest, Hungary). The individual magnets were 10 mm apart (distance between parallel axes) in the laterally plane matrix. Neighboring magnets sat in the matrix with alternating polarity. The arrangement was one-sided. Measured data along the axis of the central magnet were: 192±0.1 mT *P-P* value by 19 T/m gradient of the magnetic induction at 3 mm, 10±0.1 mT by 1 T/m at 10 mm, and 3±0.1 mT by 0 T/m at 15 mm. Typical magnetic induction values collected from a 20×20 mm area in the isocenter of the arrangement, measured at 3 mm from the magnets' surface can be seen in Fig. (**3.10**). Dosimetric measurements were carried out.

The schematics of the generator can be seen in Fig. (**3.11A**). The matrix was covered with a thin, soft tissue and was applied on the side of the face closest to the location of the pain sensation, usually between the maxilla and the mandible. The matrix was fixed on the headband of a headphone (Fig. **3.11B**), thus the patient did not have to hold the matrix to his/her face. This way the pressure of the matrix on the facial tissue was constant and limited, the maximal exerted pressure was 4.8-5.5 kPa (force measured with an American 3B Scientific (Tucker, GA, USA) dynamometer (model 10 N) divided by the area of the matrix), slightly depending on the distance between the ear pieces of the headphone. An identical looking matrix filled up with non-magnetized material of equal weight and applied to the same holder was used as a sham arrangement for the placebo-control examinations. The difference between sham and SMF-exposure devices could not be revealed by looking at, hearing, weighing the devices, or by touching with the naked hand.

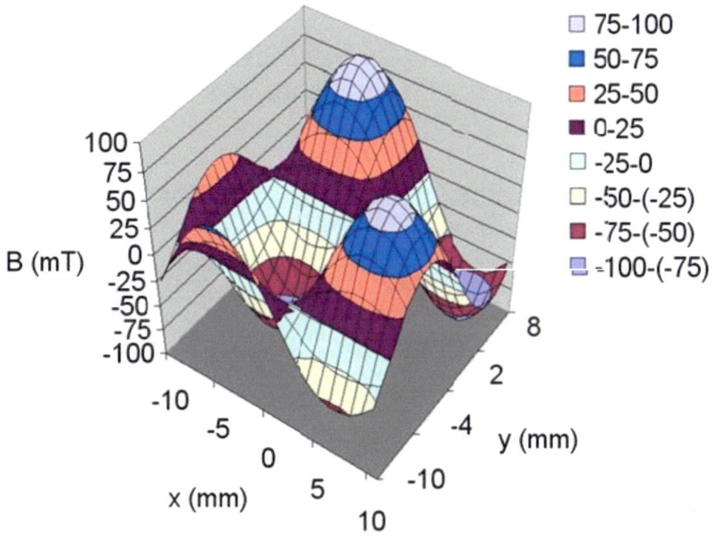

Fig. (3.10). Typical magnetic induction values collected from the isocenter of the 20×20 mm magnet arrangement at a distance of 3 mm above the magnet surface.

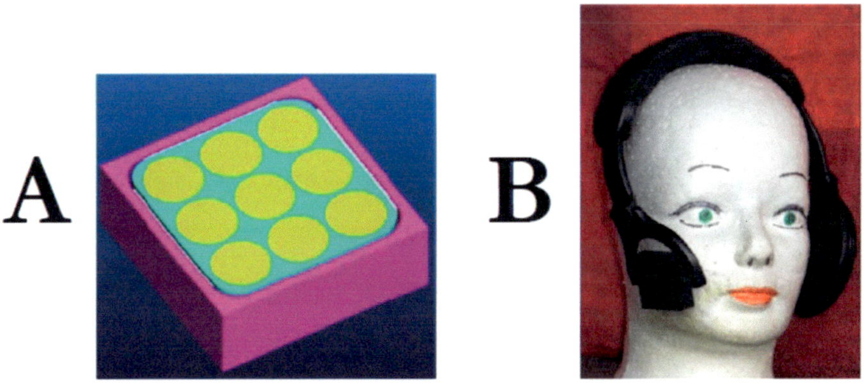

Fig. (3.11). A) Computer model of the 3×3 inhomogeneous SMF matrix. **B)** Photo of the device fixed on a headband.

GENERATOR 20

Fig. (**3.12**) shows a magnetically screened, commercially available Philips

Achieva 3 T MR tomograph. The B_0 SMF component of such a device was used in **Clinical MRI**. The dominant 3 T SMF is a homogeneous SMF within the bore of the device; it is horizontal and parallel to the axial symmetry axis of the bore. Neither the gradient, nor the radiofrequency scanning was used during our measurements. However, we performed life sciences tests at locations around the MR where only stray field components occurred in the lab and at the service area. At these locations the dominant SMF component was horizontal with a magnetic induction of 0.1, 0.5, or 3 mT.

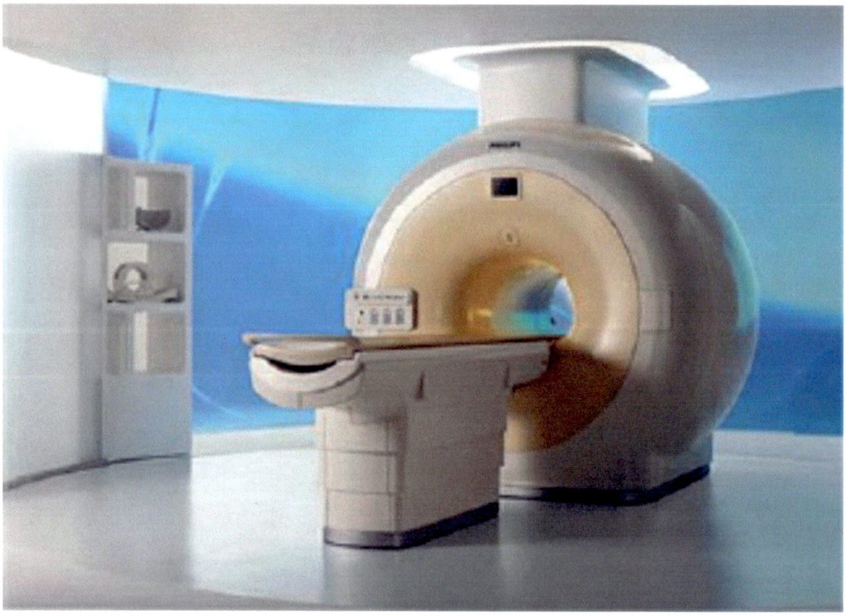

Fig. (3.12). The photo of a 3 T clinical MRI similar to the one used in the experiments (photo downloaded from http://www.mricenters.com/tesla.html).

GENERATOR 21

Fig. (**3.13**) shows this specially designed generator. This arrangement was meant to provide the advantages of (i) higher magnetic induction through the cage (to be positioned between the magnets), similarly to generator 13 and 14 but with longer magnets, (ii) using the high gradients of the checkerboard configuration of generator 11, and (iii) loosening the closed packing similarly to generator 12 and 14.

GENERATOR 22

This generator (Fig. **3.14**) furnished us with the highest achievable homogeneous, vertical magnetic induction in a lab. It contained 2 pieces of NdFeB N35 block magnets a size of 140×100×50 mm. These were fixed facing each other with opposite poles in a box made of 30 mm thick iron plates (weighing cca. 48 kg). The exposure chamber was similar in size to those in generators 1-16 (**Generators 1-16**). This generator basically created a uniform SMF of 420±3 mT inside its exposure chamber.

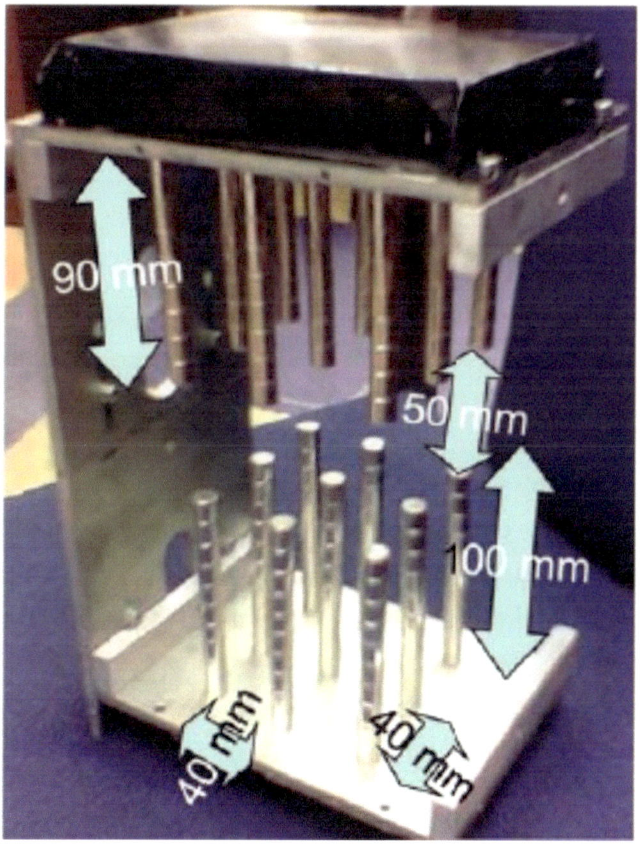

Fig. (3.13). The animal cage was inserted between the magnetic columns.

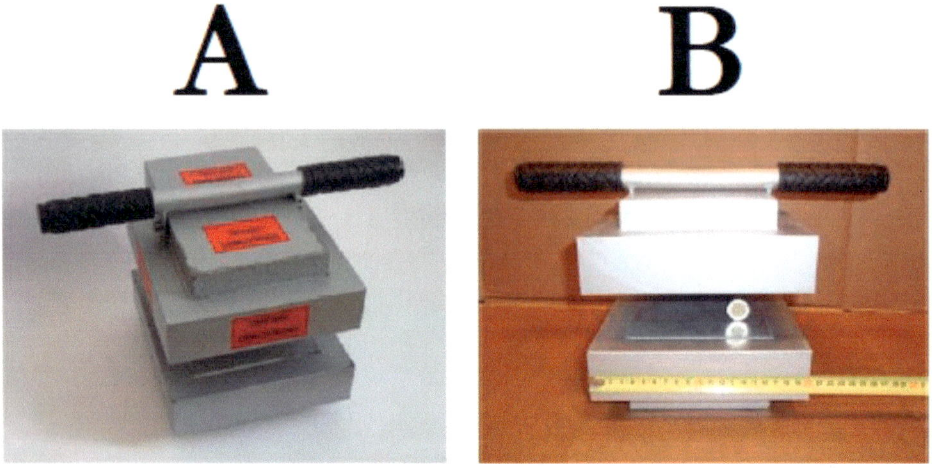

Fig. (3.14). Labels in panel **(A)** are warnings of strong magnetic field. In panel **(B)**, there is a 100 HUF coin inside the exposure chamber. The tape line is in units of cm.

In terms of mobility, this generator caused some problems. A special wooden block had to be shaped to fully fit the exposure chamber in order to prevent the generator of "sucking" in all ferromagnetic materials around it. This block was removed only during the experiments, when the animal cage was inserted in its place.

SUMMARY

The development of the SMF-generating device in the course of an acute visceral pain model experimental series will be detailed in **Optimization of SMF parameters**. The main factor in optimizing the device was how effective it could be in its *AE*. The general conclusion was drawn that the stronger and the more inhomogeneous the SMF, the higher the *AE*. A homogeneous SMF is expected to be efficient only if its magnetic induction is orders of magnitude higher (*e.g.* generator 20) than that of the *P-P* value of a strongly inhomogeneous SMF.

Generators 17a-e served the purpose of identifying whether the horizontal gradients of the vertical component of the magnetic induction affect the biological response in the same test. When using these generators, the problematic question was raised what the contribution of the self-motion-induced electric currents in the extent of the response was.

Generator 18 was a more promising model for generating stronger inhomogeneous SMF in the halving plane between the matrices than generators 1-3 and 7-15.

Generator 19 was developed for the special purpose of executing human trials. Here the main considerations were the low weight, the comfortable wearing, and the self-support of the device.

Generators 21 and 22 were also tried out in the writhing tests.

Now let us see how exposure to SMF generators 11 and 16 affected the viability of different microorganisms.

CHAPTER 4

In Vitro Experiments on Microorganisms

Keywords: *Bacillus circulans*, *E. coli*, *Micrococcus luteus*, *Pseudomonas fluorescens*, *Saccharomyces cerevisiae*, *Salmonella enteritidis*, *Serratia marcescens*, *Staphylococcus aureus*.

STATIC MAGNETIC FIELD-EXPOSURE FAILS TO AFFECT THE VIABILITY OF DIFFERENT BACTERIA STRAINS

Preliminaries

As mentioned in the **Introduction**, the proliferation of magnetic resonance imaging (MR) and the ever increasing need to achieve better graphical resolution of the image brought about the necessity of the examinations of bacteria under strong SMF again. This does not happen exclusively because of the possible adverse side effects microorganisms can cause during imaging, *e.g.* direct effect on bacterial growth [47] and/or changes in the antibiotic resistance in case of bacterial diseases [48], but also their possible long lasting effects, *e.g.* altering the DNA repair processes [49].

Several authors used bacterial strains and plant cells to study the effects of SMF-exposure. Stasiuk already in 1974 [50] exposed *Mycobacterium tuberculosis* to 180 mT SMF and found that though exposure of up to 1 h did not change the bacterial growth, but longer exposure (2 h and more) resulted in significant inhibition in their growth. No changes were observed on the sensitivity to antibiotics or growth in tissues in infected animals. Khar'kova *et al.* [51] studied the effect of long exposures of *Staphylococcus* in a 5 mT SMF. Permanent changes in the color of colonies (after 16 days), changes in their morphology and in the fermentation of proteins and hydrocarbons were observed by 18 months. After 8 months, the sensitivity to antibiotics increased significantly. The mortality increased in mice upon their infection with SMF-exposed *Staphylococcus*. More recently, Grosman *et al.* [52] studied the effect of 0.5-4 T SMF-exposure on

János F. László

Escherichia coli (*E. coli*) and *Staphylococcus aureus* with 30-120 min exposure times. They found no effect on growth. Benson *et al.* [53] observed enhancement of the effect of the antibiotic gentamicin to *Pseudomonas aeruginosa* exposed to 0.5-2 mT for 20 min. They could not claim with all certainty that the decreased growth might have been influenced by the different light conditions. Stansell *et al.* [48] exposed *E. coli* to 8-60 mT for 19.5 h and studied the effect of the antibiotic piperacillin. SMF-exposure increased the resistance to the antibiotic. Kohno *et al.* [54] examined *Streptococcus mutans*, *Staphylococcus aureus*, and *E. coli* determining growth rate, maximum numbers of bacteria, and (3H)-thymidine incorporation in the exposure of ferrite block magnets of inductions 30, 60, 80, and 100 mT. Although no effect of SMF-exposure on (3H)-thymidine incorporation and on the growth of *E. coli* cultures could be identified, the magnetic induction was found to inhibit both the growth rate and the maximum number of *Streptococcus mutans* and *Staphylococcus aureus* when cultured under anaerobic conditions. There was no effect under aerobic conditions. Binhi *et al.* [55] used *E. coli* cells for exploring effects by studying anomalous viscosity time dependencies. They found that within the range of 0 to 110 μT the spectrum showed several extremes. They explained the effect by the rotation of magnetically active complexes, such as Ca^{2+}, Mg^{2+}, and Zn^{2+}. Zhang *et al.* [56] concluded that the growth of *E. coli* was inhibited due to the presence of SMF. They modified field intensity and applied the Series Piezoelectric Quartz Crystal (SPQC) sensing technique. By relating 3 kinetic growth parameters, *i.e.* the asymptote, the maximum specific growth rate, and the lag time to the SMF-exposure, they established a response model for the frequency shift. Piatti *et al.* [57] found that the exposure of *Serratia marcescens* to 8±2 mT SMF inhibited the growth of the bacteria. For *Hordeum vulgare*, they observed a decreased viability, whereas for *Rubus fruticosus*, SMF remained ineffective. Potenza *et al.* [47] devoted a series of experiments to *E. coli* under the influence of 300 mT SMF. Their focus was on biomass growth of different strains of bacteria in 3 different media when exposed to SMF for up to 50 h. They could not identify a difference in growth between *E. coli* in the standard medium and the unexposed control. Triampo *et al.* [58] investigated cell division of *Leptospira interrogans serovar canicola* under the influence of long exposure to a 140±5 mT SMF. Their data showed a somewhat lower density of the bacterium under SMF treatment than the control; however, no statistical analysis was provided. The subject of the study of Gao *et al.* [59] was *Shewanella oneidensis*. This strain was exposed to 14.1 T SMF for 12 h and the post-exposure growth was observed for another 18 h. They found no difference between treated and control cells in terms of optical density, colony forming unit, or post-exposure growth of cells. Morrow *et al.* [60] used *Streptococcus pyogenes* to reveal potential differences in growth rate between 0.3-0.5 T SMF-exposure for 8 h and control. They correlated a significant decrease in growth rate to 0.3 T as well as a significant increase to 0.5 T exposure provided the growth was under anaerobe conditions. The contradictory data of the literature regarding the potential of SMF-exposure to promote or inhibit cell growth are summarized in Table **4.1**.

Table 4.1. Summary of literature regarding the potential of SMF-exposure to promote or inhibit cell growth in different bacterium strains.

reference	**subject**	**SMF**	**exposure time**	**findings**
Grosman *et al.* [52]	*E. coli, Staphylococcus aureus*	0.5-4 T	30-120 min	no effect on growth
Kohno *et al.* [54]	*Streptococcus mutans, Staphylococcus aureus, E. coli*	30, 60, 80, 100 mT	?	
Piatti *et al.* [57]	*Serratia marcescens*	8±2 mT	24 h ?	growth inhibition
	Hordeum vulgare			
	Rubus fruticosus			no effect on growth
Potenza *et al.* [47]	*E. coli*	300 mT	50 h	
Triampo *et al.* [58]	*Leptospira interrogans*	140±5 mT	1, 2, 3, 4, 5, 6 d	growth inhibition, but no statistics
Gao *et al.* [59]	*Shewanella oneidensis*	14.1 T	12 h	no effect on growth
Morrow *et al.* [60]	*Streptococcus pyogenes*	300 mT	8-15 h	growth inhibition
		500 mT		growth promotion

Goals

We decided to start at an early phase of phylogenesis. We considered the question whether we can establish the boundary of biological development under which an observable reaction to external SMF-exposure can be expected at all? Experiments on the viability of bacteria *in vitro* seemed to be an adequate method to test the level of development of bacteria from the viewpoint of having evolved magnetic sensors.

Materials and Methods

Magnetic Exposure Conditions

For homogeneous SMF (hSMF) generator 16 (**Generators 1-16**) was used. As a reminder for the Reader, the features of generator 16 are repeated in Table **4.2**. For an inhomogeneous SMF (iSMF) generator, generator 11 was used (Table **4.3**).

Table 4.2. Specifications of the homogeneous SMF-exposure after Generators 1-16 (generator 16).

16.18	**average *P-P* value (mT)**	**z=3 mm**	ferrite	**material**	**individual magnets**
0.78	**average surface roughness (T/m)**		n/a	**grade**	
83.75	**average *B* value (mT)**		0.40	***B*r, remanent induction (T)**	
6.99	**average *P-P* value (mT)**		n/a	**radius (mm)**	
4.98	**average surface roughness (T/m)**	**z=10 mm**	25	**height (mm)**	
0.9	**average *B* value (mT)**		70	**length (mm)**	
81.57	**average *P-P* value (mT)**		50	**width (mm)**	
1.03	**average surface roughness (T/m)**		unidir.	**polarity**	**magnet arrangement**
1.55	**average *B* value (mT)**	**z=15 mm**	2	**number of matrices**	
0.03	**average *P-P* value (mT)**		yes	**magnetic coupling**	
81.86	**average surface roughness (T/m)**		n/a	**matrix constant (mm)**	
0.37	**average *B* value (mT)**				

In order to test several magnetic inductions and corresponding lateral gradients simultaneously in a single chamber so as to minimize the enormous sample sizes, we planned our experiments by using layers in the case of inhomogeneous SMF. We had 4 layers, 1-3 different and 4 control of 2.

Table 4.3. Specifications of the inhomogeneous SMF-exposure after Generators 1-16 (generator 11).

783.22	**average *P-P* value (mT)**	**z=3 mm**	NdFeB	**material**	**individual magnets**
74.16	**average surface roughness (T/m)**		N50	**grade**	
212.90	**average *B* value (mT)**		1.47	***B*r, remanent induction (T)**	
191.62	**average *P-P* value (mT)**		5	**radius (mm)**	
108.68	**average surface roughness (T/m)**	**z=10 mm**	10	**height (mm)**	
10.69	**average *B* value (mT)**		n/a	**length (mm)**	
200.62	**average *P-P* value (mT)**		n/a	**width (mm)**	
25.01	**average surface roughness (T/m)**		bidir.	**polarity**	**magnet arrangement**
1.46	**average *B* value (mT)**	**z=15 mm**	2	**number of matrices**	
0.15	**average *P-P* value (mT)**		yes	**magnetic coupling**	
201.08	**average surface roughness (T/m)**		10	**matrix constant (mm)**	
0.29	**average *B* value (mT)**				

The diameter of the Petri dishes was 90 mm. Three Petri dishes were stacked on top of each other. A positioning mold made of plastic was used to hold stacks in place on the matrices. In case of iSMF the Petri dish at the bottom of the stack was denoted as layer 1. Similarly, the middle of the stack was layer 2 dish, and the top of the stack was layer 3 dish. The height of one Petri dish (12 mm) defined the distance between the layers. Therefore, the actual distance from the magnetic surface was z_1=3 mm for layer 1, z_2=15 mm for layer 2, and z_3=27 mm for layer 3. The magnetic induction (the vertical component) and the gradient (of the vertical components of the inductions) values were 476.7±0.1 mT and 47.7 T/m, 12.0±0.1

mT and 1.2 T/m, and 2.8±0.1 mT with 0.3 T/m for layer 1, 2 and 3, respectively. A 4th layer was also introduced at z_4=39 mm for control reasons; measured magnetic values at this distance should agree with those in layer 2.

We also worked with various SMF-exposure times: 10, 30, and 50 min in all situations; plus 24 h in some cases where suspicion arose that we may have missed the sensitive time periods of the microorganisms.

Microorganism

Bacillus circulans B 01115, *E. coli* ATCC 35218, *Micrococcus luteus* B 01072, *Pseudomonas fluorescens* B 01102, and *Saccharomyces cerevisiae* NCAIM Y 00151 were derived by National Collection of Agricultural and Industrial Microorganisms (Budapest, Hungary). *E. coli* ATCC 35218 originated from American Type Culture Collection (Manassas, VA, USA). The Department of Microbiology and Infectious Diseases, Culture Collection at Faculty of Veterinary Science, Szent István University (Budapest, Hungary) provided *Salmonella enterica serovar Enteritidis* 359/07, *Serratia marcescens* 15/2/7/2, and *Staphylococcus aureus* 52/03.

In vitro Assay, Method of Detection

These groups of microorganisms all need aerobe fermentation at 30°C for 24-48 h. We let them grow on a modified nutrient agar consisting of 28.0 g Nutrient agar (NA from Difco, Becton, Dickinson, Sparks, MD, USA), 5.0 g D(+) glucose, 5.0 g saccharose, and 3.0 g yeast extract (from Becton). The final pH of the agar was 7.2. It was then sterilized by autoclaving at 121°C for 15 min. The bacteria were grown on this modified NA agar. We added 1 ml distilled water to the agar slant of bacteria and washed the bacterial concentrate off the agar. These concentrated slants were diluted by introducing water to create 10^{-7}, 10^{-8}, and 10^{-9} diluted sample portions per 0.1 ml of water. The 0.1 ml inoculums were later spread over the freshly prepared agar with a sterile glass rod, and the dishes were placed in the SMF generator. Following the 10, 30, 50, and in some cases 1440 min SMF-exposure, the Petri dishes were incubated at 30°C for 24-48 h.

After 24 h, the number of colonies was optically examined. If colonies have not yet developed (as was the case *e.g.* for the yeast), incubation continued and the dishes were reexamined after another 24 h. The growth of colonies in a Petri dish is a positive test for the appearance of cells. The colonies in the plate were counted and the results were expressed as cell counts per ml of the concentrated bacterial sample, taking into account the corresponding dilution factor.

In order to verify the assumption that the microorganisms may be sensitive to SMF, but their sensitivity period of the day does not even partially match the time of a shorter (10-50 min) period of exposure, we carried out experiments on some strains (*Bacillus circulans, E. coli, Salmonella enteritidis, Serratia marcenses,* and *Staphylococcus aureus*) with a longer (24 h) exposure time in the hSMF setup. As for the 24 h experiment in the iSMF setup, we restricted the examinations to *Serratia marcenses* due to the time-consuming nature of the experiments.

Statistical Analysis

A minimum of 3 parallels were used for each average value (shown in the figures). Single-factor ANOVA was used to assess *p* values for multiple sets of data. Dunnett's test was applied in pairwise comparison when samples of equal number were compared. In case of comparison of unequal number of data, Bonferroni correction was used. Series of data were regarded significantly different if $p \leq 0.05$.

We defined viability as the survival probability of a strain compared to an untreated sample (control); thus $v=100(<x>/<y>)\%$ where $<x>$ and $<y>$ are the average numbers of cells in the treated and sham control group, respectively.

In order to show the data in the clearest and most concise form possible, the results of the tests are summarized in graphs with stacked columns representing average values and error bars designating negative standard errors of the mean (SEM).

Results

Effect of hSMF on Cell Number

The average cell number±SEM of *Saccharomyces cerevisiae*, *Serratia marcescens*, *Salmonella enteritidis*, *E. coli*, *Staphylococcus aureus*, *Bacillus circulans*, *Micrococcus luteus*, and *Pseudomonas fluorescens* in units of 10^8/ml as a function of homogeneous exposure duration in min can be seen in Fig. (**4.1**). (For the shading codes see Fig. **4.2**). The odd-number columns indicate SMF-exposed samples, the even-numbered columns sham control for all 4 exposure durations. The number of independent samples (*n*) was 8 for the 10-50 min and 6 for the 1440 min exposure time for each strain. We could not reveal any significant difference between SMF-exposed and control cell numbers at the 95% confidence level for any strains for any exposure times with the exception of *Saccharomyces cerevisiae* 30 min (* $p<0.05$).

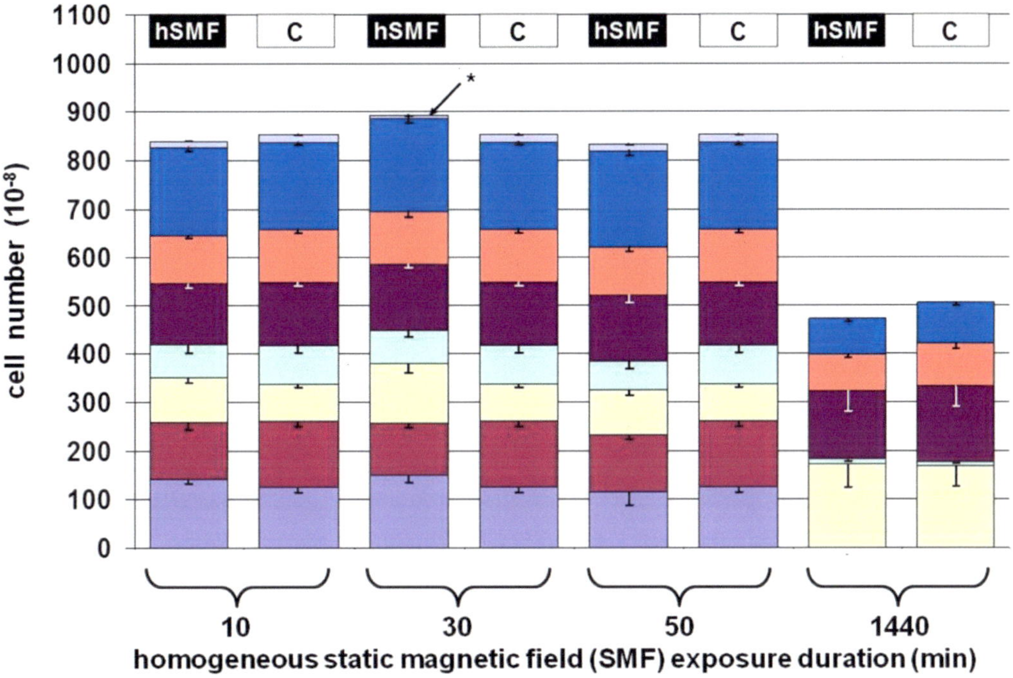

Fig. (4.1). The average cell number±SEM of *Saccharomyces cerevisiae*, *Serratia marcescens*, *Salmonella enteritidis*, *E. coli*, *Staphylococcus aureus*, *Bacillus circulans*, *Micrococcus luteus*, and *Pseudomonas fluorescens* in units of 108/ml as a function of homogeneous static magnetic field (hSMF: 159.2±13.4 mT) exposure duration in min. SEM values are designated by negative error bars. The odd-number columns denote exposed samples (SMF), the even-numbered columns sham control (C) for all 4 exposure durations. The number of independent samples (*n*) was 8 for the 10-50 min and 6 for the 1440 min exposure time for each strain. * means $p<0.05$ statistically significant difference between SMF-exposed and control cell numbers at the 95% confidence level.

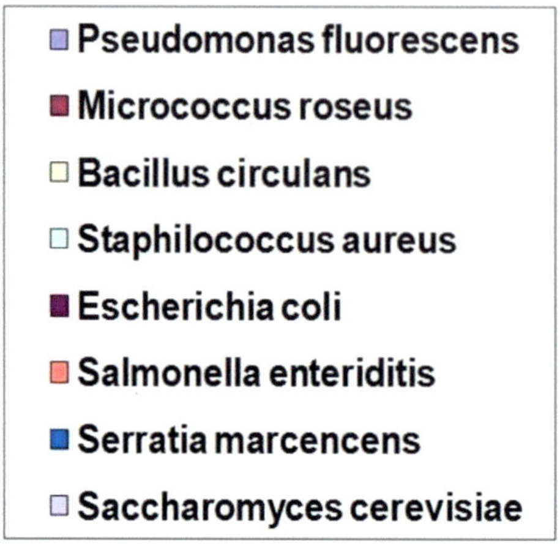

Fig. (4.2). Shading codes to Fig. (**4.1**) and Fig. (**4.3**).

Effect of iSMF on Cell Number

The average cell number±SEM of *Serratia marcescens*, *Salmonella enteritidis*, *E. coli*, *Staphylococcus aureus*, *Bacillus circulans*, *Micrococcus luteus*, and *Pseudomonas fluorescens* in units of 10^8/ml as a function of inhomogeneous exposure duration in min can be seen in Fig. (**4.3**). The independent variable axis also distinguishes between layer numbers (1 through 4) defining different magnetic inductions and corresponding lateral gradients as described in the Materials and methods section. The number of independent samples was n=8, except for *Micrococcus luteus* n=7 (50 min, layer 3); *Serratia marcescens* n=16 (30 min) for all layers and control, and n=3 (1440 min). Results obtained from *Staphylococcus aureus* and *Bacillus circulans* for 1440 min exposure time are hard to accept without reservations due to the high SEM values. There is no significant difference between SMF-exposed and sham cell numbers at the 95% confidence level for any strains for any exposure times for any layers with the exception of *Pseudomonas fluorescens* 30 min 2nd layer (** p<0.001),

Bacilluscirculans 30 min layer 3 (* $p<0.05$) and 4 (*), and *Echerischia coli* 50 min layer 1 (*).

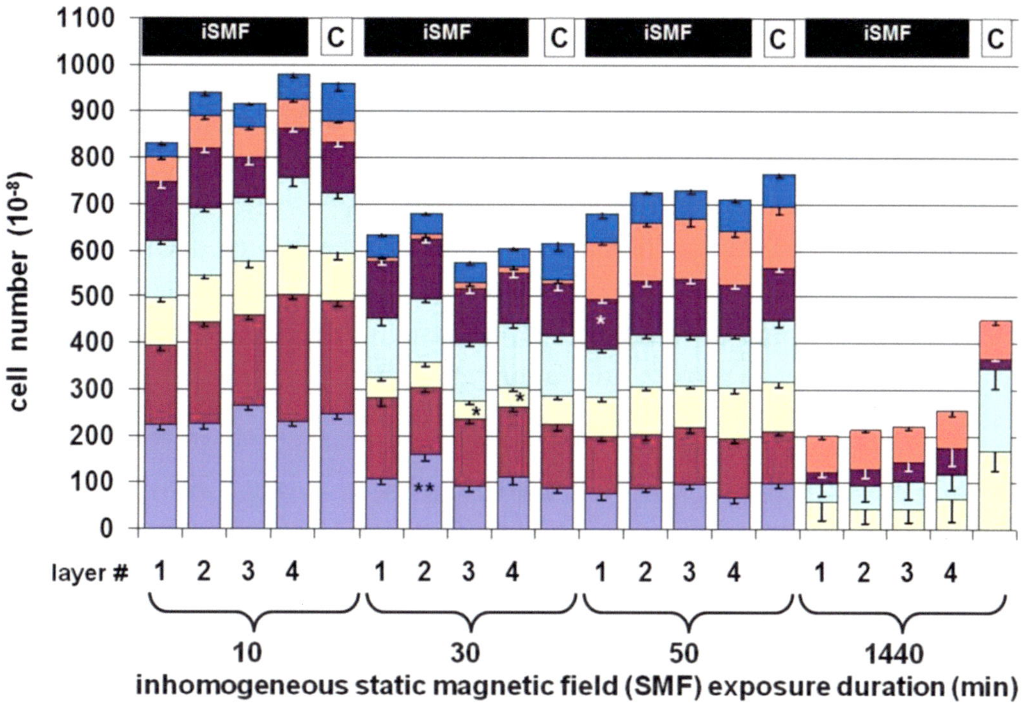

Fig. (4.3). The average cell number±SEM of *Serratia marcescens*, *Salmonella enteritidis*, *E. coli*, *Staphylococcus aureus*, *Bacillus circulans*, *Micrococcus luteus*, and *Pseudomonas fluorescens* in units of 108/ml as a function of exposure duration in min. SEM values are designated by negative error bars. The independent variable axis also distinguishes between layer numbers (1 through 4) defined by different magnetic inductions and corresponding lateral gradients (iSMF: layer 1: 476.7±0.1 mT with 47.7 T/m, layer 2: 12.0±0.1 mT with 1.2 T/m, layer 3: 2.8±0.1 mT with 0.3 T/m, and layer 4: similar to #2 layer). The number of independent samples was n=8 except for *Micrococcus luteus* 50 min, n=7 (layer 3); *Serratia marcescensn*=16 (30 min) for all layers and control, and n=3 (1440 min). * and ** mean $p<0.05$ and $p<0.001$, respectively statistically significant difference between SMF-exposed and control cell numbers at the 95% confidence level.

Comparison of Control Layers 2 and 4 in the iSMF Arrangement

We also checked the cell numbers obtained for layer 2 and layer 4 that were supposed to result in similar growth values due to the similarity of the magnetic inductions and the corresponding lateral gradients. Overall, the average cell number difference between layer 2 and layer 4 for 10, 30, 50, and 1440 min exposure times was within 14%. This seemed to be an acceptable agreement between layer 2 and 4.

Discussion, Conclusions

Our present findings; namely, the lack of positive effect of SMF on bacterium viability, supports the idea of Grosman *et al.* [52], Kohno *et al.* [54], Potenza *et al.* [47], and Gao *et al.* [59]. Even the results of Morrow *et al.* [60] could be verified as the induction in the present experiment lay between 0.3 and 0.5 T. The growth inhibition found by Triampo *et al.* [58] may have been due to the special strain of bacteria they used. In the case of Piatti *et al.* [57], the induction was only comparable to our measurements on layer 2 and 3 in the iSMF arrangement. In these cases, we found a growth promotion rather than inhibition induced by SMF-exposure for 10 min; however, no effect for 30 or 50 min.

The only bacterium type that is known to react to external SMF-exposure is magnetotactic bacteria (see *e.g.* Lefèvre *et al.* [61] and Pósfai *et al.* [62]). Nevertheless, in experiments with this type of bacteria, it is not the cell number that was modulated by the exposure, but rather the direction of motion (magnetotaxis) by the alignment and swimming along magnetic field lines. In our case, the magnetic induction was a minimum of 5 orders of magnitude bigger than that of the geomagnetic field (not mentioning the difference in the lateral gradients). Still, optical detection of the grown cell structures could not reveal any lateral periodicity, *i.e.* any pattern that would have reflected the checkerboard-like periodicity of iSMF.

In summary, it seems likely that the level of biological development where we could expect magnetic receptors lies above that of microorganisms. Every statistically significant difference between cell numbers of SMF-exposed and unexposed control samples even for 24 h exposure times that we revealed in this study, seemed more like an exception than a rule. In the forthcoming chapter, we shall be devoted to SMF-exposure experiments concerning a higher class of biological creatures, first invertebrates and then, mammals.

CHAPTER 5

In Vivo Animal Experiments

Keywords: Behavioral test, Capsaicin-sensitive, *Cepaea nemoralis*, Circadian cycle, Epsom salt challenge, *Helix pomatia*, Hot plate test, Mechanical hyperalgesia model, Mice, Morphine, Neuropathic, Opioid-receptor, Preterm birth, Resiniferatoxin, Serotonergic system, Writhing test.

MODELS AND ASSAYS

Table **5.1** summarizes the animal models, the assays, and the corresponding (pre)-treatments (if any) we shall focus in this chapter.

Table 5.1. Animal models, tests, and corresponding (pre)-treatments (if any) discussed in this chapter.

Animal	Invertebrates	Vertebrates				
	Land snail	Mouse				
	Helix pomatia	BALB/c	CD1	C57BL/6	CFLP	CSJLF1
Test						
Hot plate	naloxone serotonin tryptamine					
Elevated plus maze					morphine	
Locomotor activity					morphine	
Rotarod		×				
Seltzer		×				
Timed-pregnancy				lipopoly-saccharide		
Von Frey		carrageenan formalin resiniferatoxin	strepto-zotocin			
Writhing					β-funaltrexamine morphine naloxone naltrindole norbinaltorphimine	

János F. László

The professional expectations in *in vivo* experimental models are:

i. The model should reflect a pathological condition including symptoms similar to that occurring in humans,
ii. the model should be specific, sensitive, valid, reliable, and reproducible [63].

Supposing that all these requirements are met, data derived from observation of *in vivo* experiments are of utmost importance with regard to the therapeutic method under investigation since the psychosomatic/placebo effects can be excluded under experimental conditions.

Preclinical pain models can be separated into 3 functional divisions based on their potential mechanisms. Nociception can be induced acutely by thermal, mechanical, or chemical stimulus (*e.g.* hot plate test, or tail flick test), it can be based on tissue injury (*e.g.* writhing, formalin, inflamed joint, or paw test), or can originate in nerve injury [64].

In the experiment, detailed in this section, we used an animal cage made of Plexiglas with air holes on all sides, except on the bottom. The size of the cage was 140×140×46 mm. The 2 opposite side walls of the cage were transparent, the other 2 and the top were covered with opaque, air permeable material. Similar environmental conditions could be actualized for both SMF- and sham-exposed animals. The support under the cage was always plane and stable.

No efforts were ever made to magnetically shield the experimental setup from the geomagnetic field. Creatures throughout the hundred millions of years of phylogenesis on Earth have adapted to this field. Therefore, shielding might have introduced unwanted effects (*c.f.*, [27]).

ETHICAL ISSUES

All experimental procedures described in Chapter 5 were carried out according to the European Communities Council Directives (86/609/ECC) complying with the

i. Hungarian Act for the Protection of Animals in Research (law 1998/XXVIII, par. 32),
ii. edict 243/1988 of the Hungarian Parliament on Animal Protection and

Consideration Decree of Scientific Procedures of Animal Experiments,

iii. recommendations of the International Association for the Study of Pain [65], and the

iv. Helsinki Declaration.

Each study was approved by one of the following committees.

a. Animal Care and Protection Committee at the University of Debrecen (No.: IV/1813-1/2002 or No.: 7/2011/DE MAB),
b. Animal Care Committee of Semmelweis University, Budapest (No.: 1810/003/2004),
c. Ethics Committee on Animal Research of the University of Pécs according to the Ethical Codex of Animal Experiments (No.: BA02/2000-16-2006), and
d. Hungarian Ethical Committee for Animal Research at Debrecen University (No.: 26/2007).

MATERIALS

Chemicals were purchased from (in alphabetical order) Invitrogen (Carlsbad, CA, USA), Merck (Whitehouse Station, NJ, USA), Molecular Probes (Eugene, OR, USA), Pharmacy of the University of Pécs, Sigma-Aldrich (St. Louis, MO, USA), and Tocris Bioscience (Bristol, UK). Beyond those inbred, animals were provided by Charles River (Budapest or Isaszeg, Hungary) and Toxicoop (Budapest, Hungary). Kits and devices came from (in alphabetical order) Abcam (Cambridge, UK), Bio-Tek Instruments (Winooski, VT, USA), Experimetria (Budapest, Hungary), Lab Vision (Fremont, CA, USA), Nikon (Tokyo, Japan), Osram (Munich, Germany), Photometrics (Tucson, AZ, USA), Supertech (Pécs, Hungary), Techno Plastic Products (Trasadingen, Switzerland), and Ugo Basile, Comerio, Italy).

EXPERIMENTS ON INVERTEBRATES *IN VIVO*

Pharmacological Analysis of Response Latency in the Hot Plate Test Following Whole-Body Static Magnetic Field-Exposure in the Snail *Helix Pomatia*

Preliminaries

As mentioned already in the Introduction, artificial SMF have gradually gained an increasing importance in our life. The proliferation of diagnostic devices using strong SMF, such as the magnetic resonance (MR) tomographs raises the question whether exposure to SMF increases the risk of disease. This question initiated many investigations on the effects of SMF on biological systems in the past couple of decades. There is increasing evidence that exposure to both ultra strong (>5 T) and strong (1-5 T) SMF interacts with the vestibular system of both rodents and humans, thus, inducing changes in locomotor and visual behavior [66]. Moderate-intensity SMF (<1 T) is able to influence a number of biological systems, particularly those whose function is closely linked to membrane ion channels as part of the peripheral nerve conduction system [67], neuromuscular activity, and synaptic transmission [68, 69] (for a review see [70]). However, the mechanisms underlying the observed effects are not entirely clear.

Snails possess a simple nervous system, display a simple behavioral repertoire; therefore, are optimal subjects for *in vivo* behavioral and neuronal investigations (for a review see [71]). Thus, the possible biological effects of different SMF-exposure have been studied at the neuronal level in snails in order to contribute to the understanding of the induced effects in mammals. These studies revealed that exposure to SMF in the mT range is able to change the bioelectric properties of selected neurons in isolated CNS preparations from the snail *Helix pomatia* and *Helix aspersa* [72, 73]. However, the mechanism of the observed effects could not be explained. Behavioral studies applying SMF exclusively have not been performed on snail. SMF, in these studies, served only as one component of combined magnetic fields. The combination of 78 mT SMF and 30, 60, or 120 Hz, 299 or 141 mT (*P-P*) low frequency electromagnetic fields (LFEMF) was used in a *Cepaea nemoralis* hot plate test and was found to reduce analgesia [74]. Analgesia was induced by an enkephalinase inhibitor that increased the level of endogenous opioid peptide enkephalin [75]. Enkephalins are known to exert *AE via* μ- and δ-opioid receptors in a manner analogous to the antinociceptive responses reported in mammals [76, 77]. Prato *et al.* [74, 78] demonstrated that this reductive effect on the analgesia depenfds on the plane and direction of the SMF. They combined 299±1 μT (*P-P*), 60 Hz LFEMF with 78±1 μT SMF and varied the angle between ELF and SMF components between 0° and 90°. The maximal reducing effect (50%) could be observed when the angle was between 50° and 70°.

LFEMF usually decreases analgesia in snails. Heat stress [79], novelty [80], or darkness [81] was observed to induce analgesia mediated *via* μ- and *x*-opioid receptors in *Cepaea nemoralis* [82]. Both the prototypical opiate antagonist naloxone and LFEMF blocked the induced *AE* [82] (for a review see [83]). An extremely low frequency, weak magnetic field complemented with a special, patented, pulsed magnetic field was shown to either increase or decrease analgesia depending on the environmental conditions [74, 77]. The induced *AE* involved mainly δ- and partly μ-opioid receptors; naloxone reduced, but could not eliminate the *AE* [77] (for a review see [83]).

It was also suggested that SMF-exposure enhances neurotransmission and the liberation of transmitters and modulators [84 - 86]. Serotonin has both transmitter and modulator roles in the different behaviors of invertebrate animals (for a review see [71, 87 - 89]). To fill in some gaps that arose in previous studies with regard to SMF-exposure combined with naloxone and serotonin, we investigated the possible interactions of the opioid system and the serotonergic system in SMF-exposure induced analgesia.

Goals

In the present study we aimed to clarify whether whole-body SMF-exposure leads to the modification of the thermo-nociceptive threshold in *Helix pomatia*. We used both hSMF- and iSMF-exposure conditions. Because of its clinical relevance (the main component (B_0) in medical diagnostic devices (MRI)), we primarily applied hSMF-exposure in this study. The reason for testing with iSMF-exposure as well was to reveal whether their biological response changed due to the Faraday currents occurring in their body. Snails' average speed of locomotion is notoriously low, hindering the effect of hSMF-inducible Faraday currents in their body. However, in case of iSMF-exposure, the motion of snails results in sampling different magnetic induction vectors giving rise to potential induced electric effects. We asked, if exposure implied an effect, then how this effect depended on exposure duration. We also tested the hSMF effect on snails pretreated with naloxone to investigate whether opiate receptors were involved in the hSMF-induced effects on the thermal nociceptive thresholds. Also, the role of interaction between different transmitters and the opioidergic systems in the SMF-induced analgesia has not been investigated so far. Therefore, our goal was also to study in the present series of experiments the role of the serotonergic system in the response of snails to the thermal challenge following hSMF-exposure. Since in a previous study it was suggested that the *AE* caused by an electromagnetic field in *Cepaea nemoralis* was circadian rhythm dependent [81], we wanted to provide further evidence that the response, indeed, depended on the circadian rhythm.

Materials and Methods

Magnetic Exposure Conditions

Generators 11 and 16 were used (see Table **5.3** and Table **5.2**, respectively). The apparatus we have seen in **Generators 1-16** is here shown with a land snail for size comparison (Fig. **5.1**). Both structures allowed us to insert a 150×100×46 mm (length × width × height) Plexiglas animal cage with air holes into the exposure chamber. An air permeable, opaque material covered the cage on 4 sides to make illumination circumstances similar in the exposure chamber and in the sham experiment. For iSMF or hSMF-exposure, 8-10 snails were put into the Plexiglas cage at a time, and then the cage containing the animals was inserted into the exposure chamber. Control (or sham-exposed) animals were neither exposed to iSMF, nor to hSMF but were placed in identical Plexiglas boxes for the same durations as their exposed mates. Neither during sham-exposure, nor during the hot plate test, was there any other SMF than the geomagnetic field at work (total field of 48.1946 μT, grown to 48.2526 μT during the time period of the experiments [3]).

The treatment involved whole-body exposure, and the animals were free to move within geometric restraints. However, since the cage was congested with animals, the average speed of self-motion was even lower than the notoriously low value (0.001 m/s) for snails [90]. This low speed together with the homogeneity of SMF must have prevented the evolution of SMF-induced Faraday currents in their body. In the case of iSMF, however, even the slow motion of snails could result in the potentiality to develop induced electric currents.

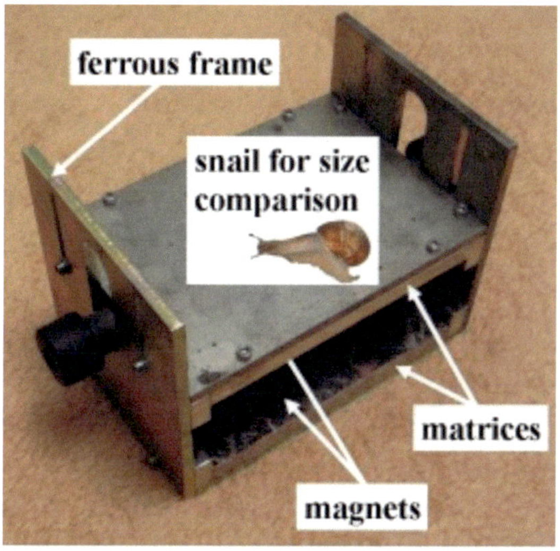

Fig. (5.1). Device for the induction of both homogeneous and inhomogeneous SMF including the photo of a Helix pomatia for size comparison. The device contains 2 magnet holding matrices, one below and another one on top of the exposure chamber (150×100×50 mm). The poles below and above the cage facing each other are of opposite polarity allowing field lines to cross the cage. Homogeneous SMF is generated by 2 ferrite block magnets (150×100×25 mm) and inhomogeneous SMF by 300 NdFeB cylindrical magnets (diameter × height=10×10 mm).

Chemical Pretreatment

The time- and dose-dependent response characteristics of different chemicals have been tested on the hot plate in *Helix pomatia* in a series of pilot tests. The chemicals diluted in *Helix* saline were injected into the body cavity of the snails right before the sham- or SMF-exposure (30 min before the thermal test). Control animals also spent 30 min under sham- or SMF-exposure preceding the thermal test. The time and dose-response characteristics of naloxone, a non-selective opioid receptor antagonist, have been tested in the hot plate test in *Helix aspersa*. The 1 μg/g dose already evoked maximal effect on the thermal nociceptive threshold that lasted for 45 min [91]. Some of the snails were, therefore, administered 50 μl, 2×10^{-4} M naloxone. Serotonin (5-HT) or tryptamine, a serotonin antagonist (5-hydroxytryptamine creatinine sulfate, tryptamine hydrochloride), was injected into the body cavity of snails in the amount of 100 μl, 10^{-4} M. Sham-exposed animals got *Helix* saline only if they were compared to chemically treated groups.

Thermal Stimulus

Land snails display a complex avoidance behavior to aversive thermal stimulus, which is analogous to that observed in rats and mice in a hot plate test. The snail's withdrawal reaction to nociceptive thermal stimulus is characterized by the elevation of the anterior portion of the fully extended foot. This response has been considered as a nociceptive one and its latency has been used to study *AE* in terrestrial snails [76, 82, 91, 92]. The response latency (time interval between placing the snail on the surface of the hot plate and the elevation of the foot until it reaches its readily discernible maximum elevation) was recorded. Preliminary experiments were run to determine the temperature at which snails displayed the withdrawal behavior in a reproducible and quantifiable manner (comfortably between 10 and 200 s) under laboratory conditions on the day of the experiment. Snails were placed on the surface of the hot plate (Model 01/1984, Farmakotechnika GMK, Budapest, Hungary) around its isocenter at temperatures ranging between 42 and 52°C. Temperature was set with an absolute accuracy of ±1°C. During the experiments, the actual hot plate temperature was 43±1°C. The sensor of a commercial digital thermometer was fixed to the center of the hot plate to serve as a control of the instantaneous temperature. All snails were allowed to fully hydrate before being tested.

Cepaea nemoralis displayed significantly greater response latency at night than during the day suggesting that the dark period of the circadian rhythm induces an *AE* in itself [81]. Our preliminary observations pointed toward the fact that SMF-exposure increased the thermal nociceptive threshold in *Helix pomatia*; consequently, the experiments were conducted during the light cycle (between 10 *a.m.* and 4 *p.m.*) to exclude potential darkness-induced *AE* unless deliberately testing the role of the circadian cycle.

The observers were blinded to the treatments. After displaying the aversive, nociceptive response, individual snails were instantly removed from the thermal surface. Each snail was tested only once to avoid a possible opioid-mediated thermal stress which would have increased the response latency to thermal stimulus as shown for *Cepaea* [79] or habituation. The hot plate did not produce any magnetic field; its surface furnished the snails with a non-magnetic, texturally acceptable, smooth metal surface.

Thermal stimulus was applied to the animals immediately following the cessation of the SMF-exposure. It will be demonstrated later in this chapter (in **Optimization of SMF parameters** Optimization of SMF parameters improves pain inhibition in mice) that the *AE* induced by 30, 20, or 10 min SMF-exposure has a prolonged effect following the cessation of the exposure for another 10, 20, or 30 min, respectively.

Animals and Groups

Individual *Helix pomatia* animals were collected from old field sites and held in a terrarium under an approximate 12-12 h light-dark cycle between 22 and 28°C. The snails had lettuce available *ad libitum*. Two experimental series were carried out, both in Tihany, Hungary in August. Animals were randomly divided into the experimental groups shown in Table **5.2**. Daily negative control (sham) groups were used every experimental day. Control measurements were carried out simultaneously by 2 observers before, during, and after the SMF tests each experimental day.

Statistical Analysis

The primary outcome measure was the difference between group averages of raw response latency data. A secondary outcome measure was the effect size in % between groups as defined by 100×[1-(average response latency in one group)/(average response latency in the other group)]. Effect size could be negative and could also exceed 100% in absolute value.

The results of the tests are presented in graphs as group averages where error bars show positive SEM values. The numbers of animals of a certain type of experiment (*n*) are also shown in the figures.

Table 5.2. Groups of Animals with Number of Animals, Treatment and Pretreatment Options, and References to Other Groups.

series	group	number of animals	SMF-exposure	time of SMF-exposure	duration of SMF-exposure	chemical treatment (amount)	reference (series, group)
	1	123					negative control (sham) group for Groups 1.2-4
	2	10			20 min		
	3	52	hSMF		30 min		
	4	10			40 min		
	5	14					negative control (sham) group for Groups 1.6-7
1	6	11	iSMF		20 min		
	7	11			40 min		
	8	30					negative control (sham) group for Groups 1.9-11
	9	11	hSMF				daily control group for Group 1.11
	10	14				naloxone (50 µl, 2×10^{-4} M)	negative control (sham) group for Group 1.19
	11	19	hSMF				
	1	28		during the day			negative control (sham) group for Group 2.2
	2	11	hSMF				
	3	9				serotonin (100 µl, 10^{-4} M)	
	4	12				tryptamine (100 µl, 10^{-4} M)	
	5	8	hSMF				
	6	15			30 min		negative control (sham) group for Groups 2.8-9
	7	10				naloxone (50 µl, 2×10^{-4} M)	positive control group for Group 2.9-10
2	8	8					positive control group for Group 2.10
	9	10	hSMF			naloxone (50 µl, 2×10^{-4} M) and serotonin (100 µl, 10^{-4} M)	
	10	25					negative control (sham) group for Group 2.11-12
	11	20	hSMF				
	12	19		during the night			negative control (sham) group for Group 2.13
	13	19	hSMF				

The F value, the critical value of F (F_{crit}) in a format of F_a=b, a=F_{crit}, and b=F, the p value, and the η^2 value wereestimated by one-way ANOVA. However, unbalanced samples warranted a double-check of ANOVA results with the Tukey's, the Fisher's, the Bonferroni, and the Dunn-Sidak methods. These methods have different strengths and weaknesses.

For *post hoc* analysis, we used Newman-Keuls, Duncan, REGWQ, and Games-Howell tests. We considered the minimum value of the modified a values for these iterative methods as $a_{min=}$min(a_N,a_D,a_R). We accepted a difference between samples significant if all tests unambiguously supported the null-hypothesis. Within experimental series, different groups have been tested at different occasions; such raw data series have not been compared to each other.

Ethics

Out of the measured 499 animals, 200 received SMF-exposure, 9 were treated with serotonin, 20 were administered tryptamine, and 43 received naloxone.

Animal suffering was minimized using as low animal numbers in groups as possible and still maintaining 80% statistical power. Moreover, short interventions were used, if any, and the hot plate test itself was also applied only for a short period of time (<2 min) at a mild temperature so as to hinder tissue damage. An animal was treated only once, and animals were not sacrificed after the experiments but were let free in the old fields where they had been collected.

Results

The Effects of hSMF- vs iSMF-exposure on Snail Nociception (Series 1, Groups 1-7)

Exposure to hSMF (Group 1 control group and Groups 2-4 exposed to hSMF for 20, 30, or 40 min, respectively) increased the response latency to thermal stimulus. The increase in response latency reached its maximum already at 20 min exposure (Group 2), which remained during longer exposures (40 min, Group 4), see Fig. (**5.2**). One-way ANOVA resulted in $F_{2.43}$=9.4, $p<0.001$, η^2=19.5%. The effect between control (Group 1, no exposure) and 20 min (Group 2), 30 min (Group 3), and 40 min (Group 4) exposure was 40.2%, 29.2%, and 41.7%, respectively.

These were all significant at the a_{min}= 0.008 level: $p<0.001$.

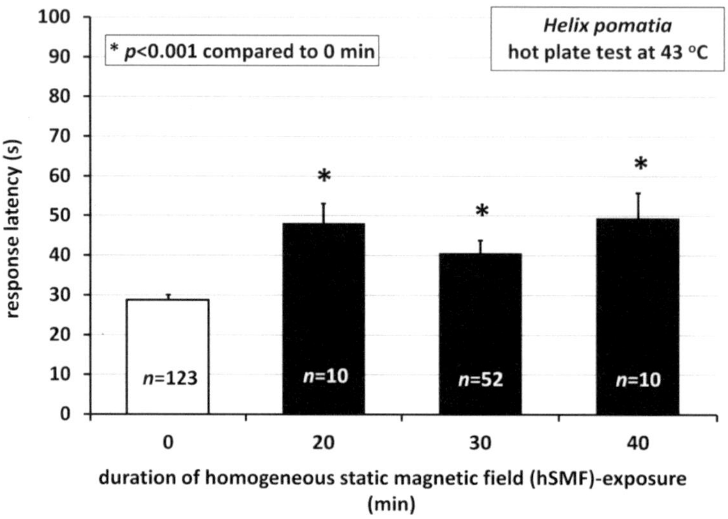

Fig. (5.2). Average response latency of Helix pomatia in the hot plate test (series 1). Some animals (dark columns) were pretreated in hSMF environment. The function parameter is the duration of hSMF-exposure in min. * denotes significant difference to negative control.

The exposure to iSMF (Group 5 control group and Groups 6-7 exposed to iSMF for 20 or 40 min, respectively) also increased the response latency to thermal stimulus. Whereas the hSMF-induced increase reached its maximum at 20 min exposure (Group 2), the iSMF-induced effect reached its maximum only after 40 min exposure (Group 7), see Fig. (**5.3**). The 20 min and 40 min exposure durations resulted in an effect of 32.7% and 46.2%, respectively with values $F_{3.28}$=11.9, $p<0.001$, a^2=41.9%. Both effects were statistically significant at the $a_{min=}$0.017 level: $p<0.05$ and $p<0.001$, respectively.

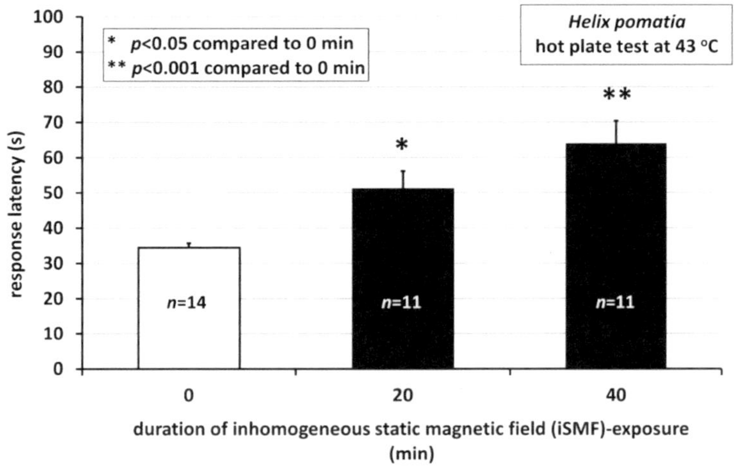

Fig. (5.3). Average response latency of Helix pomatia in the hot plate test (series 1). Some animals (dark columns) were pretreated in iSMF environment. The function parameter is the duration of iSMF-exposure in min. * or * * denote significant differences to negative control.

Opioid Receptor-involvement in hSMF-induced Antinociception in Snails (Series 1, Groups 8-11)

The injection of 1 μg/g naloxone (Group 10) evoked a significant 41.9% decrease in the response latency to thermal stimulus when compared to the control (Group 8), see Fig. (**5.4**) ($F_{4.07}$=10.75, p<0.002, η^2=20.4%, a_{min}= 0.008). Naloxone pretreatment depressed the *AE* of 30 min hSMF-exposure (Group 11) compared to hSMF-exposed animals without naloxone pretreatment (Group 3) (Fig. **5.4**). However, the exposure elevated the response latency of naloxone injected animals (Group 11) to the level of non-injected animals (Group 9): $F_{4.09}$=4.40, p<0.05, η^2=10.14%. This difference was shown not to be significant in the *post hoc* tests. There was no significant difference between the response latencies of control (Group 8) and naloxone+hSMF-treated animals (Group 11): $F_{4.05}$=1.26, p=0.27, η^2=2.62%.

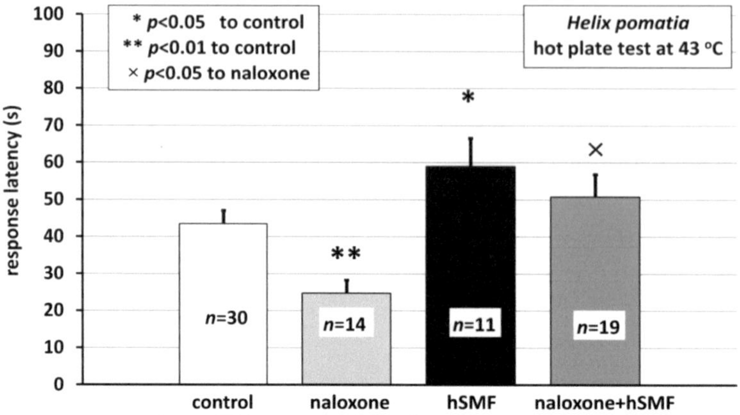

Fig. (5.4). Average response latency of Helix pomatia in the hot plate test (series 1). Some animals (columns 3 and 4) were pretreated in hSMF environment for 30 min. Some animals received 1 μg/g naloxone injection (columns 2 and 4). * and ** denote significant differences (p<0.05 and p<0.01, respectively) to negative control, × denotes significant difference (p<0.05) to naloxone-treatment.

The Role of the Serotonergic System on SMF-induced Response Latency (Series 2, Groups 1-5)

Fig.(**5.5**) presents the average values of response latency. One-way ANOVA resulted in F=17.08, p<0.001, F_{crit}=2.52 significant difference in the multiple group analysis.

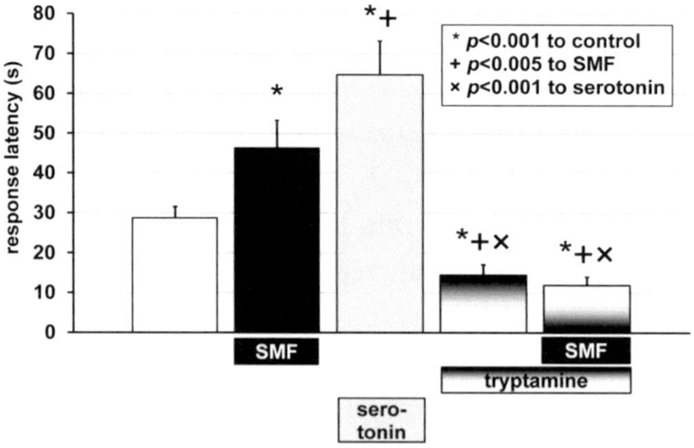

Fig. (5.5). Average response latency of Helix pomatia in the hot plate test (series 2). Groups: Open column: Negative control (n=28), dark column: SMF-exposure (n=11), grey column: Serotonin treatment (n=9), gradient filled columns: Tryptamine treatment without (n=12) or with SMF (n=8). Error bars denote positive SEM. *, +, and × designate significant differences to negative control, to SMF, and to serotonin, respectively as assessed by Games-Howell post hoc analysis.

The injected serotonin (10^{-4} M) increased response latency significantly (effect size 55.7%, $p<0.001$), even compared to SMF-exposure (28.2%, $p=0.004$). Higher concentrations of the injected 5-HT (10^{-3} M, 10^{-2} M) induced vigorous locomotion and frequent brief retractions of the head, but not the lift-up of the sole; therefore, these animals could not be used for evaluation. Serotonin antagonist tryptamine, on the other hand, decreased response latency (-97.8%, $p<0.001$). Even if combined with otherwise response latency-raiser SMF-exposure (38.2%, $p<0.001$), tryptamine kept response latency down thus reversing the SMF-induced effect (-21.3%, $p<0.001$).

The Interaction between Serotonergic and Opioid System in SMF-induced Response Latency (Series 2, Groups 6-9)

Average response latencies are shown in Fig. (**5.6**). One-way ANOVA resulted in $F=5.05$, $p=0.005$, $F_{crit}=2.85$ significant difference in the multiple group analysis.

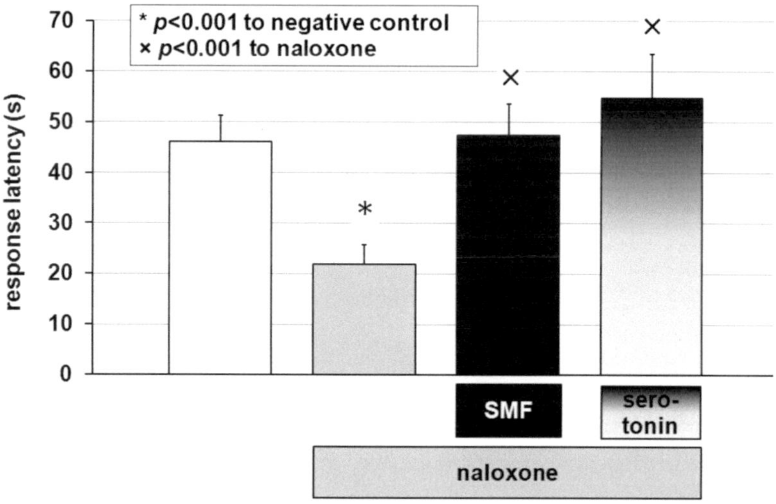

Fig. (5.6). Average response latency of Helix pomatia in the hot plate test (series 2). Groups: Open column: Negative control (n=15), dark column: SMF-exposure (n=10), grey column: Naloxone treatment (n=8), gradient filled column: Serotonin treatment (n=10). Error bars denote positive standard error of the mean. * and × designate significant differences to negative control and to naloxone treatment, respectively as assessed by Games-Howell post hoc analysis.

Naloxone administration (2×10^{-4} M), as an exclusive treatment, completely and significantly diminished the response latency compared to negative control

(-52.5%, $p<0.001$). Serotonin combined with naloxone reversed the effect of naloxone alone; the response latency went back to slightly over the negative control (-19.0%, $p=0.105$ to negative control, (150.2%, $p<0.001$ to naloxone). Trend-wise, SMF-exposure had a similar effect to that of serotonin. Combined with naloxone, however, the response latency-decreasing effect of naloxone could be reversed (-3.1%, $p=0.724$ to negative control, (116.9%, $p<0.001$ to naloxone).

The Role of the Circadian Cycle on SMF-induced Response Latency (Series 2, Groups 10-13)

Average response latencies are depicted in Fig. (**5.7**). One-way ANOVA resulted in $F=17.49$, $p<0.001$, $F_{crit}=2.72$ significant difference in the multiple group analysis.

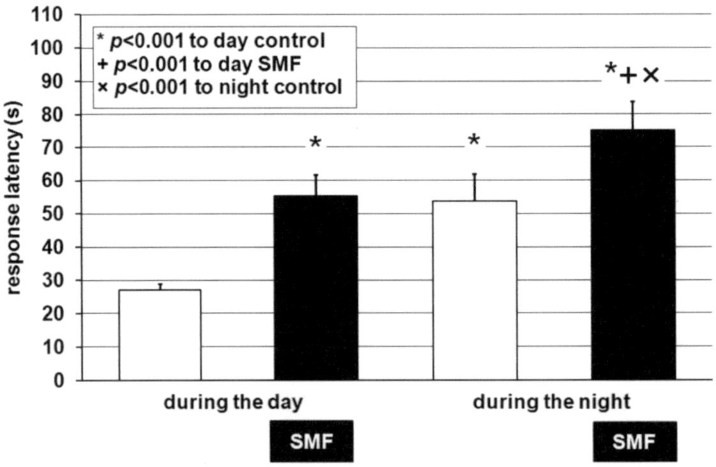

Fig. (5.7). Average response latency of Helix pomatia in the hot plate test (series 2). Groups: Open columns: Negative control during the day (n=25) or during the night (n=19), dark columns: SMF-exposure during the day (n=20) or during the night (n=19). Error bars denote positive standard error of the mean. *, +, and × designate significant differences to day control, to day SMF, and to night control, respectively as assessed by Games-Howell post hoc analysis.

SMF-exposure significantly increased response latency of *Helix pomatia* during the day as well as during the night compared to corresponding control in the hot plate test. As a nocturnal animal, this snail species had significantly higher response latency during the night than during the day (51.2%, $p<0.001$). This trend also held for the SMF-exposure (28.6%, $p<0.001$).

Discussion, Conclusions

In this study, we demonstrated that exposure to either homogeneous or inhomogeneous SMF (in the mT range) increased the thermal nociceptive threshold in the snail *Helix pomatia*, suggesting that SMF-exposure induces *AE* in snails. Both hSMF and iSMF-exposure (20-40 min) increased the response latency to thermal stimulus. hSMF-exposure reached its maximal effect (40.2%) in the response latency already after 20 min of exposure, whereas iSMF reached its maximal effect (46.2%) later, only after 40 min of exposure.

Naloxone, a prototypic opioid antagonist decreased the threshold of thermal nociceptive response in *Helix pomatia* similarly as it did in *Helix aspersa* [91]. In snails, different forms of stress, such as tail pinch [93], heat [79], or even novelty [80, 94] were able to induce opioid-mediated analgesia which could be reversed by naloxone (for a review see [83]). In contrast, cold stress-induced analgesia was insensitive to naloxone treatment, indicating that such analgesia was mediated by non-opioid mechanisms [82]. Therefore, the hot plate effect in *Helix* may be regarded as a stress-induced opioid-mediated analgesia. In our experiments, naloxone also depressed the SMF-induced analgesia, suggesting that the *AE* of hSMF-exposure on the thermal nociceptive response has a naloxone-sensitive component which is mediated *via* opiate receptors. Findings that opioid receptor agonists (μ- and *x*-receptor specific morphine and dynorphin) increased the response latency which was depressed by naloxone in *Helix aspersa* support this suggestion [91]. However, naloxone was not able to fully reverse, only reduce the pulsed magnetic field-induced analgesia in *Cepaea* implying that the induced analgesia also had a naloxone-insensitive component [95]. This would explain our observation according to which SMF-exposure increased the response latency in naloxone-pretreated animals to the control level but not beyond that; SMF-induced analgesia seems to have a naloxone-insensitive component in *Helix* as well.

It is not clear, though, whether the opioid system of snails (i) is sensitive to SMF-exposure, and this exposure induces the liberation of opioid peptides as we shall propose in **Pharmacological analysis** in mice, or (ii) induces direct membrane changes in cells, leading to the modulation of ion channel and opiate receptor functions [96, 97]. Opioid peptides have been identified, isolated, and sequenced from a variety of invertebrate species (for a review see [98]). Studies in which numerous enkephalin immunolabeled neurons were shown in the CNS of *Helix* [99], and in which strong nociceptive stimuli induced the liberation of opioid peptides in the snail *Planorbarius* [100], confirm the idea that endogenous opioid peptides are, indeed, present in snails and are liberated in response to stress or noxious stimuli. Opioid peptides were also shown to suppress different transmitter-induced responses in snail neurons [101 - 103]. 10 mT SMF-exposure hyperpolarized the bursting neuron in isolated *Helix* CNS [73] similarly to met-enkephalin [101], resulting in a decreased firing activity of the neuron. Furthermore, behavioral experiments showed that the sensitivity of defensive behavior to mechanical stimuli in the mollusk *Clione* and *Helix* can be suppressed by opioid peptides [104, 105]. The foot sole of *Helix*, coming in contact with the hot surface, is tufted with receptor cells sending axon to the pedal ganglia [106], which have a sensory information processing center [71]. Therefore, we suggest that hSMF exerts both central and peripheral effects leading to the decreased effectiveness of nociceptive sensory inputs which manifests itself in increased response latency.

The injected 10^{-4} M serotonin increased response latency significantly even when compared to SMF-exposure. The application of serotonin antagonist tryptamine (10^{-4} M), on the other hand, markedly decreased response latency. The tryptamine effect could not be antagonized by the latency-raiser effect of the SMF-exposure, which observation indicates that the liberated serotonin is necessary to the production of SMF-induced effects. Tryptamine is a potent antagonist of 5-HT excitation on *Helix* neurons suggesting the antagonist role of serotonin receptors mediating excitation. 5-HT receptors could not be classified in terms of vertebrate subtypes of 5-HT receptors [107]; therefore, we propose that tryptamine markedly decreases the activity of a still unknown type of neurons which liberate key molecules necessary to perform SMF-induced effects.

Similarly to SMF-exposure, serotonin administration could reverse the effect of naloxone and even increase the response latency above that of negative control. However, compared to positive control naloxone, both SMF-exposure and serotonin caused significantly higher response latency. These observations tell us that 5-HT does not only plays a role in the thermo-nociceptive circuits but is also required to the execution of the naloxone-sensitive opiate receptor-mediated effect of the latency-raiser SMF-exposure.

Naloxone, as an opiate receptor antagonist in an amount of 2×10^{-4} M, significantly diminished the response latency compared to negative control-like tryptamine. In contrast to tryptamine, though, the naloxone-induced effect could be fully antagonized by SMF-exposure indicating a naloxone-sensitive *AE* of SMF-exposure.

The role of opiates in stress-induced analgesia is well-documented in both vertebrates and invertebrates. Investigations on the snail *Cepaea nemoralis* demonstrated that some stress factors (high temperature) as well as administration of enkephalin induced reversible increase in the latency of the thermal nociceptive response [79, 94, 108].

In hot plate experiments, leu- and met-enkephalin attenuated the retraction response in the snail *Cepaea nemoralis*. The 5-HT antagonist methysergid counteracted the *AE* of enkephalins, indicating that the enkephalin-induced responses are dependent on endogenously released 5-HT, which findings support the co-liberation and synergistic effects of enkephalins and 5-HT in the nociceptive circuits [109]. The coexistence of 5-HT and enkephalin could be demonstrated in different ganglia of *Cepaea nemoralis*, including the pedal ganglia [110] confirming the above mentioned synergic effect in the nociceptive circuits. When the extracellular 5-HT level was increased by 5-HT reuptake inhibitors, the *AE* of μ agonists was enhanced [111]. Even the reuptake inhibitors themselves were able to produce weak *AE* in rhesus monkeys [112] indicating that opioids and serotonin had synergic effects also in the nociceptive circuits of mammals. Studies claiming that opioid receptors were expressed in numerous neurons of the brainstem antinociceptive circuits and part of them displayed coexistence with 5-HT [113] is in accordance with the above observations.

In the pedal ganglia of the pulmonate snail *Megalobulimus*, 5-HT immuno-reactivity increased in separated groups of 5-HT neurons following nociceptive thermal stimulus, which supposes that the thermal nociceptive stimulus increases both the liberation and the synthesis of serotonin [114]. The hot plate challenge induces antinociception by releasing endogenous opioids [79, 94] which suggests that the released opioids affected the liberation of 5-HT. This is in harmony with the finding that opioids caused an increase in release, synthesis, and turnover of 5-HT in the rat diencephalon [115]. In the snail *Helix pomatia*, the central distribution of both serotonin [116, 117] and met-enkephalin [99] immunoreactive neurons have been described. According to these sources, the majority of immunolabeled serotonergic neurons are located in the pedal ganglia; whereas, the majority of met-enkephalin immunolabeled neurons are distributed in the cerebral and in the pedal ganglia. These neuroanatomical observations allow for the interaction of the opioid and the serotonergic system in the antinociceptive circuits of *Helix*.

In snails, the serotonergic modulatory neurons, contrary to motor *vs* sensory neurons, maintain their activity and liberate 5-HT even after the cessation of the stimulus. Moreover, they increase the activity of the 5-HT reuptake system [118, 119]. Consequently, these 5-HT cells in the pedal ganglia have been suggested to maintain their increased activity following the thermal stimulation, leading to increased serotonin immunoreactivity in the pedal serotonergic neurons. The above findings can help us make sense of the fact that SMF-induced *AE* persists in snails following the SMF-exposure. Snails and mice exhibit a similar reaction in this respect, as we shall see in an acute visceral pain model in mice in **Optimization of SMF parameters**. These pedal 5-HT cells of the snail are claimed to constitute a part of the circuits processing the nociceptive thermal afferents in the pedal ganglia [114].

Considering that both SMF-exposure and serotonin decreased the nociceptive sensitivity of *Helix* in the hot plate test, similarly to opiate mediated analgesia, we can not exclude that SMF-exposure exerts its *AE* partly through the central and peripheral liberation of serotonin. The centrally liberated serotonin can modulate the nociceptive information processing in the pedal ganglia leading to the attenuation of nociceptive response. On the other hand, the peripherally liberated 5-HT may decrease the activity of the peripheral nociceptive receptor cells leading to the attenuation of nociceptive sensory inputs.

The pedal serotonergic neurons build a dense network of immunolabeled fibers in the pedal ganglia implying that serotonergic neurons take part in the pedal sensory information processing [117]. Not only do pedal serotonergic neurons densely innervate the foot musculature [117], but serotonin labeled fibers protrude along the primary sensory neurons of the foot sole indicating modulatory contact with them [120]. The foot sole makes contact with the hot plate; therefore, the possible modulatory effects of serotonin on the activity of nociceptive receptor cells of the foot sole might play an important role in the peripheral modulation of the activity of thermo-nociceptive response.

Spoont [121] pointed out serotonin's general modulatory role in the control of sensory reactivity by altering the ongoing processing of sensory input in mammals. She reviewed accumulated evidence that increasing 5-HT decreased reactivity to sensory stimuli and protected against overstimulation; whereas, low 5-HT states elicited an exaggeration of signal saliency and amplified signal passage.

Animals had significantly higher nociceptive response latency during the night than during the day (effect size 51.2%, $p<0.001$) suggesting a circadian cycle-dependent mechanism of *AE*. SMF-exposure significantly increased response latency during both the day and the night periods (28.6%, $p<0.001$) compared to corresponding control in the hot plate test. Each snail was tested only once to avoid possible opioid-mediated thermal stress or habituation, which again would have increased the response latency to thermal stimulus as had been found for *Cepaea* [79].

In Kavaliers *et al.*'s study [81], *Cepaea nemoralis* displayed significantly greater response latency at night than during the day indicating that the dark period of the circadian rhythm induces an *AE*. Our results on *Helix pomatia* serve as evidence for the assumption that the peripheral thermal nociceptive threshold decreases at night. Both *Cepaea* and *Helix* are nocturnal animals; conversely, these findings are indicative of the fact that during the dark period, when the animals are active, the liberation of transmitters and modulators change, leading to the attenuation of nociceptive inputs.

In *Aplysia*, the haemolymph 5-HT level slowly increased during the afternoon and reached its maximum during the dark period of the day; moreover, was able to modulate the feeding behavior of the animal. In constant darkness, the 5-HT level remained constant at this high level suggesting that light decreases the haemolymph level of 5-HT [122]. In the light period, the elevated haemolymph 5-HT modulated the locomotion and the feeding latency in *Helix pomatia* [106]. Therefore, we suspect that darkness increases both the activity of the serotonergic system and the liberation of serotonin in *Helix*, leading to the attenuation of nociceptive response at night. The exclusion of trouble sensory inputs might help the successful foraging and matting of the animals in the long run.

In contrast to the hSMF-induced *AE*, low frequency electromagnetic fields induced nociception or decreased opioid-induced analgesia in snail [82] (for a review see [83]) indicating that the 2 types of magnetic fields initiate opposite processes in the opiate system: SMF-exposure may induce the liberation of opiates or activate opioid receptors, whereas low frequency electromagnetic fields initiate opposite effects. Although the hSMF-exposure induces a well visible naloxone-sensitive effect on the nociceptive threshold *via* opiate receptors, the magnetic field sensing/transduction mechanism remains to be established.

In principle, when a snail moves in a SMF environment, its body is subject to lateral gradients of the SMF and; consequently, to abrupt time derivatives. The effect is identical to the application of LFEMF to a static (*e.g.* anesthetized) living object as discussed recently by Jokela and Saunders [123]. However, taking into account that (i) snails move with a notoriously low speed as well as (ii) in our experiments several snails were SMF-exposed in a cage at the same time hindering each other's locomotion, we presume that the electric current-inducing effect of hSMF-exposure is negligible. This assumption coincides with computer simulated results [124]. On the other hand, the stimulus generated in the subject moving in an iSMF may influence pain perception in both rodents and humans [125]. In the present experiments, as a snail moving in the external iSMF could sense a fast changing magnetic induction in all 3 directions, we expected a difference between responses due to hSMF and iSMF. Interestingly however, no significant differences were identified between snail responses under these different conditions. In other words, induced electric effects may not have played an important role. This problem will be under scrutiny in more detail in the section **Clinical MRI** 3 T clinical MRI significantly inhibits pain in mice where we shall see how the SMF of a clinical MRI (**Generator 20**) and how different inhomogeneous SMF arrangements (**Generators 17a-e**) in the section **Lateral gradients** influence visceral nociception.

Meanwhile let us investigate whether the behavior of rodents changes under SMF-exposure conditions.

EXPERIMENTS ON MAMMALS *IN VIVO*

HEALTHY ANIMALS

Locomotor activity and anxiety behavior in healthy mice

Inhomogeneous Static Magnetic Field-Exposure Fails to Influence Locomotor Activity and Anxiety Behaviour in Mice

Preliminaries

The behavioral patterns (cognitive performance, avoidance, and learning) of rodents under the influence of static magnetic field (SMF) have recently drawn the attention of researchers due to the following reasons: i) To understand animal behavioral patterns, including navigation and corresponding reception mechanisms as evolved during phylogenesis in the geomagnetic field of Earth; ii) to reveal potential adverse effects of strong SMF-exposure, primarily because of the proliferation of MRI technology.

The effects of static magnetic fields (SMF) on several behavioral patterns and neural functions, such as conditioned taste aversion [126], vestibular activation [127], and induction of locomotor activity [66] have been described recently. Data available on the effects of SMF-exposure on nociceptive processes are still somewhat contradictory. Some authors have reported that acute exposure of mice to SMF suppressed stress and morphine-induced analgesia [128, 129] and increased nociceptive heat sensitivity [130]. Other papers demonstrate inhibitory actions on nociception in murine models [27, 131]. The reason for this contradiction might be the differences between the species and the characteristics of the SMF (*e.g.* induction) as well as the duration of the exposure in acute or chronic disease models.

Mice were studied by Davis *et al.* [132] who checked the behavior of adult mice that were continuously exposed to a 1.5 T SMF for up to 72 h. They focused on the effect of SMF-exposure on electroshock-motivated passive avoidance task, on general locomotor activity, and on pentylenetetrazol-induced seizures. They found no behavioral alterations in the SMF-exposed mice as compared to control. Levine and Bluni [133] and Levine *et al.* [134] exposed mice to SMF up to 2 T for up to 100 min. They found that left-right discrimination learning ability decreased following the SMF-exposure, but since a "spin-echo" MRI sequence completed the test, the effect of the time-varying gradient fields could not be ruled out. Tsuji *et al.* [135] reported decreased food and water intake in mice exposed to a 5 T magnetic field for 24 or 48 h as compared to control. Exposure to a 9.4 T magnetic field used by Nolte *et al.* [126] resulted in a conditioned taste aversion in rats. Using c-Fos immunohystochemistry, it was found that the rats' visceral and the vestibular nuclei in the brain stem were responsible for this aversion [126]. Lockwood *et al.* [136] exposed restrained and unrestrained mice to an SMF of 14.1 T. All mice developed conditioned taste aversion and a significant number of them produced tight circling and suppression of rearing. Unrestrained mice exhibited larger effects than those that were restrained, supporting the view that these responses are consistent with vestibular stimulation as well as the reports of vertigo and nausea in human beings during movement in very strong SMF. It is noteworthy that such effects are consistent with Schenck's claim [17], according to which small head movements in a strong SMF could induce vestibular stimulation through the action of magnetohydrodynamic forces on the fluid within the semicircular canals. The special, very low frequency magnetic field applied by Choleris *et al.* [137], induced a reduction in the general locomotor activity of mice. The SMF-exposure increased self-grooming and spin turns. The same group [130] published that exposure to this same special magnetic field increased the nociceptive sensitivity of mice.

On the basis of important contributions [66, 138 - 147], we may conclude that the effect of SMF-exposure has brought positive results (*e.g.* conditioned taste aversion, some moderate changes is locomotion, and inhibition of Sidman avoidance response) in only few behavioral tests. Saunders [148], in his review, concluded that: "No consistently demonstrable effects of exposure to fields of approximately 1 T and above have been seen on other behavioral or cardiovascular endpoints... Overall, however, far too few animal studies have been carried out to reach any firm conclusions."

The development of MR also brought with it the tendency to search for possible adverse (side) effects of strong magnetic fields. It turned out, though, that some of the side effects may even be beneficial. An increasing number of evidence shows that SMF-exposure can induce analgesic action under experimental conditions [27, 131, 149].

Goals

The aim of the present work is to reveal whether SMF-exposure affects:

- Locomotor activity and anxiety behavior in mice,
- morphine-induced analgesia and hyperlocomotion.

Materials and Methods

Magnetic Exposure Conditions, Special Drug

SMF was generated by generator 11 (**Generators 1-16**) specified in Table **5.3**. Morphine was given *s.c.* in an amount of 10 mg/kg, 20 min preceding the acetic acid challenge.

Behavioral Tests

Since SMF-exposure *in situ*, during the behavioral tests was not possible, mice were exposed to the inhomogeneous SMF with their whole-body for 30 min before starting the test. Control animals were placed in identical cages for 30 min, but were not exposed to SMF.

Elevated plus maze (EPM) was used to study whether SMF-exposure would induce an anxiogenic or anxiolytic effect in the mice. The apparatus consists of 2 open arms "O" (500×150 mm) and 2 closed arms "C" (500×150 mm with a 100 mm surrounding wall). The 2 open arms and the 2 closed arms are extended from a central platform (150×150 mm) and are opposite to each other forming the shape of a plus sign. The whole apparatus is elevated to a height of 700 mm. It is set in an isolated dark room, only the arms are illuminated. The number of entries into the open and closed arms and the time spent in each was recorded. The observation period was 5 min.

Locomotor activity following SMF-exposure was tested with a "Conduct a System for behavioral and activity studies". The apparatus consists of black-painted testing boxes (400×500×500 mm) set in an isolated room (see the box in Fig. **5.8**). Conducta detects movements of the experimental animals by high-density arrays of infrared diodes. The time spent with the following variables was recorded: Horizontal activity (ambulation-walking, running), vertical activity (rearing), and immobility. In **Lateral gradients** we shall discuss locomotion of mice in a little more details apropos of ambulation models.

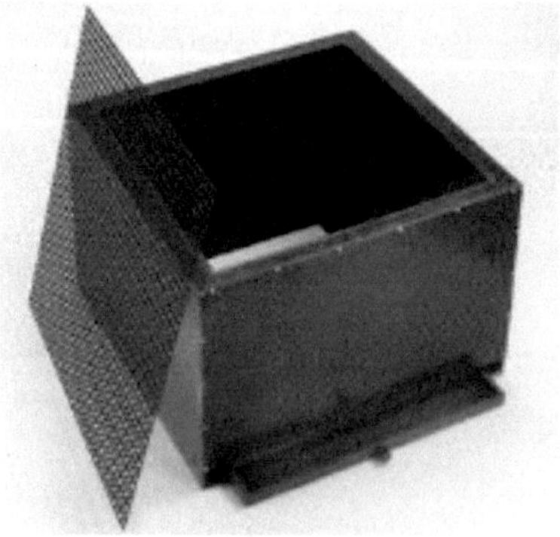

Fig. (5.8). Conducta System for behavioral and activity studies (400×500×500 mm).

Both the spontaneous locomotor activity and the hyperlocomotion inducing effect of morphine (MO, 10 mg/kg) were checked following the SMF-exposure. The animals were divided into 4 groups:

Group 1: Treated with saline, not exposed to SMF,
Group 2: Treated with saline and exposed to SMF,
Group 3: Treated with MO, not exposed to SMF,
Group 4: Treated with MO and exposed to SMF.

MO (or saline) was administered *s.c.* to the mice just before they received the SMF-exposure. After the 30 min exposure the observation started immediately and lasted for 40 min.

Statistical Analysis

One-way ANOVA followed by Dunnett's *post hoc* and Mann-Whitney U test was performed in the locomotor activity test and in the EPM test, respectively.

Results

The Effect of Inhomogeneous SMF-exposure on the Behavior Pattern of Mice in the Elevated Plus Maze Test

Fig. (**5.9**) shows the results obtained in the EPM test. SMF failed to influence the times spent either in the open or in the closed arms, *i.e.* there was no statistically significant difference between control and SMF-treated animals. The averages of 10 animals in each group are shown with SEM values.

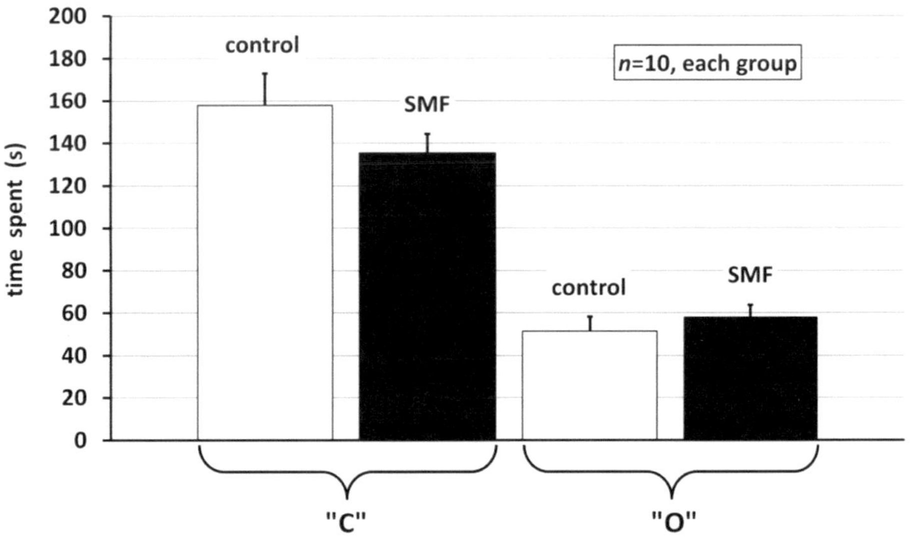

Fig. (5.9). Time± SEM (s) spent in the closed (C) and in the open (O) arms of the elevated plus maze. SMF: Animals were exposed to an inhomogeneous static magnetic field for 30 min immediately before the observation.

<u>*The Effect of Inhomogeneous SMF-exposure on the Locomotor Activity of Mice*</u>

Fig. (**5.10A - 5.10C**) shows the results concerning locomotor activity. As expected, morphine in a dose of 10 mg/kg enhanced ambulation and reduced immobility. One-way ANOVA analysis revealed significant differences in both parameters ($p<0.001$ for ambulation and $p<0.001$ for immobility).

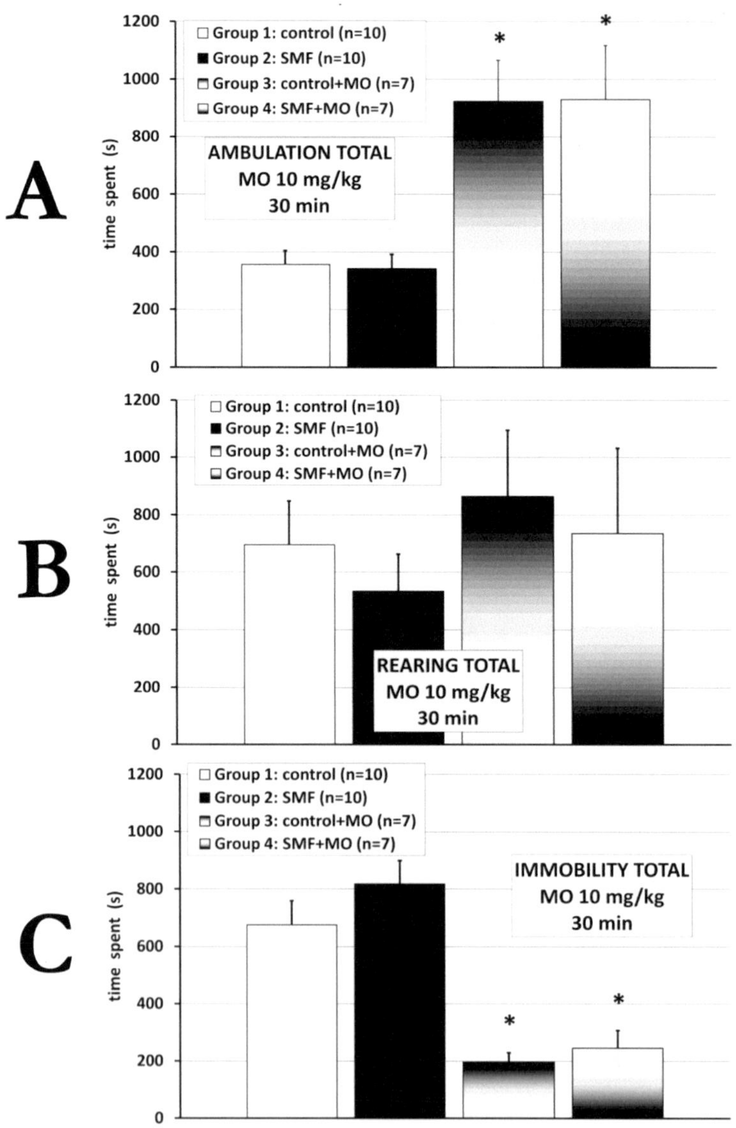

Fig. (5.10). Time± SEM spent **A)** with ambulation, **B)** with rearing, or **C)** in immobility in the locomotor activity test. Open column: Group 1: Treated with saline, not exposed to static magnetic field (SMF); dark column: Group 2: Treated with saline and exposed to SMF; gradient shaded (90°) column: Group 3: Treated with morphine (MO), not exposed to SMF; gradient shaded (270°) column: Group 4: Treated with MO and exposed to SMF. SMF: Exposure of mice to an inhomogeneous static magnetic field for 30 min immediately before starting the observation. Treatment: MO 10 mg/kg or saline s.c. before placing the animals into the cages. The number of animals is indicated in parentheses. * $p<0.05$ (one-way ANOVA followed by Dunnett's post hoc test between Group 1 and 3, as well as between Group 2 and 4).

According to Dunnett's *post hoc* statistical testing there was no difference between Group 1 and 2 as well as between Group 3 and 4, indicating that SMF-exposure failed to influence either the spontaneous locomotion or the MO induced hyperlocomotion. Neither SMF-exposure, nor morphine treatment affected the vertical activity.

Discussion, Conclusions

Hyperlocomotion in mice is also a characteristic behavioral effect of morphine; however, there are important differences in the molecular mechanisms involved in morphine induced hyperlocomotion. Whilst the antinociceptive action is mediated first of all by μ-opioid receptors, but both *x*- and δ-opioid receptors are also involved in the processes. The hyperlocomotion is mediated by the activation of mesolimbic dopamine (DA) receptors. The stimulation of μ- and δ-opioid receptors enhances the mesolimbic DA release and increases the locomotor activity. However, in contrast to the antinociception, *x*-opioid receptor agonists decrease the locomotor activity [150] and suppress the locomotor-enhancing effect of morphine [151] *via* reducing the mesolimbic DA release. In addition, the DA-independent hyperlocomotion inducing effect of δ-opioid receptor agonists was also published [152]. This was the authors' reason to check the effect of SMF-exposure on the locomotion in mice. The other behavioral test (EPM) was chosen to assess, whether SMF-exposure induces effects in the brain, which may provoke anxiety.

The literature shows an equivocal picture of the behavioral effects of SMF-exposure in rodents. While Davis *et al.* [132], Innis *et al.* [138], Weiss *et al.* [144], and Trzeciak *et al.* [145] failed to find behavioral alterations in the SMF-exposed mice as compared to control, Choleris *et al.* [137] observed a reduction in the general locomotor activity of mice in the special, very low frequency magnetic field they applied.

The behavior of mice was tested immediately after 30 min SMF-exposure in either test of ours. The results suggest that no vestibular stimulation occur at these levels of velocities, magnetic inductions, and gradients. In the EPM test there was no significant difference between times mice spent in the open or closed arm, indicating that SMF-exposure failed to induce either anxiogenic or anxiolytic effect.

In the locomotor activity test the time mice spent with horizontal activity (ambulation), vertical activity (rearing), and immobility was monitored. As shown in Fig. (**5.10**), the SMF treatment failed to induce any change in the spontaneous locomotor activity of the mice. Neither was the hyperlocomotion inducing effect of morphine in a dose of 10 mg/kg influenced by a preceding 30 min long SMF-exposure. In contrast, Kavaliers and Ossenkopp reported in 1986 that a rotating magnetic field significantly reduced the locomotor effects of morphine in mice [153].

In summary, the present paper showed that SMF-exposure failed to affect either locomotor activity, or morphine induced hyperlocomotion. Now let us investigate, whether SMF-exposure would have a clinically significant effect under different peripheral pathological conditions induced in mice.

PAIN AND INFLAMMATION

Pain and Analgesia

The pain processing neural apparatus in mammals is quite elaborated. It is well documented that neural activities evoked by various noxious stimuli in peripheral receptors are conducted by C and Aδ primary afferents to the spinal dorsal horn [154]. Most of the C and Aδ fibers terminate in laminae I and II, where they activate second order sensory neurons and initiate a complex, as yet mostly unidentified, information processing mechanism. After processing by spinal neural circuits, nociceptive impulses are finally conveyed to cells of origin of ascending sensory pathways that transmit the impulses to higher brain centers including various nuclei in the brain stem, diencephalon, telencephalon, and cortical areas like somatosensory, anterior cingulate or insular cortices [155, 156]. Due to multiple interactions among the activated cortical and subcortical areas, the nociceptive signals finally generate complex behaviors with sensory-discriminative, motivational-affective and autonomic components that are generally defined as pain [155 - 157].

Pain as a complex state involves both central and peripheral mechanisms. Even nowadays morphine and aspirin (and related compounds) serve as the most prevailing painkillers even, if both groups of analgesics are known to have a number of considerable adverse effects. Efforts have been made to develop a safer painkiller. Development of selective cyclooxygenase-2 inhibitors (*e.g.* coxibs) promised a safer alternative to traditional NSAID. However, because of the unforeseen increase in cardiovascular morbidity and mortality, some of these, for example, rofecoxib have been withdrawn from the market.

Although the mechanisms by which SMF-exposure mediates its great variety of actions are unknown [136, 148], modification of the endogenous opioidergic system as shown by Kavaliers and Ossenkopp [158] and in **Experiments on invertebrates *in vivo*** has been suggested. The section **Pharmacological analysis** will provide further evidence. Also several findings indicate the ability of exposure to relatively weak SMF to diminish neural excitability by the inhibition of Ca^{2+} and Na^{+} currents [96, 97, 159].

Capsaicin-sensitive, Transient Receptor Potential Vanilloid 1 (TRPV1) receptor-expressing sensory nerves play an important role in several inflammatory and nociceptive processes *via* the release of pro-inflammatory/pro-nociceptive sensory neuropeptides such as substance P (SP) and calcitonin gene-related peptide (CGRP) into the innervated area [160, 161]. The TRPV1 receptor is a non-selective cation channel, which is activated by exogenous vanilloid compounds (*e.g.* capsaicin or resiniferatoxin), as well as noxious heat and several endogenous chemical stimuli, such as protons, bradykinin, and leukotrienes produced in the inflamed tissues [161, 162]. TRPV1 receptors will be demonstrated to contribute to SMF-exposure induced antinociception in **Peripheral action**.

Beside human data preclinical studies support the clue that SMF-exposure induces *AE* under experimental conditions [153]. This whole **Pain and analgesia** including both acute and chronic disease models is devoted to prove this hypothesis. A pulsed magnetic field was shown to exert *AE* against thermal stimuli in different species, for example, in snails, rats, mice [131, 163, 164]. A little more in details, animal experiments were performed in different species in order to circumvent subject awareness, when biological responses to painful stimuli were studied. *AE* against thermal or chemical stimuli have been observed, for example, in snails [74], rats [149], and mice [130, 165]. Mice will be our own subjects as well in **Pain and analgesia**. Moderate SMF has proven to be effective in treating inflammatory agonist induced edema in rats [166], yet seemed to reduce the cognitive performance [167, 168]. Prato *et al.* [27] investigated the *AE* in CD-1 mice due to magnetic field shielding and concluded that there was a robust effect of the shielding on analgesia. Pain response modulation is successfully realized by shielding the external geomagnetic induction, and the stress induced *AE* in mice has been reduced upon pre-stress treatment in a shielded environment [129]. Possible molecular mediators of analgesic modulation include series of endogenous signal transducing peptides such as β-endorphin, substance-P, and serotonin [169]. The magnetic induction in currently applied SMF therapies typically ranges from 1 to 400 mT [29, 42] and an *AE* of exposure to such SMF on the visceral pain of mice will be demonstrated in **Visceral action: The writhing test**. Rogachefsky *et al.* [170] studied the effect of a mattress with permanent magnets on osteoarthritis in dogs and found that osteoarthritis developed in the medial femoral condyle might have been inhibited by SMF-exposure.

The *AE* of SMF-exposure in mice in chemically induced pain assays has been extensively studied. Applying external inhomogeneous SMF does not tend to influence the anxiety and behavioral pattern of mice (ambulation, rearing) and furthermore, does not affect the morphine induced hyperlocomotion and antinociception as we already demonstrated in **HEALTHY ANIMALS Locomotor activity and anxiety behavior in** healthy mice. The *AE* will be shown to remain detectable several minutes subsequent to the cessation of SMF-exposure (**Optimization of SMF parameters** improves pain inhibition in mice).

In most experiments (with the exceptions discussed in **Lateral gradients significantly enhance static magnetic field-induced inhibition of pain responses in mice – a double blind experimental study**), mice are constrained to either SMF- or sham-exposure conditions without the possibility of free locomotion between sham and SMF side.

ACUTE MODELS

Peripheral action

Static Magnetic Field Induced Anti-Nociceptive Effect and the Involvement of Capsaicin-Sensitive Sensory Nerves in this Mechanism

Goals

The aim of the present series of experiments was to elucidate the effects of SMF-exposure on acute inflammatory nocifensive behaviors and inflammatory mechanical hyperalgesia in mice using generator 11 (see **Generators 1-16** and Table **5.3**). Furthermore, the involvement of capsaicin-sensitive sensory fibers in SMF induced actions was also investigated.

Materials and Methods

Animals

Experiments were performed on male BALB/c bred and kept in the Laboratory Animal Centre of the University of Pécs under standard pathogen free conditions at 24-25°C and provided with standard rat chow and water *ad libitum*.

Resiniferatoxin Induced Mechanical Hyperalgesia Model

Mechanonociceptive threshold of the hind paws was determined by aesthesiometry (Dynamic Plantar Aesthesiometer 37400). Previous studies have revealed that this method is the most appropriate to study mechanical hyperalgesia in mice [171]. Measurements were performed before and 30 min after *s.c.* injection of the ultrapotent capsaicin receptor VR1/TRPV1 agonist resiniferatoxin (RTX, 20 μl/mouse; 0.1 μg/ml) into the plantar surface of the left hind paw (in short intraplantar or *i.pl.* administration). Hyperalgesia in each mouse was expressed as percentage decrease of the mechanonociceptive thresholds compared to the control values. Mice were placed into the SMF-exposure chamber for 30 min directly before measurements. In the control group animals were placed into the same Plexiglas cage, but were not exposed to the artificial SMF (sham-exposure).

Formalin Test

Formalin (50 μl per mouse, 2.5%) injected *i.pl.* into the left hind paw induced nocifensive reactions in 2 phases, the first of which (0-5 min) is thought to be due to a direct chemonociceptive effect of formalin, while the second (20-45 min) is mainly mediated by inflammatory reactions [172]. Nocifensive behavior was quantitatively evaluated by the total duration of paw liftings and lickings in each examination period [171]. Mice were placed into the exposure chamber for 5 min before and throughout the whole experimental period.

Carrageenan-evoked Inflammatory Mechanical Hyperalgesia Model

Mechanonociceptive threshold of the hind paws was determined by aesthesiometry as described earlier. Measurements were performed before and 3 h after *i.pl.* injection of λ-carrageenan (50 μl/mouse; 3%) into the left hind paw, which induces a mixed-type acute inflammatory reaction reaching its maximum at 3 h [171]. Inflammatory hyperalgesia in each mouse was expressed as percentage decrease of the mechanonociceptive thresholds compared to the control values. Mice were placed into the SMF for 30 min directly before measurements.

Resiniferatoxin Desensitization

The function of capsaicin-sensitive primary sensory fibers was selectively abolished by pretreatment with RTX. Mice were given 30, 70 and 100 μg/kg RTX *s.c.* on 3 consecutive days [173] and they were studied in the formalin test 5 days later. As a consequence of repeated high dose RTX treatment, intracellular Ca^{2+} concentration increases and Ca^{2+} accumulates in the mitochondria evoking metabolic damage of the cells. This is accompanied by ultrastructural changes like disorganized, swollen mitochondria [174].

Rotarod Test

Mice were studied in Ugo Basile 7750 accelerating rotarod in order to examine if SMF-exposure influences coordination or motor function [175]. Three mice were placed simultaneously on the rotating drums; the counter started at the same time for all 3 animals, and the rod was set to accelerate from 4 to 40 rpm every 20 s. Mice were trained in the equipment on 3 consecutive days for 3 trials per day before the experiment. Their rotarod performance was evaluated on the basis of the duration of time (s) spent on the rotating drum. They were examined before and after they had been placed into the SMF-exposure chamber or in the control group into the same Plexiglas cage without exposure (sham-exposure) for 30 min. Each measurement was repeated 3 times; means with standard errors (SEM) were calculated.

Drugs and Chemicals

Formalin (*formaldehydum solutum* 37%; Ph.Hg. VII.) was obtained from the Pharmacy of the University of Pécs and acetic acid from Merck. Resiniferatoxin and λ-carrageenan were purchased from Sigma-Aldrich. A 1 mg/ml stock solution of RTX was prepared with 96% ethanol and diluted further with saline.

Statistical Analysis

For statistical evaluation data analysis of variance (single factor ANOVA) followed by Bonferroni's modified Dunnett's test was used. In all cases $p<0.05$ was considered statistically significant.

Results

Effect of SMF on RTX Induced Mechanical Hyperalgesia

The TRPV1 receptor agonist RTX (20 μl per mouse, 0.1 μg/ml) decreased mechanical touch sensitivity of the hind paw from 8.4± 0.2 g to 3.6±0.3 g in the control group 30 min after the *i.pl.* injection. In mice which were placed into the SMF-exposure chamber for the 30 min period between RTX administration and measurement, a significantly smaller hyperalgesia developed, the mechano-nociceptive threshold changed from 8.0±0.4 g to only 4.9±0.4 g (Fig. **5.11**).

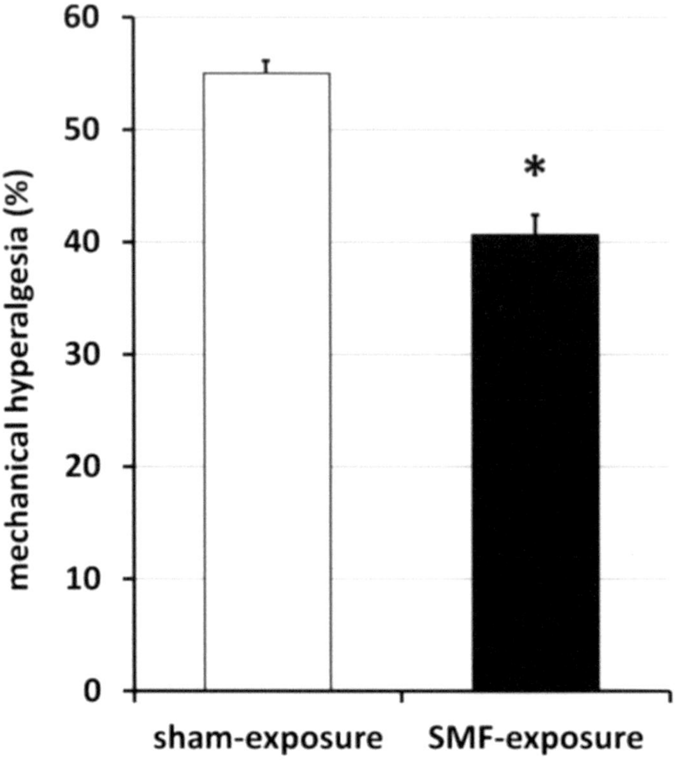

Fig. (5.11). Effect of a 30 min SMF-exposure on i.pl. RTX induced mechanical hyperalgesia of the mouse hind paw. In the control group animals were placed into the same cage for the same time period without SMF (sham)-exposure. Each data point represents the mean±SEM mechanical hyperalgesia (%) compared to the respective basal thresholds of n=11 animals/group. * $p<0.05$ SMF- *vs* sham-exposure (ANOVA followed by Bonferroni's modified Dunnett's test).

Effect of SMF on Formalin Induced Acute Nocifensive Behavior; Mediator Role of Capsaicin-sensitive Fibers

The effect of SMF-exposure was assessed on the characteristic 2 phases of the formalin test. Nocifensive behavior (total duration of paw lickings and liftings) throughout 5 min periods was significantly diminished in mice placed into the SMF-exposure chamber 10 min before and during the whole examination period both in the early phase (0-5 min) referring to acute chemono-ciception and in the late phase (20-45 min) evoked by the inflammatory reaction (Fig. **5.12A**).

However, in mice which were pretreated with RTX 5 days before the formalin test in order to inactivate capsaicin-sensitive sensory nerves, SMF-exposure did not induce significant inhibitory action (Fig. **5.12B**).

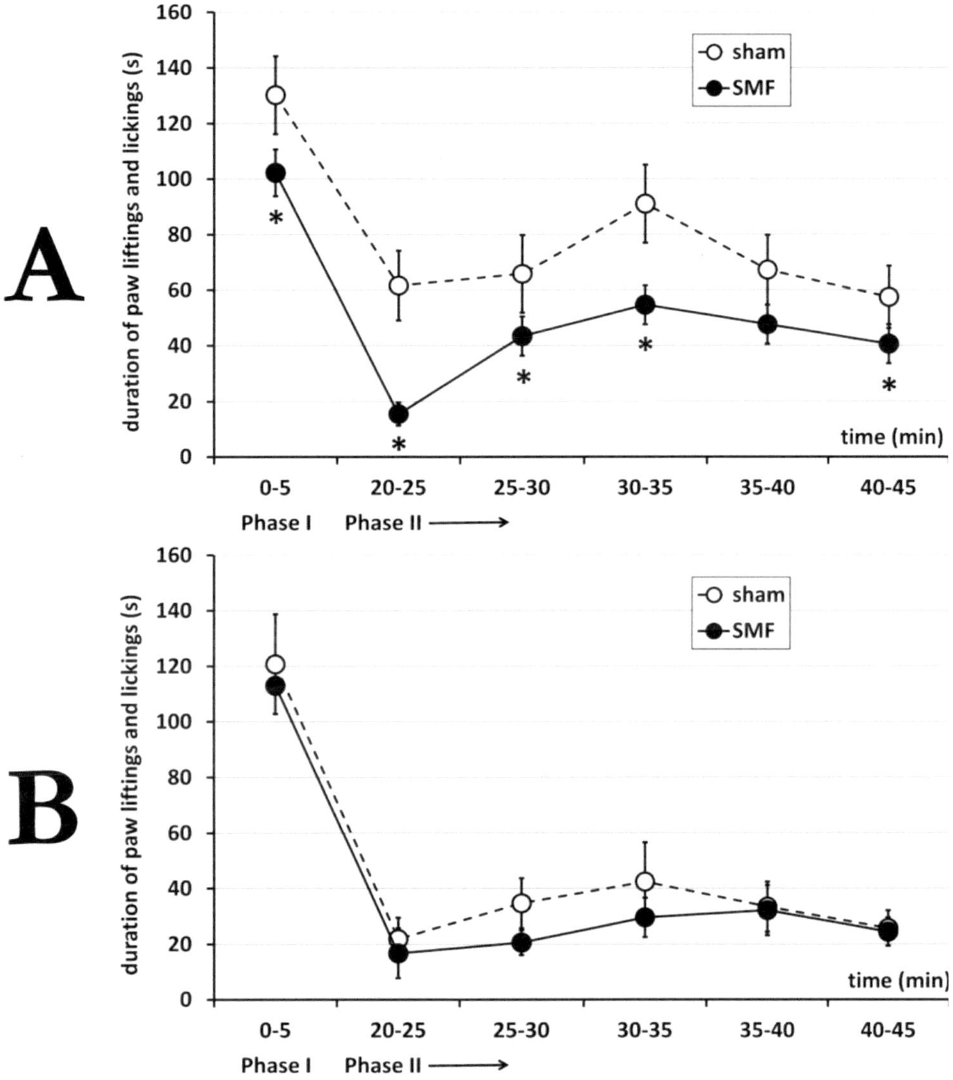

Fig. (5.12). A) Inhibitory effect of SMF-exposure on formalin induced nocifensive behaviors in mice. **B)** No effect of SMF-exposure on formalin induced nocifensive behaviors in mice after inactivation of capsaicin-sensitive sensory nerves by RTX pretreatment. In both cases mice were exposed to SMF or sham starting 5 min before formalin injection and lasting until the end of the experimental period. Results are shown as total duration of paw lickings and liftings (s) (means±SEM of n=10 animals/ group). * $p<0.05$ SMF- *vs* sham-exposure (ANOVA followed by Bonferroni's modified Dunnett's test).

Effect of SMF-exposure on Carrageenan Induced Acute Inflammatory Mechanical Hyperalgesia; Mediator Role of Capsaicin Sensitive Fibers

In the control group mechanonociceptive threshold of the left hind paws was 8.7±0.2 g before the induction of the inflammation, which decreased to 5.5±0.2 g 3 h after carrageenan injection. In mice SMF-exposed for the 30 min period before measurement significantly less hyperalgesia developed, the mechano-nociceptive threshold changed from 8.9±0.3 g to only 7.4±0.7 g. Although in mice pretreated with RTX to inactivate capsaicin-sensitive sensory nerves carrageenan induced hyperalgesia was about 30% smaller, it did not prove to be statistically significant. Furthermore, the inhibitory action of SMF-exposure observed in untreated mice was absent in the RTX pretreated group (Fig. **5.13**).

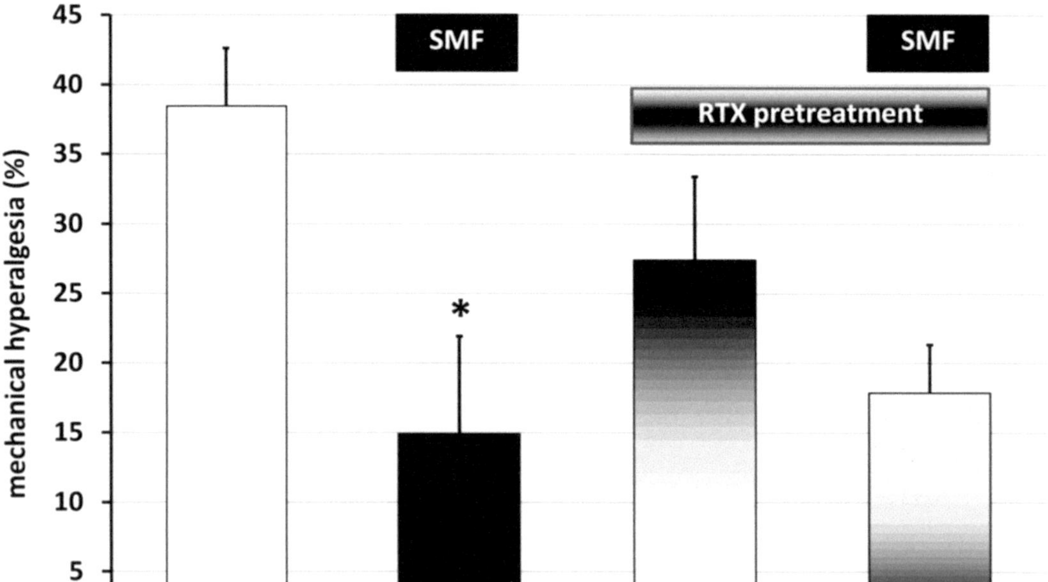

Fig. (5.13). Inhibitory effect of a 30 min SMF-exposure on i.pl. carrageenan induced inflammatory mechanical hyperalgesia of the mouse hind paw, which was prevented by inactivation of capsaicin-sensitive sensory nerves by RTX pretreatment. In the control groups animals were placed into the same cage for the same time period without SMF (sham cage). Each data point represents the mean±SEM mechanical hyperalgesia (%) compared to the respective basal thresholds of n=6-8 animals per group. * $p<0.05$ SMF *vs.* sham cage (ANOVA followed by Bonferroni's modified t-test).

SMF-exposure Fails to Affect Rotarod Performance

The rotarod performance after exposure to SMF for 30 min did not alter compared to that before exposure; they stayed on the accelerating drum for 50.7±5.5 and 63.6±10.7 s, respectively. Results of the animals in the control group were similar; their performance values were 46.5±8.1 s and 65.9±7.8 s, respectively before and after being in the same cage for the same time without SMF-exposure. No significant differences could be detected either between the 2 groups or between performances before and after the 30 min period.

Discussion, Conclusions

Phase I of the formalin test is due to the direct chemical stimulatory action of the compound, in phase II inflammatory mechanisms are involved [172]. Nocifensive reactions in phase II, but not in phase I were reduced in control (sham-exposed) mice after selective inactivation of capsaicin sensitive sensory fibers by RTX pretreatment; SP and CGRP released from these fibers are likely to be involved in the development of this inflammatory reaction. SMF-exposure diminished nocifensive behaviors in both phase I and phase II. The extent of the inhibition in the late phase was similar to that observed after RTX pretreatment. This inhibition was prevented after the destruction of peptidergic sensory fibers by RTX pretreatment.

Carrageenan, a polysaccharide derived from seaweeds, produces a subacute local inflammation which is a very commonly used model in pharmacological research. Edema and mechanical hyperalgesia reach their maximum 3 h after injection [171, 176]. Both neurogenic and non-neurogenic mechanisms with several mediators such as inflammatory neuropeptides, cytokines, and cyclooxygenase products are involved in this process [177, 178]. Carrageenan induced mechanical hyperalgesia was reduced, but not significantly following RTX pretreatment, which suggests that capsaicin-sensitive nerves do not play a predominant role in this type of edema formation. Similarly to the other models, SMF-exposure exerted a marked, about 70% inhibitory action on this inflammatory mechanical hyperalgesia, which was also prevented after the destruction of peptidergic afferents by RTX pretreatment.

These results reveal that capsaicin-sensitive sensory fibers are involved in the mediation of the SMF induced antinociceptive action. One potential mechanism for the inhibition in phase I might be a direct inhibition of sodium influx and action potential generation at the level of capsaicin-sensitive nerve terminals. In the SMF induced inhibitory effect in phase II decreased Ca^{2+} influx and consequently diminished sensory neuropeptide release mediating the local neurogenic inflammatory response can also be considered. This theory is supported by data on the ability of SMF-exposure to diminish neural excitability by the inhibition of Ca^{2+} and Na^{+} currents [70, 96, 159]. Reduced visual evoked potential and lower spontaneous discharge have been observed in the lateral geniculate body of the cat brain following SMF-exposure, which could be the result of slow reorientation of aligned groups of diamagnetic phospholipid molecules in the cell membrane distorting ion channel functions [70].

SMF-exposure also diminished inflammatory mechanical hyperalgesia induced by the *i.pl.* injection of the TRPV1 receptor agonist RTX. In response to the activation of this cation channel on capsaicin-sensitive sensory nerve terminals by RTX, pro-inflammatory neuropeptides such as SP and CGRP are released in the innervated area, which produce a local neurogenic inflammatory reaction in the plantar surface of the hind paw of mice with a consequent drop of the mechanonociceptive threshold. Since the development of mechanical hyperalgesia in this model involves peripheral mechanisms, one explanation for the antinociceptive action of SMF might be the inhibition of activation induced cation influx into the nerve terminals leading to a decreased release of pro-inflammatory/pro-nociceptive neuropeptides. On the other hand, neither inhibition of central sensitization, nor decreased synaptic transmission can be excluded.

Exposure of mice to SMF for 30 min did not alter their rotarod performance, therefore impairment of motor function cannot be considered as a factor influencing their nocifensive behaviors.

In conclusion, this study is the first to provide experimental evidence for the involvement of capsaicin-sensitive sensory nerves in the SMF induced anti-nociceptive action, but the precise mechanism needs further investigation. Our focus in the next some sections will be on the effect of SMF-exposure on mice that are experiencing acute visceral pain.

Visceral Action: The Writhing Test

Materials and Method

In this rodent model pain is elicited by the intraperitoneal (*i.p.*) injection of a slightly irritating agent. The pain sensation manifests itself in a characteristic stretching, writhing movement of the animal, the number of writhings per time period reflects pain intensity. Both opioid and non-opioid analgesics are able to exert *AE* in this pain model. This animal model is widely spread and it counts as a good predictor of human studies [63]. The method was described first by Wende and Margoli [179] and modified by Witkin *et al.* [180]. Male CFLP mice (24-26 g) were used in the experiments (Toxicoop, Budapest, Hungary). Numerous agents have been described to cause abdominal pain [181] and depending on the irritant, inflammatory or non-inflammatory pain can develop [182]. The visceral pain was elicited by the *i.p.* injection of acetic acid ($C_2H_4O_2$, 0.2 ml/mouse, 0.6%) or Epsom salt ($MgSO_4$, 0.2 ml/mouse, 2%). Since pain sensation is known to be socially modulated in mice [44], the same number of mice (2) was placed simultaneously in the cage both in the control (sham-) as well as in the SMF-exposed cases. Mice could freely move in their cage. Mice were exposed to SMF with their whole body during the experiment. The number of writhings was monitored in the 0-5, 6-20, 21-30, and sometimes in the 31-40 min intervals after the injection of acetic acid or Epsom salt. The nociceptive reaction was measured during the exposure of mice to SMF for 10, 20, or 30 min as well as after the cessation of SMF-exposure for 30, 20, or 10 min in order to determine the effect of the duration of exposure on nociception.

In all experiments a daily control was used, *i.e.* every experiment was completed with a control, where the mice got an *i.p.* injection with acetic acid or Epsom salt, were placed in identical cages as their SMF-exposed mates, but were not exposed to SMF. This sham apparatus assured the same dimensions and conditions as the SMF-exposure chamber but the animals inside were not exposed to either inhomogeneous or homogeneous SMF beyond that of Earth. Negative control animals received physiological salt solution *i.p.* and were considered unchallenged.

To reduce experimental stress, mice were handled and placed in the plastic cage (where they were kept during the experiments) for 30 min for 4 consecutive days before the experiment in the course of an adaptation period. Mice were sacrificed 48 h after the experiments, meanwhile their behavior and appetite was checked: No difference between treated and untreated mice could be observed. Neither morbidity, nor mortality was observed. Animals were housed in groups of 5, the room was held under a 12:12 light/dark cycle at 20±2°C.

OPTIMIZATION OF SMF PARAMETERS

Optimization of SMF Parameters Improves Pain Inhibition in Mice

Goals

Although 2254 patents with the key phrase "magnetic therapy" are available in the patent office (http://v3.espacenet.com) in February of 2014, most of which are electromagnetic applications, we still lack a trustworthy recipe how to achieve optimal results in analgesia/antinociception with SMF-exposure. The following study is devoted to this problem through a reliable animal model. Another aim of the presents work was to find out, whether *AE* induced by SMF-exposure could be in fact demonstrated; if yes, what the dynamics is, how long the prolonged effect holds following the cessation of the exposure.

Materials and Methods

Magnetic Exposure Conditions

Generators 1-16 were used throughout the first set of experiments, generators 17-22, but 19 throughout the second set of experiments (see **Generators 1-16**).

Statistical Analysis

We defined the *AE* of a treatment in a given time interval as $AE=100(1-\bar{x}/\bar{y})\%$, where $\bar{x}$ is the average of the number of writhings for the treated and $\bar{y}$ is that for the control animals. As some treatments were applied in several experiments on different days with different numbers of animals, they had more than one observed value of *AE*. For such treatments we calculated a pooled *AE* based on all experiments in which the treatment occurred. For pooling we applied weighted averages with weights inversely proportional to the variances of the particular *AE* estimates. This is optimal in the sense that it results in a minimum variance pooled estimate (Handbook [183], *pp*. 401-402). From a general result about the variance of a ratio estimate (Handbook [183], *pp*. 63-64), the asymptotic variance of *AE* is

$\sigma^2 = \frac{\bar{y}^2}{\bar{x}^2}\left(\frac{\sigma_x^2}{\bar{x}^2} + \frac{\sigma_y^2}{\bar{y}^2}\right)$, where σ_x^2 and σ_y^2 are the variances of the number of writhings for the treated and control animals, respectively. Thus, the pooled *AE* for a treatment that occurred in *m* different experiments with n_j number of treated and u_j number of control animals on the *j*th date ($1 \leq j \leq m$), can be obtained as $100\frac{\sum_{j=1}^{m} w_j\left(1-\frac{\bar{x}_j}{\bar{y}_j}\right)}{\sum_{j=1}^{m} w_j}\%$, where $\bar{x}_j = \frac{1}{n_j}\sum_{i=1}^{n_j} x_{ij}$ and $\bar{y}_j = \frac{1}{u_j}\sum_{i=1}^{u_j} y_{ij}$ are the average values of the number of writhings for the treated and control animals on the *j*th day of measurement, respectively. The weights w_j are inversely proportional to the variance estimates from the particular experiments, *i.e.* $w_j = \frac{1}{\sigma_j^2} = \frac{1}{\left(\frac{\bar{x}_j}{\bar{y}_j}\right)^2\left(\frac{\sigma_x^2}{\bar{x}_j^2} + \frac{\sigma_y^2}{\bar{y}_j^2}\right)}$. This definition of the *AE* has the advantages that

i. it is based on comparisons between treated and control animals examined on the same day and

ii. it takes into account different sample sizes correctly.

To achieve the best possible transparency of the data, we summarized the results of the writhing tests in Table **5.3** including SEM, *e.g.* for treated animals on the *j*th date: $SEM_j = \sqrt{\frac{\sum_{i=1}^{n_j}\left(x_{ij}-\bar{x}_j\right)^2}{\left(n_j-1\right)n_j}}$ with $n_j = \sum_{i=1}^{m} n_i$ number of animals of a certain type of experiment and *AE* for all 3 time periods, plus for the whole 30 min interval. The *p* values were computed from the 30 min interval (in **boldface** in Table **5.3**) using 2-sample heteroscedastic Dunnett's tests. For experiments carried out on several different dates, the highest *p* value is reported. We also carried out a joint analysis of all experiments using a mixed model ANOVA with the date of experiment as a random factor. Due to the large number of data, this resulted in extremely small *p* values ($p<0.001$), so we found it more informative to report the *p* values from the Dunnett's tests. Note that although the headline of Table **5.3** displays pooled number of writhings based on all control groups together, *p* values were calculated by comparing treated and control groups investigated on the same day. Altogether 378 mice participated in 17 types of experiments.

Table 5.3. Summarized data of the writhing tests for the first 5 min, from 6 to 20 min, and from 21 to 30 min; boldface values Stand for the whole 30 min time interval for generators 1-16. Detailed in Chapter 3 (Generators 1-16).

generator	0-5 min		6-20 min		21-30 min		0-30 min		
	control: $\bar{y}_j$ =8.52 ±0.37; treated: $\bar{x}_j \pm SEM_j$	analgesic effect (%)	control: $\bar{y}_j$ =34.91 ±0.63; treated: $\bar{x}_j$ ±SEM_j	analgesic effect (%)	control: $\bar{y}_j$ =27.54 ±0.58; treated: $\bar{x}_j$ ±SEM_j	analgesic effect (%)	control: $\bar{y}_j$ =70.97 ±1.08; treated: $\bar{x}_j$ ±SEM_j	analgesic effect (%)	*ANOVA*, number of animals control: $u=\sum_{j=1}^{m} u_j$ =109
1	2.34±0.26	89.04	19.22±0.67	55.37	16.58±0.50	46.70	**36.30 ±1.79**	**54.07**	$p<$ **0.003, *n*=76**
2	10.18±0.82	-0.55	38.64±2.43	-2.92	26.55±1.59	7.71	**75.36 ±4.17**	**1.40**	$p>$ **0.883, *n*=11**
3	4.73±1.00	40.25	28.18±4.49	26.91	23.73±2.92	17.81	**56.64 ±7.59**	**24.39**	$p>$ **0.104, *n*=11**
4	8.11±1.67	-102.78	39.33±1.44	0.84	33.44±0.75	-2.91	**80.89 ±2.94**	**-6.20**	$p>$ **0.216, *n*=9**
5	6.08±0.73	42.61	27.50±2.48	24.66	18.42±0.95	36.05	**52.00 ±3.13**	**31.49**	$p<$ **0.001, *n*=12**
6	2.50±0.40	66.93	18.70±0.88	52.16	18.00±1.10	45.71	**39.20 ±1.70**	**50.21**	$p<$ **0.013, *n*=10**
7	3.15±0.37	67.32	19.81±0.89	48.74	18.73±1.03	39.92	**41.69 ±1.89**	**47.54**	$p<$ **0.001, *n*=26**
8	2. 70±0.47	76.86	15.80±0.74	59.94	14.00±1.90	55.07	**32.50 ±2.89**	**59.81**	$p<$ **0.001, *n*=10**

(Table 5.3) contd.....

generator	0-5 min		6-20 min		21-30 min		0-30 min		
	control: $\bar{y}_j$ =8.52 ±0.37; treated: $\bar{x}_j$ ± SEM_j	analgesic effect (%)	control: $\bar{y}_j$ =34.91 ±0.63; treated: $\bar{x}_j$ $\pm SEM_j$	analgesic effect (%)	control: $\bar{y}_j$ =27.54 ±0.58; treated: $\bar{x}_j$ $\pm SEM_j$	analgesic effect (%)	control: $\bar{y}_j$ =70.97 ±1.08; treated: $\bar{x}_j$ $\pm SEM_j$	analgesic effect (%)	*ANOVA*, number of animals control: $u=\sum_{j=1}^{m} u_j$ =109
9	2.00±4.17	72.72	24.00±0.67	41.78	18.89±1.75	46.13	**44.89 ±1.93**	**46.05**	$p< 0.001$, $n=9$
10	2.33±0.51	76.61	15.75±1.56	68.02	9.75±1.16	70.45	**27.83 ±2.46**	**68.07**	$p< 0.002$, $n=12$
11	1.00±0.21	89.07	8.60±1.96	79.97	5.30±0.93	89.48	**14.90 ±2.28**	**83.40**	$p< 0.001$, $n=10$
12	0.30±0.15	92.50	9.00±1.20	77.31	6.50±0.76	80.00	**15.80 ±1.76**	**79.26**	$p< 0.001$, $n=10$
13	0.33±0.24	91.89	8.44±0.82	78.20	6.11±0.72	80.94	**14.89 ±1.55**	**80.75**	$p< 0.003$, $n=9$
14	0.22±0.22	89.47	6.56±2.06	83.82	7.22±0.98	79.18	**14.00 ±2.40**	**81.81**	$p< 0.003$, $n=9$
15	13.64±2.96	44.11	34.00±4.06	35.71	24.91±1.00	18.76	**72.55 ±7.04**	**27.57**	$p> 0.077$, $n=11$
16	8.56±1.70	21.38	34.56±3.91	16.09	21.56±1.93	25.62	**64.67 ±5.97**	**19.98**	$p> 0.084$, $n=9$

Results for Generators 1-16

From now on we present the results sorted around problems and their solutions regarding characteristics of the specific magnetic arrangements (*i.e.***Generators 1-16**).

The results presented in Table **5.3** time-resolve the experiment; they are split into 3 parts: From 0 to 5, from 6 to 20, and from 21 to 30 min. The last columns (0-30 min, in **boldface**) denote the weighted averages of all 3 previous columns.

On AE Caused by SMF-exposure (Generator 1)

In this set of experiments mice were exposed to a medium SMF produced by individual magnets (NdFeB cylindrical magnets of grade N35, *R*=5 mm, *L*=10 mm) arranged in a checkerboard configuration with alternating polarity (bidirectionally). The average *P-P* value was 389 mT and the average surface roughness was 39 T/m (these were measured 3 mm from the surface of an individual magnet along its axis), see generator 1 in Table **3.3** and Table **3.4**. The raw data of the number of writhings for this situation are collected in Fig.(**5.14**). The data corresponding to the 0-5, 6-20, and 21-30 min intervals are deliberately scattered in the time coordinate in a random manner in 5 min intervals around 5, 20, and 30 min, respectively for better comprehension. Arrows show the averages. The derived results are shown as generator 1 in Table **3.3**. The overall *AE* was found to be over 54%. There is a significant *AE* caused by this SMF-exposure.

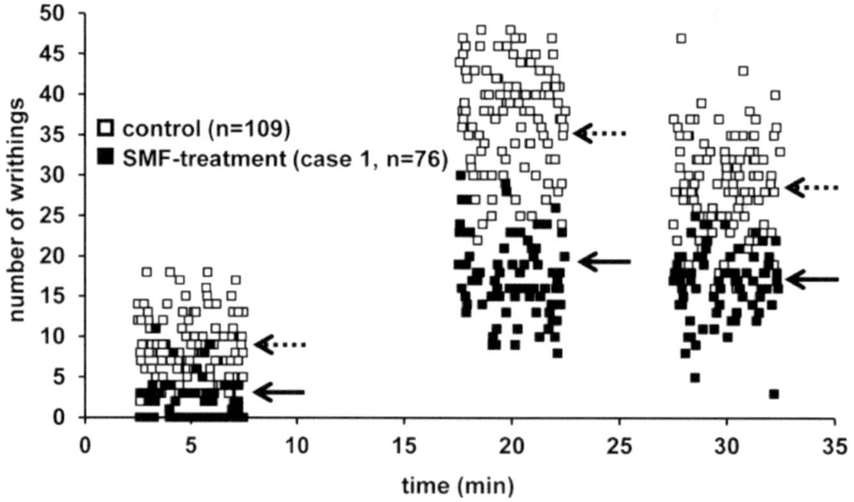

Fig. (5.14). Raw data of the number of writhings due to visceral pain elicited by i.p. injection of acetic acid in mice. For better comprehension data corresponding to the 0-5, 6-20, and 21-30 min time intervals are deliberately scattered in the time coordinate in a random manner in 5 min intervals around 5, 20, and 30 min, respectively. Solid and dashed arrow shows the SMF- and sham-exposed average values, respectively. SMF was provided by generator 1.

On the Reproducibility of the Experiments

In these examinations the magnetic arrangement was again identical to generator 1 (*c.f.*, Table **3.3** and Table **3.4**). The average number of writhings is illustrated in Fig. (**5.15A**) and Fig. (**5.15B**) as a function of the time of the experiments in weeks. Solid lines in the figures between markers guide the eye only. The sham-exposed results (headline in Table **5.3**) are shown in Fig. (**5.15A**), the results of SMF-exposure (generator 1 in Table **5.3**) in Fig. (**5.15B**). In Fig. (**5.15A**) the average value of writhings for the 0-30 min interval was 70.97. The linear trend line fitted to the 0-30 curve had a slope of 0.29. In Fig. (**5.15B**) these were 36.30 and 0.07, respectively. Since the slopes of the trend lines were small, the experiments could be regarded as stable and a sufficiently good reproducibility was achieved and maintained. The residual standard deviation was 11.24, the standard deviation due to the random factor (the date) was 6.76. Accordingly, the variance within a date was 126.34, while the total (including all dates) was 147.30.

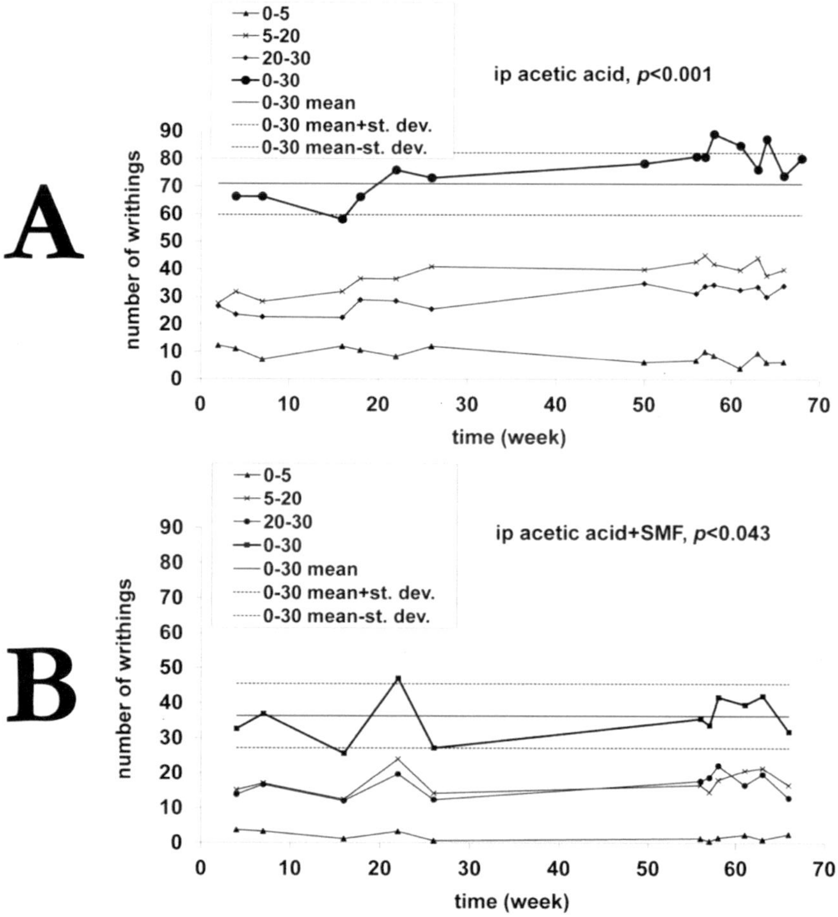

Fig. (5.15). Measured average number of writhings originating from the **A)** sham-exposed (control) group (headline in Table **5.3**) and the **B)** SMF-exposed group as a function of the date of the experiment (generator 1 in Table **5.3**). The mean and the standard deviations are also designated. Solid lines between markers guide the eye only.

This nice test-retest reliability is why we accepted the averaging over similar types of experiments executed on different days (see Statistical analysis section above). The experiments proved to be reproducible. The differences between SMF- and sham-exposed animals were always statistically significant ($p<0.003$).

On the Effect of the Instrument (Generator 2)

The next set of experiments was executed with "placebo" matrices that did not contain magnets; otherwise the experimental setup looked exactly like the one with magnets. The results are presented as generator 2 in Table **5.3**. The placebo effect furnished us with the same results as the control group within experimental error. In other words the experimental setup did not significantly influence the results as shown in the significance test; the probability was $p>0.883$.

On the Single Sided Arrangement of Magnets (Generator 3)

The arrangement was similar to generator 1 with the only exception that there was no matrix on top of the cage; see Table **3.3**, Table **3.4**, and Table **5.3**. *AE* became far less expressed (24.39%) in the case of a one sided matrix arrangement of magnets and the probability of statistical significance $p>0.1$ also suggested that there was no significant *AE* from the clinical point of view (both biological and statistical significance fail).

On the Polarity of the Individual Magnets (Generators 4, 5, and 6)

In these arrangements (see Table **3.3** and Table **3.4**) there were magnetic matrices on both sides of the cage; the magnets were of the same size, cylindrical shape, ferrite, NdFeB N35 or N50. Both the average *P-P* values and the average $\bar{\alpha}$ values were low, because of the unidirectional arrangement (with still opposite poles in the facing 2 matrices). The results are compiled in Table **5.3** (generators 4, 5, and 6). *AE* increases with increasing magnitude of the magnetic induction. The maximal unidirectional *AE* of 50.21% was achieved when the applied SMF was very strong created by individual magnets of 1.47 T remanent magnetic induction. Statistical analysis showed that ferrite magnets did not produce a significant *AE* ($p>0.216$), while for NdFeB N35 and N50 magnets the results were significant ($p<0.001$ and $p<0.013$, respectively). The negative *AE* value in the 0-5 min period for the weakest unidirectional field was due to an extremely low daily control value.

We should note here that unidirectionality strongly decreases $\bar{\alpha}$, the average surface roughness as mentioned in Chapter 2 (Fig. **2.2C** and Fig. **2.2D**).

On Average Surface Roughness, $\bar{\alpha}$ (the Inhomogeneity of the Magnetic Field) and on Average P-P values, (Generators 1, 7, and 8)

This case was studied with the help of bidirectional matrix arrangements on both sides (Table **3.3** and Table **3.4**). λ, lattice parameter (**Constraints, solutions**) was kept constant. The writhing test details can be found in cases 1, 7, and 8 in Table **5.3**. The maximal activity of 59.81% was achieved at 51 T/m surface roughness (at z=3 mm). In all 3 cases the *AE* was statistically significant (p_{max}≤0.003). The bidirectional arrangements caused higher *AE* than the unidirectional arrangement. Increasing the average surface roughness as well as increasing the average *P-P* values causes increasing *AE*.

On lattice Constant, λ (Generators 9-10 and 11-12)

The situation presented by generators 9 and 10 was such: NdFeB cylindrical magnets of grade N35, R=2.5 mm, L=10 mm at λ=5 mm were compared to λ=10 mm. Both arrangements were bidirectional and 2-sided. It seemed that introducing a gap between the magnets increased *AE*. This is in harmony with the observations in the case of the normal distributions (*c.f.*, Fig. **2.2**).

The next situation (generators 11 and 12) was, when the magnets were of grade N50, the fields were enhanced by *mc* (see Fig. **3.1**), R=5 mm, L=10 mm at λ=10 mm *vs* λ=20 mm. At first sight it might be surprising that the difference in *AE* vanished. A reasonable explanation would be though, that *AE* does not only depend on the individual magnet radii, but also on the average *P-P* values (*e.g.* at z=3 mm). The *P-P* values changed in a different manner from generator 9 to 10 and from generator 11 to 12. Dunnett's test showed a significant *AE* in all 4 cases (p_{max}≤0.002). The change of the magnet constant (λ) from 2R to 4R did not reduce *AE*.

On the Height of the Individual Cylindrical Magnets (Generators 11-14)

This question was answered on the basis of experiments with a bidirectional, both sided arrangement with NdFeB N50 magnets. The field was *mc* enhanced. λ was kept 10 mm, just the height of the individual magnets was different; L=10 mm *vs* 20 mm, *c.f.*, generator 11 and 13 in Table **3.3**, Table **3.4**, and Table **5.3**. There was hardly any difference in *AE*, which suggested that *AE* did not benefit from the slight increase in the magnetic induction due to the longer magnets. This effect may be due to a threshold in the induction that manifests itself in a saturation of the *AE* at a value somewhat over 83%. The probabilities showed a significant *AE* in both cases (p_{max} <0.001). Doubling the height of the individual magnets did not significantly contribute to the enhancement of *AE*.

Remark: If we let both height and lattice constant double, we get generator 13 and 14 for L=20 mm magnets (to be compared to generator 11 and 12 for L=10 mm) in Table **3.3**, Table **3.4**, and Table **5.3**. The high *AE* did not change.

On the Diameter of the Individual Cylindrical Magnets (Generators 1 and 9)

Again the arrangements were bidirectional and both sided. The following cases are compared: NdFeB N35 magnets with L=10 mm, R=2.5 mm *vs* 5 mm (generator 9 *vs* 1). The slimmer magnets had about the same surface induction values as the bigger ones (200.88 *vs* 201.56 mT as measured at z=3 mm from the magnets' surface, see Table **3.4**). As shown in Table **5.3** no big difference occurred between *AE* for the magnets with different radii; in both cases there was a significant *AE* (p_{max}≤0.001). Halving the radius of the individual magnets did not significantly reduce *AE*.

On Magnetic Coupling (mc) (Generators 8 and 11)

The magnets were bidirectionally arranged, NdFeB N50, R=5 mm, L=10 mm at λ=10 mm. The *AE* for the *mc* situation was found more expressed. Dunnett's test showed a significant *AE* in both cases (p_{max}≤0.001). We found the record holding highest average *AE* of 83.4% in case 11 in the course of our investigations. The effect *mc* caused (see in Fig. **3.1**) could explain this ratio of increase. In case of bidirectional arrangements, *mc* increases *AE*.

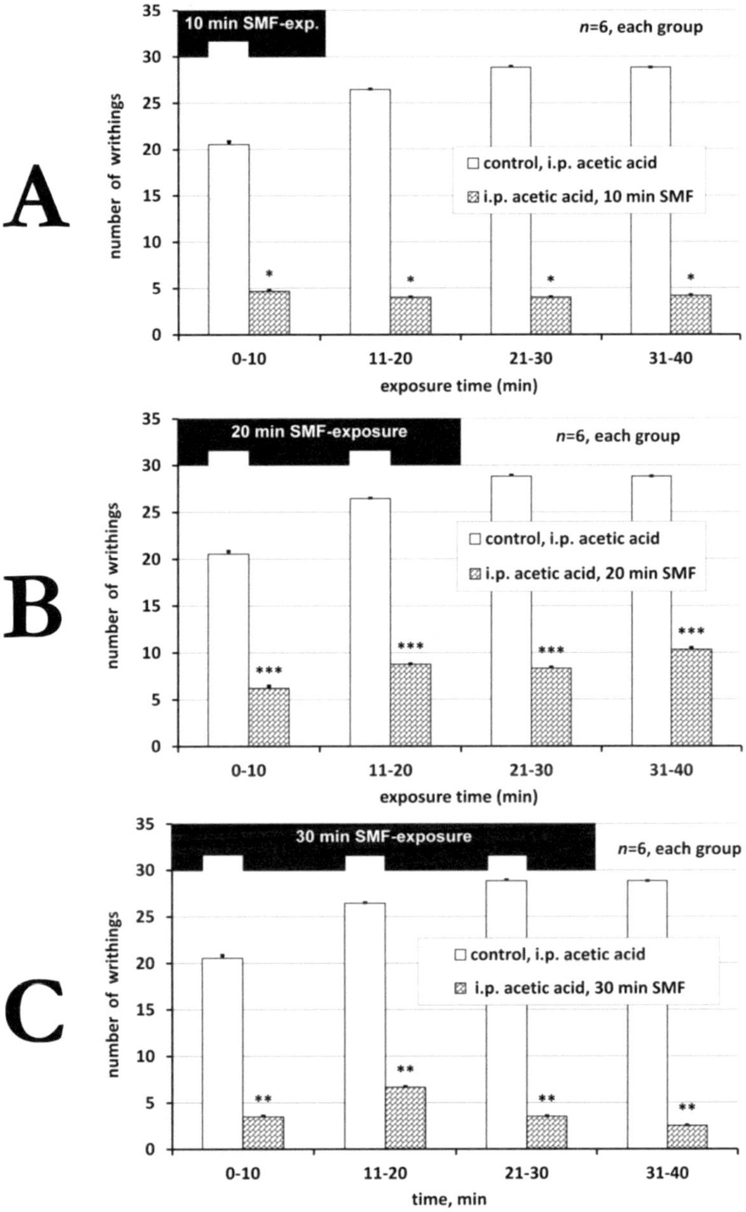

Fig. (5.16). Panels **(A)**, **(B)**, and **(C)** demonstrate the average number of writhings±SEM of mice exposed to an inhomogeneous SMF (generator 11) for 10, 20, or 30 min, respectively (stripped columns). Open columns denote the control group, where mice got the same amount of i.p. acetic acid, but were not exposed to SMF. Dark bars on top show the time of exposure. Mice were challenged with acetic acid at t=0. A probability $p<0.05$ was considered statistically significant. * $p<0.003$, ** $p<0.002$, *** $p<0.001$ assessed by Dunnett's post hoc test. The number of animals (*n*) was 6/group.

On the Form of the Magnets (Generators 15 and 16)

The arrangements in these cases were such that ferrite block magnets were used on both sides either bidirectionally or unidirectionally. The results in Table **5.3** show that both bidirectional and unidirectional cases resulted in *AE* below 30%. These can be regarded as clinically insignificant.

On the Dynamics of Action, Duration of Exposure

This series was tested with generator 11, specifically. Results are summarized in Fig. (**5.16**). It can be observed that the *AE* induced by SMF in the mouse exposed for 10 (Fig. **5.16A**), 20 (Fig. **5.16B**), or 30 (Fig. **5.16C**) min can be detected for an additional period of 30, 20, or 10 min, respectively following SMF-exposure.

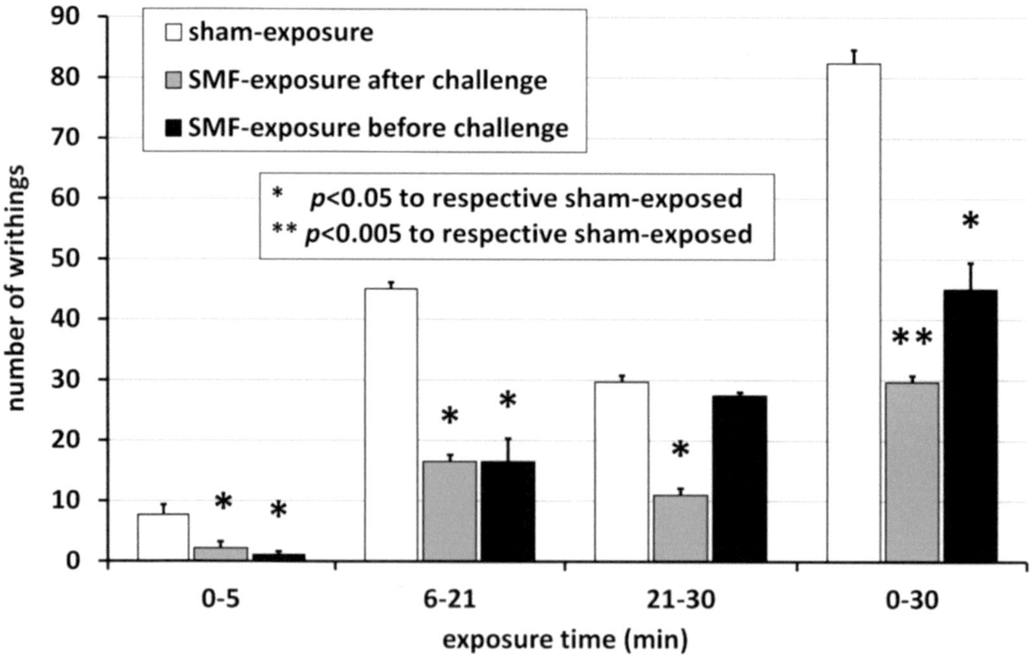

Fig. (5.17). The effect of SMF-exposure on writhing syndrome applied for 30 min either after or before the injection of 0.6% acetic acid measured in 0-5, 6-20, and 21-30 min after the acetic acid challenge. Open columns: Control animals unexposed to SMF. Grey columns: Mice exposed to SMF after the administration of acetic acid. Dark columns: Mice exposed to SMF before the administration of acetic acid. Each column represents the mean±SEM of 6 mice. * $p<0.05$, ** $p<0.005$ significant differences to respective control as assessed by one-way ANOVA.

On the Dynamics of Action, Timing of Exposure

Comparison of *AE* of SMF-exposure applied either before or after the *i.p.* injection of acetic acid is shown in Fig. (**5.17**). Inhibition of pain reaction induced by SMF-exposure did not differ in mice exposed either before or after the acetic acid challenge in the 0-5th, 6-20th min observation period. However, no *AE* could be observed in the 21-30th min period in mice exposed to SMF before the injection of acetic acid. The abdominal pain reaction during the whole 30 min observation period was inhibited by 46% ($p<0.05$) when SMF was applied before, and 64% ($p<0.005$) when SMF was applied after the *i.p.* injection of acetic acid.

Results for Generators 17-22

Table **5.4** contains time-resolved writhing responses of mice exposed to SMF in generators 17-22 (*c.f.*, **Sources of Static Magnetic Fields, Generators**, generator 19 excluded) for 30 min. Generator 19 was used exclusively in human trials.

Table 5.4. Similarly to Table 5.3, summarized data of the writhing tests for the first 5 min, from 6 to 20 min, and from 21 to 30 min for special arrangements (generators); boldface values stand for the whole 30 min time interval.

generator	0-5 min		6-20 min		21-30 min		0-30 min		
	control: $\bar{y}_j$ =7.52 ±0.44 treated: $\bar{x}_j \pm SEM_j$	analgesic effect (%)	control: $\bar{y}_j$ =40.39 ±0.76 treated: $\bar{x}_j$ $\pm SEM_j$	analgesic effect (%)	control: $\bar{y}_j$ =30.98 ±0.66 treated: $\bar{x}_j$ $\pm SEM_j$	analgesic effect (%)	control: $\bar{y}_j$ =78.89 ±1.50 treated: $\bar{x}_j$ $\pm SEM_j$	analgesic effect (%)	*ANOVA*, number of animals control: $u = \sum_{j=1}^{m} u_j$ =54
17a	3.67±0.42	51	17.00±0.86	58	18.00±0.89	42	**38.67±1.80**	51	$p<$ **0.001**, ***n*=6**
17b	5.00±1.00	33	18.33±0.56	55	17.33±0.80	44	**40.67±1.45**	48	$p<$ ***0.001*, *n*=6**
17c	1.83±0.75	76	14.83±0.70	63	9.83±0.87	68	**26.50±1.61**	66	$p<$ **0.001**, ***n*=6**
17d	1.92±0.51	75	11.75±0.79	71	11.00±0.87	64	**24.67±1.23**	69	$p<$ **0.001**, ***n*=12**
17e	4.17±0.60	45	18.50±1.06	54	15.33±1.20	51	**38.00±1.84**	52	$p<$ **0.001**, ***n*=6**
18	1.39±0.52	42	15.33±1.17	62	14.33±1.19	54	**34.00±1.94**	57	$p<$ **0.001**, ***n*=9**
20("3 T")	1.04±0.29	86	13.48±1.15	67	10.57±0.89	66	**22.08±2.32**	72	$p<$ **0.001**, ***n*=6**

(Table 5.4) contd.....

generator	0-5 min		6-20 min		21-30 min		0-30 min		
	control: $\bar{y}_j$ =7.52 ±0.44 treated: $\bar{x}_j \pm SEM_j$	analgesic effect (%)	control: $\bar{y}_j$ =40.39 ±0.76 treated: $\bar{x}_j$ $\pm SEM_j$	analgesic effect (%)	control: $\bar{y}_j$ =30.98 ±0.66 treated: $\bar{x}_j$ $\pm SEM_j$	analgesic effect (%)	control: $\bar{y}_j$ =78.89 ±1.50 treated: $\bar{x}_j$ $\pm SEM_j$	analgesic effect (%)	*ANOVA*, number of animals control: *u*= $u=\sum_{j=1}^{m} u_j$ =54
20 ("out 0.1 mT" together with "out 0.5 mT")	4.00±0.68	47	32.17±1.58	20	25.83±1.96	17	**62.00±3.20**	21	$p<$ **0.001,** n=24
20 ("in 3 mT")	2.00±4.17	42	33.17±2.51	18	25.50±1.45	18	**63.00±4.12**	20	$p<$ **0.001, n=6**
21	0.33±0.21	82	1.89±1.24	73	9.44±1.02	70	**21.72±2.40**	72	$p<$ **0.001, n=18**
22	4.33±0.83	96	6.00±0.82	85	8.33±1.12	73	**14.67±1.23**	81	$p<$ **0.001, n=6**

On the Effect of Magnetic Induction in Homogeneous SMF (Generators 4, 16, 20, and 22)

Homogeneous SMF-exposure causes a significant inhibition of pain in the writhing test in mice as presented in Fig. (**5.18**). The dominant component of the magnetic induction in the 80-450 mT range was dorsal-ventral; in the 3 T case (clinical MRI) it was cranial-caudal or dextrosinistral. Detailed description of the writhing test applied in and around the bore of a clinical MR can be found in the next point.

Discussion, Conclusions

An important concern about using SMF-exposure on the whole body of a mouse if the mouse is free to move in the field, is: What apparent SMF is manifested in the body of the mouse? By collecting models from the literature [12] and creating our own models, we concluded that the motion induced magnetic field induction is many orders of magnitude below that of the external SMF and therefore, probably does not affect analgesia. This point will be further discussed in sections **Clinical MRI** 3 T clinical MRI significantly inhibits pain in mice, **Lateral gradients** Lateral gradients significantly enhance static magnetic field-induced inhibition of pain responses in mice – a double blind experimental study, and **Pharmacological analysis**.

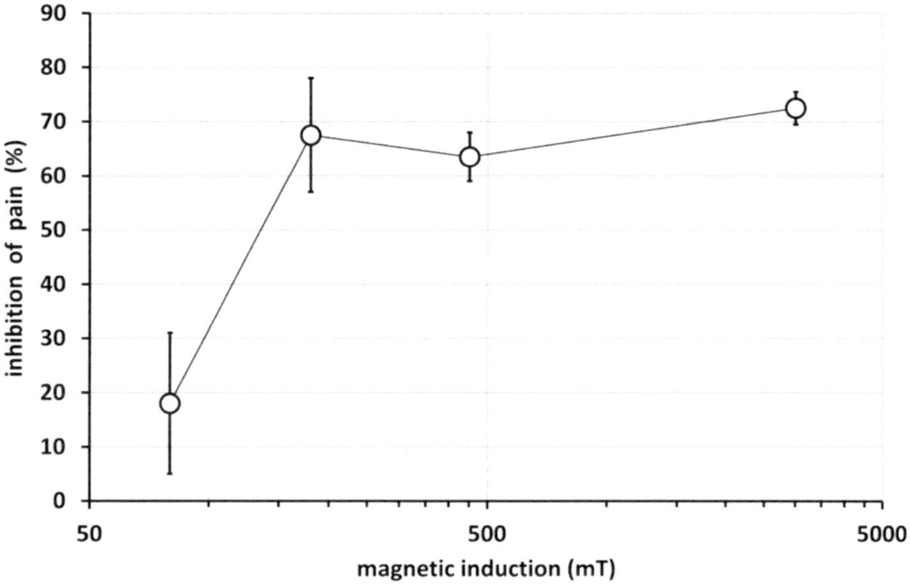

Fig. (5.18). Inhibition of pain (%) by homogeneous static magnetic field (hSMF) exposure in the writhing test in mice. Error bars represent standard errors of the mean. Linear sections between markers guide the eye only.

In an effort to provide a critical analysis of how the parameters of SMF influence the *AE* and then choose the most appropriate setup, we should first recognize the possible errors introduced in the evaluation. These were:

i. The reading error of the scans (for bigger elevations and lower inductions the scans were distorted),
ii. lateral components of SMF have not been tested in the pain assay,
iii. there was a difference between B_r values (presumably equal to the absolute value of the homogeneous magnetization vector $\vec{M}$ in the magnetic material) given in the technical specification of the magnets and the ones calculated from the surface induction value,
iv. the magnetization was neither perfectly homogeneous, nor perfectly cylindrically symmetrical in the cylindrical magnets,
v. and the experiments were not factorially designed; therefore, a complete survey may lack some experiments.

However, the following 10 trends and relationships could be identified.

1. The *AE* has a correlation of 85.61% ($p<0.001$) with the grade of the magnet so that it emphasizes the role of the grade of the magnet. Due to collinearities this also involves a strong correlation with B_r remanent induction (84.06%), with the induction measured on the magnet surface (82.96%), and with the material of the magnet (76.07%). The grade should be optimized, since constructional and budgetary viewpoints of a potential medical device contradict.
2. The *AE* correlates with the polarity of the magnet arrangement to an extent of 69.27% ($p<0.001$). Accordingly, the bidirectional arrangement should be preferred. A bidirectional SMF generates a local *P-P* value at 3 mm from the magnet surface of a minimum of 4.37 (ferrite magnets, generators 4 and 7) to a maximum of 80.39 (NdFeB N50 magnets, generators 6 and 8) times that of a unidirectional field, and contributes to the enhancement of the average surface roughness, which consequently generates a higher *AE* (-6.20% *vs* 47.54% and 50.21% *vs* 59.81%, generators 4 *vs* 7 and 6 *vs* 8, respectively).

   The cylindrical shape is better than the block shape as suggested by the 63.95% ($p<0.001$) correlation between the *AE* and the shape of the magnet.
4. The *AE* has a correlation of 57.06% to *mc* ($p<0.001$); *mc* should be included in the successful arrangement for analgesia. It enhances the *AE* by 39.44% as shown for example, between generator 8 and 11.
5. The *AE* shows a correlation to the average *B* value of the induction scan at 3 mm from the magnet surface by 52.19% ($p<0.001$). See column 5 in Table **3.4**. This may imply that the analgesia happens in the mice close to the magnet surface, in other words the point of action may be rather peripheral than central. This answers the question, what the possible relation is between the SMF generated at the source and the SMF at the target (animal) site.
6. There is a correlation of 55.99% ($p<0.001$) with the number of magnetic matrices; two is better than one. A single sided arrangement causes far less than 50% as much *AE* as a double sided.
7. We found a moderate correlation between 46.24% and 47.93% ($p_{max}<0.001$) concerning the *AE* and the surface roughness, and this was consistent for all 3 surface scans (at 3, 10, and 15 mm from the surface). See columns 3, 8 and 13 in Table **3.4**.

8. The *AE* is most expressed in the first 5 min of the experiments as suggested by the number of writhings per 5 min period (5 min writhing rate) in the treated groups. The 5 min writhing rates increase by even 16 times from the first 5 to the last 5 min of the 30 min time period.
9. A bigger matrix constant does not reduce the *AE* (by decreasing resultant induction, but increasing surface roughness) and therefore can be preferably applied from budgetary considerations.
10. Block magnets with lateral sizes exceeding or comparable to that of a mouse do not perform well in analgesia due to the laterally slowly changing magnetic field and therefore, due to small surface roughness. This phenomenon will be discussed in details in **Lateral gradients**.

A stepwise and a best subset regression were also executed to explore deeper relations between parameters of exposure. In this estimate the matrix in question consisted of number of writhings corresponding to all 17 types of experiments (carried out on 71 dates) and to 31 variables, which were not necessarily independent, *i.e.* collinearity appeared. The variables were distributed into 3 groups: Magnet arrangement, magnetic field map, and animal experiment. The magnet arrangement group (see parts in Table **3.4**) contained: Material, grade, remanent induction, shape, height, radius, side length, matrix constant, number of bonds, induction value on the magnet surface, magnetic coupling, and polarity. The field map group (Table **3.4**) contained: *P-P* value, surface roughness, mean and standard deviation of the induction at 3, 10, and 15 mm *z* values. The animal experiment group (see parts in Table **5.3**) contained: Animal identification number, period of examination, mean and standard deviation of writhings. We looked for those variables which are the best predictors of analgesia. On the basis of our experiences so far, we could not identify one or two parameters that would exclusively be responsible for the results.

Remark: There might be a chance that magnetic induction, surface roughness, matrix constant, or other quantities work in synergy only in a "window". See for example, the paper of Kirson *et al.* [184] concerning the window effect in a situation induced by an electric field. Further studies must be devoted to this question.

Summarizing the results for the 0-30 min interval in Fig. (**5.19**) the following relationships can be established. The first prize in the *AE* of SMF (category 1) goes to bidirectional magnet arrangements with *mc* with or without a gap (λ=2*R* or 4*R*). In the second category there are arrangements which consist of bidirectional or very strong unidirectional magnetic fields with no gap. Arrangements in the last class (category 3) cannot be proposed for purposes of analgesia. These include arrangements with unidirectional or block magnets, or magnets on only one side of the cage.

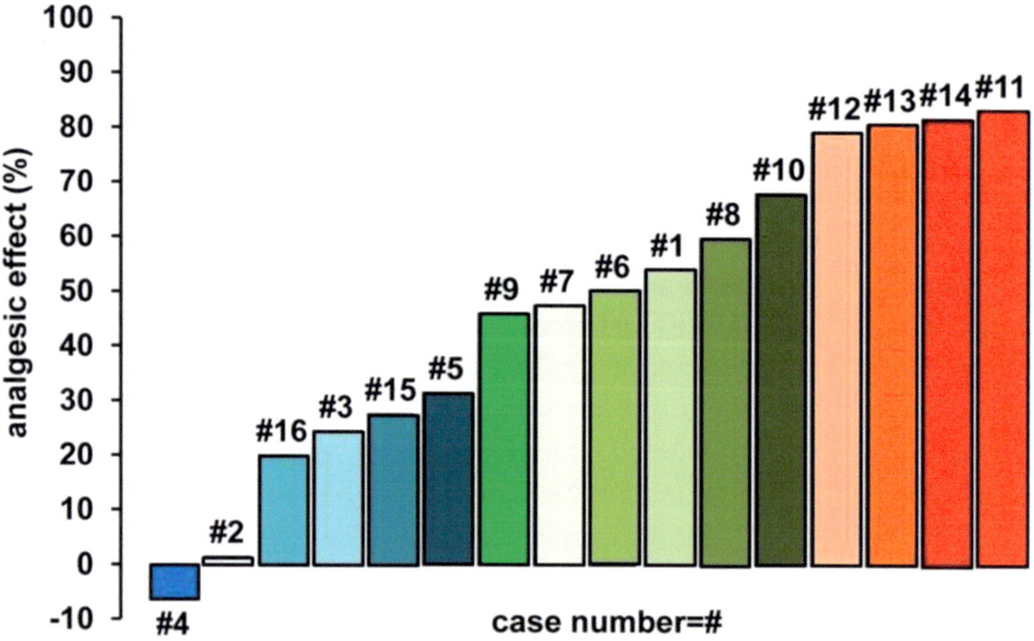

Fig. (5.19). The AE due to SMF on visceral pain elicited by i.p. injection of acetic acid in mice in the 0-30 min time interval. SMF was applied whole-body by different SMF generators; see Table **3.3**, Table **3.4**, and Table **5.3** for the generator numbers (Generators 1-16).

Having tested a number of different SMF arrangements for their *AE* in mice we concluded that the optimal arrangement for this purpose is an arrangement with 2 magnetic matrices below and above the animal cage. The separation of the 2 matrices should be kept as low as possible. The lower poles of the lower matrix and the opposite upper poles of the upper matrix should be coupled magnetically, the individual magnets must sit one next to another or at a double diameter distance from each other with alternating poles, and their material should be

NdFeB grade N50, cylindrical shape with a radius of 5 mm and height 10 or 20 mm. The best magnetic arrangement obtained (generator 11) will be used in pharmacological studies to clear up the possible mechanisms of action and the device will be adjusted to fit human experiments (**Generator 18** and **Generator 19**).

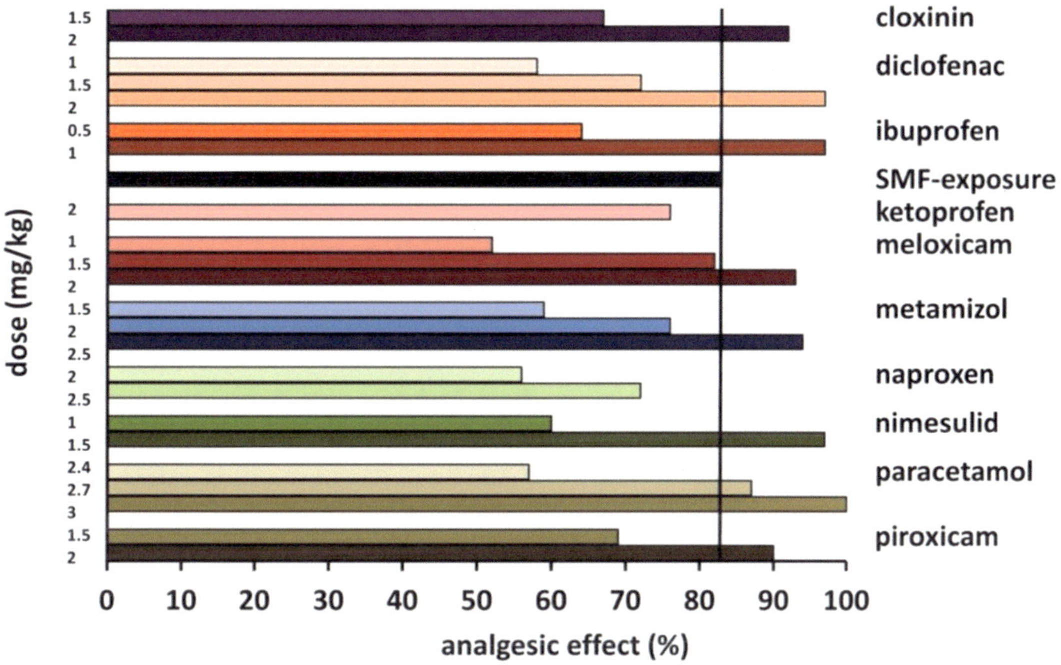

Fig. (5.20). The AE of different NSAIDs in different doses compared to SMF-exposure with generator 11 in the writhing test in mice. Solid vertical line just extends the result obtained for SMF-exposure.

Present data demonstrate the long-lasting effect of exposure to an inhomogeneous SMF for the first time: The pain-inhibitory effect of SMF could be observed well after the exposure finished. Additional experiments are needed though, since even a short, 10 min long exposure of mice to the inhomogeneous SMF may result in a statistically significant *AE* for another 30 min following the exposure (*c.f.*, Fig. **5.16A**). For an exposure of 10 min, *AE* is 91% during the exposure, and then remains still 71% in the time interval between 31 and 40 min. When mice were exposed to SMF for 20 min, *AE* was 68% during the exposure, and then it fell back to 29% in the time interval between 31 and 40 min. For an exposure of 30 min, *AE* is 82% during the exposure, then 83% in the time-interval between 31 and 40 min. It should be emphasized that the prolonged effect of SMF-exposure is of great importance in the view of potential human therapy. On the other hand, the long-lasting effect allows the detection of the effect of SMF-exposure under experimental conditions, where *in situ* application of the SMF-exposure system would be technically difficult or impossible; or where it would disturb the experiments.

In fact the writhing test was applied in a series of NSAIDs in the preclinical phase in mice [185]. The results can be seen in Fig. (**5.20**).

Now we understand that such generators can be elaborated that when mice are exposed to a clinically significant *AE* in the writhing test is mice can be observed. Is this true for an enormous high homogeneous SMF as well?

CLINICAL MRI

3 T clinical MRI Significantly Inhibits Pain in Mice

Preliminaries

MR as a diagnostic tool has become an everyday device also in the investigation of small animals. Starting with Hansen *et al.* [186], many studies have dealt with rodents in an MR. Good reviews of the state of the art can be read in the paper of Pirko *et al.* [187] and in Section 7.2.2 of the report of the WHO [12]. However, with the exception of behavioral studies, the subjects were immobilized by anesthesia in almost all experiments [188].

Beyond mammalian reproduction and development studies, most of what we know about the complex effects of MR apparatuses on rodents is as follows. Prasad *et al.* [189] examined the chromosomes in the bone marrow of mice influenced by 1 h exposure to homogeneous 0.75 T SMF in an MR and experienced no effects, no chromosomal damage. Innis *et al.* [138] performed spatial memory tests, Ossenkopp *et al.* [139] examined open field behavior and passive avoidance in mice, neither group could find any effect. Messmer *et al.* [140] executed the taste aversion paradigm in rats under the exposure of 1.89 T for 30 min. Teskey *et al.* [190] examined survival and stress reactions. They neither found any effect in the hormone levels or in the body mass of animals in a period of 13-22 months following the exposure. They could not identify any change in the survival rate. The blood brain barrier was investigated by Shivers *et al.* [191]. They observed a temporary opening of the blood brain barrier, which recovered spontaneously 15-30 min after exposure. Kwong-Hing *et al.* [192] examined the acute exposure effects of a 0.05 T MRI on dentin and bone formation in mice. They found that the exposure caused a significant increase in the synthesis of the collageneous matrix of dentin in the incisors. Prato *et al.* [8, 193] discovered a significant increase in the permeability of the blood brain barrier. Weiss *et al.* [144], later Nolte *et al.* [126] investigated the behavior of laboratory rodents in SMF equal to or greater than 4 and 9.4 T, respectively. They found that SMF stronger than 4 T may be unpleasant, may induce aversive responses and conditioned avoidance. Levine, Bluni and coworkers made efforts [133, 134] to reveal the effect of 0.3 and 2 T homogeneous SMF of an MR on the left and right discrimination learning ability and the serum melatonin levels of mice with exposure durations of 30 to 100 min. They found a significant interference of SMF with spatial discrimination learning, but no influence of SMF on serum melatonin levels. Rofsky *et al.* [194] examined the stability of chromosomal damage in regenerating liver cells. They used an MR with 1.5 T homogeneous plus gradient magnetic fields for 5-10 min. No effect induced by the MRI alone or in combination with gadopentetate dimeglumine was observed. High *et al.* [195] published a substantial contribution to the study of the effects of a strong homogeneous SMF (9.4 T) on a wide range of biological endpoints from spatial memory to gross pathologic findings in male and female rats exposed to the SMF 3 h a day, twice a week for 5 weeks. Their basic conclusion was that no adverse biological effects in either the parent rats or in their progeny could be attributed to the exposure. Later Houpt *et al.* [66, 146] confirmed these findings, when published a result on rats that could freely move through the 4 T homogeneous SMF of an MR, but avoided to enter the field. The authors related this experience to the action of the motion induced currents in the vestibular system.

There are only few papers on the low frequency magnetic field induced analgesic action in experimental animals. Ossenkopp *et al.* [196] used a combined exposure of SMF and RF fields (simulating the MRI diagnostic procedure) with 0.15 T magnetic induction for a duration of 2×22.5 min in mice and found an alteration in the day- and night-time responses to morphine in a thermal stimulus test. Mice in this experiment freely moved in their cage in groups of 5 within the bore of the magnet. The following year Prato *et al.* [197] published that the SMF component of the same MR had no evident effect on morphine induced analgesia. More recently Shupak *et al.* [131] have used a special pulsed magnetic field with *P-P* magnetic induction of 0.1 mT and frequency 60 Hz. Mice had no restraint in their cage. The authors found a statistically significant difference in the latency period of treated mice compared to control in the hot plate test. The difference was found to be equivalent to a moderate dose of morphine (5 mg/kg).

Goals

As a continuation of the previous studies, we investigated the influence of exposure to the SMF component of a clinical MR device on pain reaction. Here we prove the results already mentioned in **Clinical MRI** 3 T clinical MRI significantly inhibits pain in mice that the strong, homogeneous SMF of the MR could induce a significant antinociception in the writhing test in mice. We aim to study

i. the pain perception of mice in a clinical MR (at rest) using the writhing test; if there is an effect,
ii. the possible mechanism of *AE*.

During the experiments we had to control the potential effect of noise, vibration, and illumination stimuli. We also had to estimate the potential effect of motion induced current densities and time derivatives of the magnetic induction.

Materials and Methods

Magnetic Exposure Conditions

A commercial Philips Achieva 3 T MR with magnetic shielding (mentioned as **Generator 20**) was used in our experiments.

The lighting conditions inside the animal cage were basically independent of the cage location (locations are described in the next paragraph). The cage was illuminated with halogen lights (Model L58W/640) from above during the experiments. The shaded area was always bigger than 94×140(×46) mm during the experiments. The lamps generated a scattered light in the shaded area of the cage between 3.9-20.6 lx. The dosimetric illumination values are shown in Fig. (**5.21**).

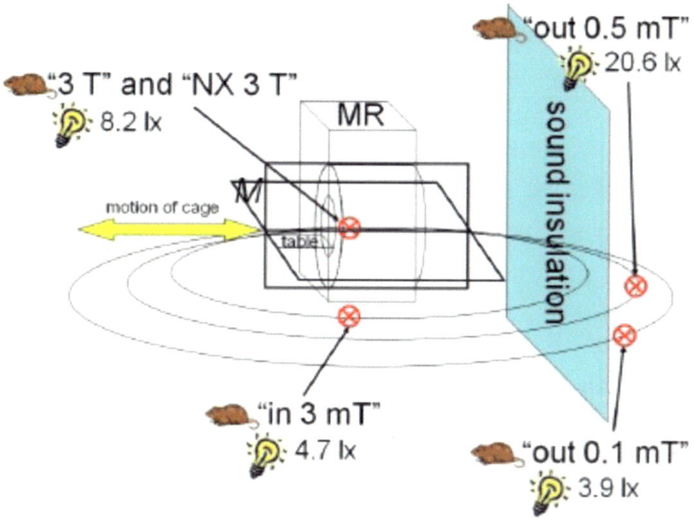

Fig. (5.21). Scheme of the experimental arrangement. We denoted locations by crossed circles, where the magnetic field has been probed: i) 0 T SMF (control, n=18), not seen in the figure, ii) 0.1 mT inside the MR lab ("in 0.1 mT", n=6), iii) 0.1 mT outside the MR lab ("out 0.1 mT", n=6), iv) 0.5 mT outside the MR lab ("out 0.5 mT", n=6), v) 3 T inside the bore of the MR ("3 T", n=18), and vi) 3 T inside the bore of the MR following naloxone pretreatment ("NX 3 T", n=6). n denotes animal numbers. Double arrow shows the motion of the cage into and out of the bore. M is the median plane of the bore. Dosimetric illumination values in units of lx are also shown.

In order to check the possible effect of noise stimulus originating from the cryogenic cold head of the helium pump of the MR regarded as background noise (64 dB equivalent continuous A-weighted sound pressure level at the isocenter, *c.f.*, [198, 199]) as a stress source for mice, 3 additional locations (tested with groups of 6 animals each) were applied. The cage was placed in the service area outside the MR lab, where the stray field had either 0.1 mT or 0.5 mT horizontal induction components denoted as "out 0.1 mT" and "out 0.5 mT", respectively, see Fig. (**5.21**). The vertical field component could be neglected since the cage was in the median plane of the bore (denoted by *M* in Fig. **5.21**). Gradient fields were not on; the only horizontal field components were the axial ones that certainly could be regarded homogeneous within the cage. In the 3rd group (denoted by "in 3 mT") animals were exposed to SMF inside the MR lab in the median plane (*M*), where the horizontal magnetic induction originating from the MR was 3 mT, but noise and vibration were similar to those in the bore. The 0.1, 0.5, and 3 mT induction values were taken from the SMF map of the MRI as provided by Phillips showing the main horizontal components of the stray field in the median plane (*M*).

In order to minimize the generation of motion induced currents in the body of the animals, the groups of mice at locations "3 T" and "NX 3 T" were moved into the experimental position in the bore along its axis (*c.f.*, double arrow in Fig. **5.21**) with a constant speed not exceeding 0.5 m/s. The way of the cage out of the bore did not influence the measurement.

In order to examine the potential involvement of an opioid component in SMF induced analgesia naloxone was injected *s.c.* in a dose of 0.2 mg/kg, 20 min before the acetic acid challenge (denoted as "NX 3 T"). Naloxone was purchased from Sigma-Aldrich (Budapest, Hungary). Altogether 60 naïve mice participated in 6 types of experiment. 24 animals were exposed to the 3 T SMF.

Statistical Analysis

The results are expressed as means of number of writhings±SEM. Statistical analysis of the data was performed by one-way ANOVA completed with Dunnett's test between pairs of data. A probability of $p<0.05$ was considered statistically significant. Equal numbers of animals were compared. In case of the comparison between "3 T" group and control, we used pooled data; in every other case we compared the treated group to the daily control. The antinociceptive (or analgesic) effect (*AE*) of a treatment in a given time interval was defined as before.

Results

The average number of writhings±SEM in different time intervals following the acetic acid (no Epsom salt in this experimental series) challenge in the writhing test in mice can be seen in Fig. (**5.22A**) and the corresponding *AE* in % in Fig. (**5.22B**). The results in Fig. (**5.22B**) are derived from Fig. (**5.22A**) according to the definition of the AE. The experiments were performed according to the following protocol:

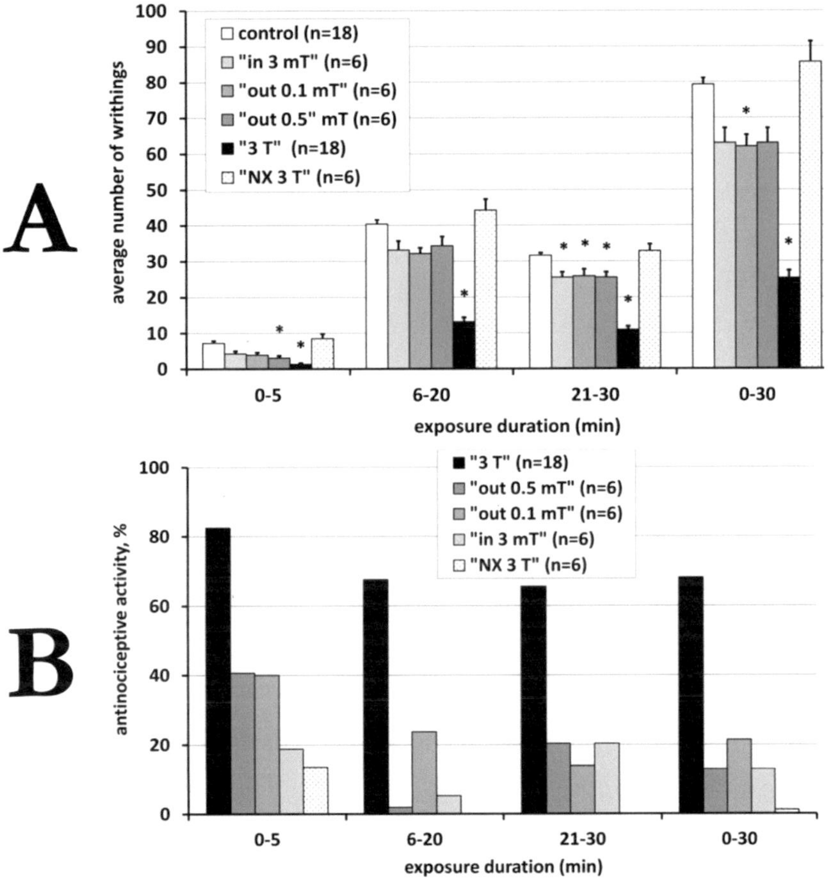

Fig. (5.22). A) The average number of writhings (mean±SEM) in mice in different time intervals following the i.p. injection of 0.6% acetic acid. The locations, where SMF has been probed are the same as summarized in Fig. (**5.21**). n denotes animal numbers. Statistical analysis of the data was evaluated by means of one-way ANOVA completed with Dunnett's test between pairs of data. A probability of $p<0.05$ was considered statistically significant. ANOVA resulted pmax<0.001 by $F_{min}>18.7$, $F_{crit}=2.4$ for the 4 the time intervals 0-5, 6-20, 21-30, and 0-30 min. The p and η^2 values of the pairwise comparisons are listed in Table **5.5**. **B)** AE in the same test. These results are derived from those in panel (A) according the definition of the AE. The AE in group "NX 3 T" proved to be -1% and 0% in the 6-20 and 21-30 min time interval, respectively and thus remain hidden in the graph.

- No SMF (control or sham-exposure, *n*=18),

- 3 mT inside the MR lab ("in 3 mT", n=6),
- 0.1 mT outside the MR lab ("out 0.1 mT", n=6),
- 0.5 mT outside the MR lab ("out 0.5 mT", n=6),
- 3 T inside the bore of the MR ("3 T", n=18), and
  3 T inside the bore of the MR following naloxone pretreatment ("NX 3 T", n=6).

The "NX 3 T" group achieved an average *AE* of -1% and 0% in the 6-20 and 21-30 min time interval, respectively and thus these values remain hidden in Fig. (**5.22B**). ANOVA resulted p_{max} <0.001 by F_{min}> 18.7 and F_{crit} =2.4 for the 3 time intervals 0-5, 6-20, and 21-30 min. The p and η^2 values of the pairwise comparisons with the control can be seen in Table **5.5**. If we did not pool the results for group "3 T" and control, we would have 68±5%, p_{max} <0.001 as the average *AE* for 3 groups of 6 mice each instead of the pooled 68±2% (p<0.001, n=18).

Table 5.5. ***P*** **and η^2 2 values as assessed with Dunnett's test for pairwise comparisons between different treated groups and control. In case of the comparison between group "3 T" and control, we used pooled data (n=3*6), in every other case we compared the group to the daily control (n=6). * denotes significant difference at the 5% risk level (p<0.05).**

time period (min)	"3 T" (n=18)		"in 3 mT" (n=6)		"out 0.1 mT" (n=6)		"out 0.5 mT" (n=6)		"NX 3 T" (n=6)	
	P	η^2	*P*	η^2	*P*	η^2	*P*	η^2	*P*	η^2
0-5	<0.001*	0.2	>0.1	0.1	>0.1	0.1	<0.05*	0.0	>0.1	0.2
6-21	<0.001*	0.3	>0.5	0.1	>0.1	0.0	>0.5	0.1	>0.5	0.2
21-30	<0.001*	0.4	<0.01*	0.1	<0.05*	0.1	<0.05*	0.1	>0.5	0.1
0-30	**<0.001***	**0.3**	**>0.05**	**0.1**	**<0.05***	**0.1**	**>0.05**	**0.1**	**>0.5**	**0.2**

Discussion, Conclusions

It was previously shown that an inhomogeneous SMF with 783±8 mT (mean± SEM) maximum *P-P* magnetic induction and 10 mm lateral periodicity (generator 11, see in **Generators 1-16**) caused an *AE* in the acetic acid- as well as in the Epsom salt induced writhing tests in mice (**Optimization of SMF parameters**). Since the SMF induced *AE* was reversed by the opioid receptor antagonist naloxone in the snail, an opioid-mediated mechanism was raised (**Pharma-**

cological analysis). Moreover, capsaicin-sensitive nerves were also demonstrated to be involved in the *AE* of the same inhomogeneous SMF in formalin-, and carrageenan induced hyperalgesia in mice (**Peripheral action**). Namely, mice were pretreated with resiniferatoxin in order to desensitize the C fibers. In this group the anti-hyperalgesic effect of the inhomogeneous SMF was shown to be abolished.

Our earlier investigations including homogeneous SMF (**Optimization of SMF parameters**) showed that a homogeneous SMF of 84±3 mT could be associated with an *AE* of 50±2% ($p<0.05$, $n=10$) in the writhing test in mice during a 30 min observation period. In the present experiment the 3 T homogeneous SMF of a clinical MR caused an *AE* of 68±2% ($p<0.001$, $n=18$) in the same test.

In our present experiments naloxone pretreatment reversed the pain-inhibitory effect of SMF-exposure confirming the suspicion that an opioid component is involved in the action also in mammals. Since the dose of naloxone (0.2 mg/kg *s.c.*) has been considered selective for μ-opioid receptors, we might conclude that μ-opioid receptors play a role in the *AE* of MR's SMF.

If we compare the results of the writhing test in the group of mice close to the bore of the MR ("in 3 mT"), or in the proximity of the MR, but outside the range of the background noise ("out 0.1 mT" and "out 0.5 mT"), we can conclude that noise stimulus did not significantly affect pain-inhibition. Even if it did, noise has never been shown to produce analgesia. (A practical concern that occurs is rather noise protection.)

The effect of vibration stimulus that is known to produce anesthesia (*e.g.* [200]) and analgesia (for references see [201]) could be excluded, since the vibration of the table at rest (without imaging sequence) is negligible. The magnets' mass was 6 tones, while the moving table is less than 20 kg. We optically checked this by simply positioning a glass of water at the spot of measurement on the table and watched for surface waves. We failed to find any sign of vibration. This control was reliable in the frequency range between 10 and 100 Hz.

Another potential confound was the effect of illumination. It has been long known that light can be a source of aversive stimulus for rodents [202 - 204], even an anxiety model [205], and a light/dark test [206] were proposed on this basis. Garcia *et al.* [207] published that 3 lx seemed to be the threshold of aversion in the exploratory behavior of rats in an EPM test, but not in their locomotor activity. Some animals use the polarization of sunlight for their orientation, even the million-time dimmer polarization of the moonlight proved to be a sufficient source to orient the African dung beetle [208]. Therefore, in our experiments care was taken to produce similar illumination at all experimental locations: Inside the bore of the MR and outside. A big enough dimmed (<20.6 lx) area was produced inside the cage by screening light emitted from halogen lamps above the cage. The highest illumination was provided at the location of the control experiments.

One parameter of the circadian cycle is the change of lighting. Rodents are subject to the circadian cycle in almost all areas of their life (*e.g.* [209]). The experiments were therefore carried out in the same period of time of the day, between 9 and 12 *a.m*.

Although we cannot exclude the possibility that pain perception of mice was influenced by motion induced currents in their body, we believe that this effect is also negligible from the viewpoint of the present study. From the **Relevant interactions in biology**, where the Reader was introduced to the possible mechanisms between SMF and living tissue, we know that magnetohydrodynamic forces are related to the power product: Induction × gradient of the SMF in the direction of the field (see *e.g.* [17, 210]. Motion induced currents in a homogeneous SMF are usually regarded quite small [124]. The difference between magnetic susceptibilities (or relative magnetic permeabilities) at interfaces of biological materials are small and therefore, may not have an effect [17, 211]. The question at hand is rather the movement of the cage (and the mice inside) into the bore of the MR, along which the induction changes from practically zero to 3 T. In order to control the effect of the induced currents due to the gradient of the SMF, we moved the cage along the axis of the bore with a constant speed not exceeding 0.5 m/s. By accepting the numerical results extrapolated from the literature [212] and applying a size conversion from human to mouse according to the inverse-square law (*e.g.* [213]), we found a potentially inducible current of 0.6 mA/m^2 in mice. The threshold is currently considered to be 480 mA/m^2 for humans. This threshold value has been extensively discussed in the past 2 decades (*c.f.*, [15], Section 8.3 in [214], [215 - 220]). The size-corrected value for mice is 1.6 mA/m^2. On the other hand, motion induced effects, primarily on peripheral nerve stimulation (PNS) are closely related to the time derivative of the induction [210, 221 - 223]. Although this effect is often connected to gradient switching in MR, it should also be estimated when moving the cage into this very strong SMF. The threshold for PNS is accepted to be at 40 T/s [16, 210, 221, 224]. Since in our experiments this derivative never exceeded 1.5 T/s, this effect could be ignored. Also, it is difficult to imagine that induced currents would decrease pain perception, data of the literature suggest the opposite (*e.g.* [125]). There is also evidence that exposure to SMF greater than 1 T induces flow potentials around the heart and major blood vessels, nevertheless; the physiological consequences of this remain unclear [218]. Several hours of exposure to very high inductions of up to 8 T in the heart region however, did not result in any cardiovascular effects in pigs [225]. Neurobehavioral studies report that the movement of laboratory rodents in SMF equal to or greater than 4 T may be unpleasant, inducing aversive responses and conditioned avoidance [66, 126, 144, 146]. We did not experience any efforts of the mice to avoid the 3 T SMF in the bore of the MR; mice made no attempts to escape from the cage. Van Rongen *et al.* [226] wrote about all so far animal studies: "In all these cases however, the endpoints are rather labile, a situation that may have been complicated by pharmacological manipulation, including anesthesia in some cases and immobilization."

The present study shows that the 3 T homogeneous SMF of a clinical MR induces a significant pain-inhibitory effect in the writhing test in mice. Since the *AE* for the whole 30 min observation period is 68% ($p<0.01$, $n=18$), MR's SMF should be regarded as a potential tool for therapy. Naloxone pretreatment reverses the pain inhibitory effect of SMF indicating that the effect is likely to be mediated by opioid receptors. Noise, vibration, lighting stimuli, as well as motion induced effects were estimated not to contribute to pain sensation in a significant manner in the present experiments. We have seen in **Optimization of SMF parameters** that strongly inhomogeneous SMF are the best choice for inhibiting acute visceral pain in mice. Thus tells us that SMF gradients play a significant role in the development of the AE. The next section will discuss this topic in due details.

LATERAL GRADIENTS

Lateral Gradients Significantly Enhance Static Magnetic Field-Induced Inhibition of Pain Responses in Mice – a Double Blind Experimental Study

Goals

Reminding the Reader of **Locomotor activity and anxiety behavior in healthy mice**, where we were dealing with SMF-exposure of healthy mice, we here investigate

i. the possible aversive effect of SMF-exposure on mice with and without induced abdominal pain,
ii. the cognitive recognition of the benefits of *AE* of SMF, and
iii. the role of other external contributing factors that may further improve *AE* of SMF, particularly the role of lateral SMF gradients in a half-SMF, half-sham-exposure chamber.

Using this specific exposure chamber unlike so far, animals are allowed to move unhindered between the SMF- and sham-exposed areas; thus, making a comparative analysis of their site preference and long-term pain response possible. Our working hypothesis in these experiments was that SMF-exposure is aversive to mice and they are able to recognize *AE* of SMF, which would be reflected in their locomotion pattern. We also planned to tackle the issue of motion induced electric current density, MR-equivalent switching, and slew rate in the mouse ambulating freely while exposed to an inhomogeneous SMF. Do these quantities correlate with the response to visceral pain? Can they be made responsible for peripheral nerve stimulation (PNS)?

Materials and Methods

Animals

One hundred and twenty three, 6 week-old, male CFLP mice were on standard rodent pellet and tap water was provided *ad libitum*. The animals were randomly selected and distributed into experimental groups with the nomenclature:

Groups 1-7, s: Sham, h: Homogeneous, i: Inhomogeneous SMF-exposure, *M*: Partition number, detailed in Table **5.6**. In order to minimize animal suffering, animal numbers were kept as low as possible. Animal numbers in groups varied between 3 and 12 (6 on average). The smallest number was allowed for the replication of earlier, previously published experiments (**Optimization of SMF parameters**) and for measurements where the measured quantity on 3 animals already provided acceptable standard deviations.

Table 5.6. Overview of results of the 30 min long writhing test in mice in different cages and under different exposure conditions.

animal group	exposure type	cage size	animal number	partition	number of writhings (mean±S.E.M.)	I (%)	F_{crit}	F	p	η^2 (%)	significance	subject of testing
1s	sham	single	3	-	63.00±5.13	62	7.71	55.70	<0.002	93	yes	sham *vs* inhSMF in single cage
1i	inhSMF		3	1	23.67±1.20							
2s	sham		6	-	50.67±4.18	64	4.96	36.41	<0.001	78		sham *vs* hoSMF in single cage
2h	hoSMF		6	1	18.00±3.44							
3s	double sham	double	6	-	44.33±2.29	60	4.96	28.31	<0.001	74		sham *vs* hoSMF in double cage
3h	double hoSMF		6	1	17.83±4.42							
4h	hoSMF&sham		3		1.67±0.33 *vs* 9.00±2.08	81	7.71	12.10	<0.03	75		hoSMF *vs* sham side within double cage
5i	inhSMF&sham		6		7.50±1.54 *vs* 29.67±2.79	75	4.96	48.36	<0.001	83		inhSMF *vs* sham side within double cage
5i	inhSMF&sham		6		7.50±1.54	68	5.59	45.64	<0.001	87		inhSMF side in double *vs* inhSMF in single cage
1i	inhSMF	single	3		23.67±1.20							
2h	hoSMF		6		18.00±3.44	91	5.59	10.53	<0.02	60		hoSMF side in double *vs* hoSMF in single cage
4h	hoSMF&sham	double	3		1.67±0.33							
3h	double hoSMF		6		17.83±4.42	91	5.59	6.23	<0.05	47		hoSMF side *vs* full hoSMF in double cage
4h	hoSMF&sham		3		1.67±0.33							
5i	inhSMF&sham		6		7.50±1.54	78	5.59	6.60	<0.05	49		inhSMF *vs* hoSMF exposure in double cage SMF side
4h	hoSMF&sham		3		1.67±0.33							
4h & 5i	inhSMF&sham and hoSMF&sham		9		5.56±1.40	90	4.49	154.68	<0.001	91		sham side of inhSMF together with that of hoSMF in double cage *vs* corresponding pooled sham groups in single cage
1s & 2s	sham	single	9	-	54.78±3.70							
1s	sham		3	-	63.00±5.13	9	5.59	1.26	>0.29	15	no	cage size effect under sham exposure
6s	sham	double	6	-	57.50±2.43							
2h	hoSMF	single	6	1	18.00±3.44	1	4.96	0.001	>0.98	0		cage size effect under hoSMF exposure
3h	double hoSMF	double	6		17.83±4.42							
7s	sham	single	12	-	69.67±4.66	71	4.30	103.52	<0.001	82	yes	sham for all in single cage (identical to 1s)
7i	inhSMF		12	1	20.33±1.34							identical to 1i
7M2i	inhSMF		6	2	38.67±1.80	45	4.49	20.75	<0.001	56		different homogeneous partitions in inhomogeneous SMF (M=2, 3, 4, 5, 6)
7M3i	inhSMF		6	3	40.67±1.45	42	4.49	18.37	<0.001	53		
7M4i	inhSMF		6	4	26.50±1.61	62	4.49	40.51	<0.001	72		
7M5i	inhSMF		12	5	24.67±1.23	65	4.30	87.20	<0.001	80		
7M6i	inhSMF		6	6	38.00±1.84	45	4.49	21.62	<0.001	57		

Magnetic Exposure Conditions

Inhomogeneous SMF (inhSMF) Exposure

Type 1) InhSMF was induced with generator 11 (**Generators 1-16**, Table **5.3**). The front iron wall of the exposure chamber was removed in order to allow a better view for the observer. Fig. (**5.23**) shows the schematic arrangements plus scanned magnetic induction maps of the vertical components in the isocenter of the magnetic arrangements at 3 mm from the lower magnets' surface. In the isocenter the asymmetric induction from the matrix edges do not distort the map. The custom-fabricated inhSMF&sham chamber was similar to the inhSMF chamber with the difference that the ferrous plates were twice as wide and consequently, the exposure chamber was 140×280×46 mm. Half of the exposure chamber in width did not contain magnets. The typical magnetic induction values were similar to that in panel A of Fig. (**5.23**), but the induction was close to zero in the non-magnetic side of the chamber (only the horizontal components of the geomagnetic field needed to be taken into account).

Type 2) Inhomogeneous SMF was also generated by the exposure system described in **Generators 17a-e**. As a reminder to the Reader this special arrangement called *M*-SMF denoted that generator 11 was modified in the sense that some magnets sat in the matrix with identical polarity in quadratic groups, whereas the neighboring groups were of opposite polarity. We used the square root of the number of magnets (*M* partitioning number) in each group for distinguishing between partitionings. The notation of these arrangements follows the rule: 2×2 for the quadratic groups of 4 magnets (M=2), 3×3 for groups of 9 magnets (M=3), *etc*. The original inhomogeneous SMF corresponds to 1×1 (M=1) in this notation. These SMF types were only tested with Cage 1 (140×140×46 mm), see Fig. (**5.23B**).

It is noteworthy that the switching rate of an MR machine is often connected to the time-varying gradient field component. We defined a similar quantity termed MR-equivalent switching rate (*MEWR*). Its definition is the maximum *P-P* amplitude of the magnetic induction at the boundary of 2 partitions, divided by the average duration it takes the mouse to move through the boundary. This boundary means a distance of 10 mm, if M=1; 20 mm, if M=2, *etc*. for a mouse crossing it perpendicularly. We also termed a quantity similar to MR's slew rate, the MR-equivalent slew rate (*MESR*). This is similar to *MEWR*, but instead of the *P-P* amplitude of the magnetic induction it has magnetic induction gradient between 2 partitions in the numerator.

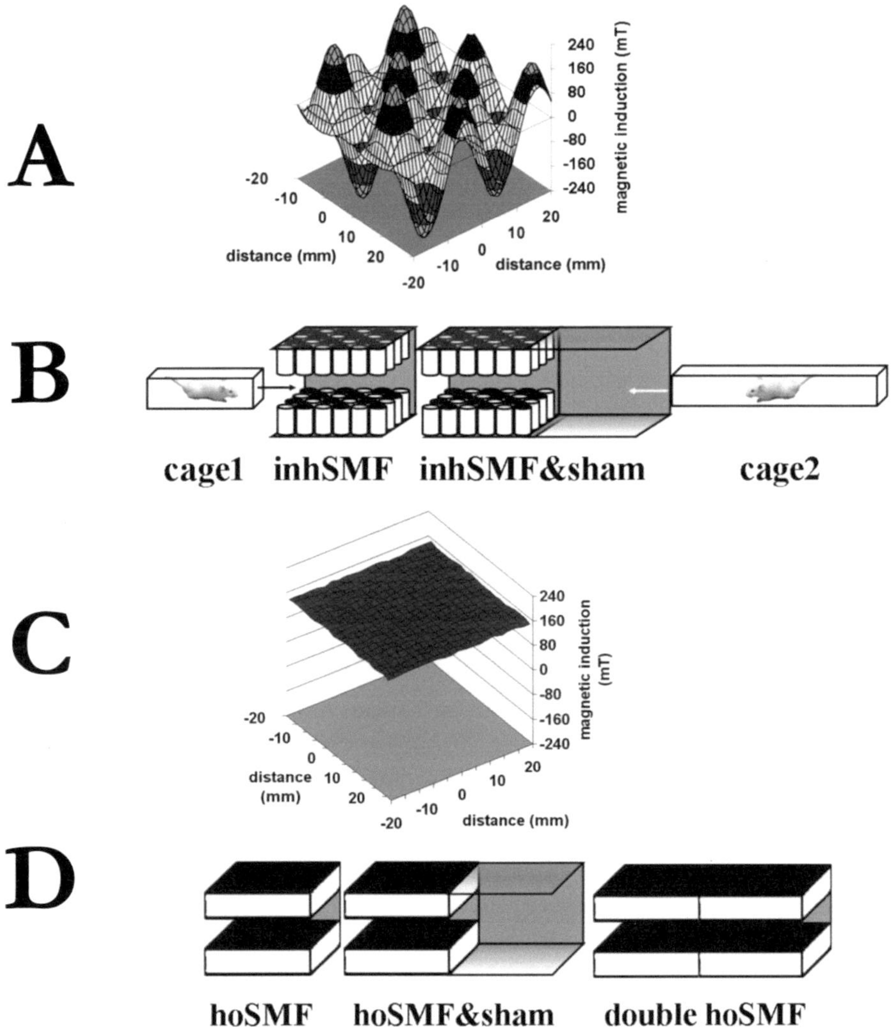

Fig. (5.23). Panels **(A)** and **(C)** demonstrate line-scanned magnetic induction maps of vertical components of SMF from an area of 40×40 mm in the isocenter of magnetic arrangements at a distance of 3 mm from the magnets' surface. Panel **(A)** shows the inhomogeneous SMF and panel **(C)** shows the homogeneous SMF. Panels **(B)** and **(D)** show the schematics of inhomogeneous and homogeneous SMF generators, respectively; the animal cages are shown in panel (B) (panels are not to scale). The ferrous house is shown in gray, and the magnets are white with a black or white top, distinguishing between magnetic North and South poles.

Homogeneous SMF (hSMF) Exposure

The hSMF generator was similar to generator 16 (**Generators 1-16**, Table **5.3**), just the magnetization of the single-block ferrite magnets was different. The average hSMF value in the exposure chamber was 145±5 mT. The hSMF&sham chamber in this arrangement contained magnets similar to those in the hSMF chamber but the size of the ferrous housing was double than in the inhSMF&sham chamber. The magnetic induction value in the non-magnetic side was close to zero (geomagnetic field).

The double hSMF chamber also contained ferrite block magnets and was double the size in width of the hSMF&sham chamber but the full length of the exposure chamber was equipped with ferrite block magnets on both sides. The magnetic induction was again 145±5 mT on both sides.

The exposure chambers allowed us to insert either a single-sized Cage 1 or a double-sized (140×280×46 mm; Cage 2) perforated Plexiglas animal cage with air holes into the exposure chambers (see Fig. **5.23**). An air-permeable opaque material covered the cage on 4 sides to provide similar illumination conditions in the exposure chamber and in the sham experiment; only the front side of the cages was transparent to visible light. The support under the cage was always flat and stable. In the sham-only arrangement, we used a chamber that looked exactly like the hSMF generator but contained no magnets, that is, there was no magnetic induction, only the geomagnetic field (by approximately 4 orders of magnitude lower than the induction measured in the generator). In the double-length chamber arrangements (inhSMF&sham and hSMF&sham), one side of the exposure chamber was considered inhSMF or hSMF, and the other sham; in the case of double hSMF, both sides were hSMF.

Experiments were recorded with a high resolution video camera (Model Power Shot G9, Canon, Tokyo, Japan). The numerical evaluation of the results was carried out on the basis of these video clips, where SMF and sham-exposure systems were disguised, thus providing a double-blinded manner.

The exposure was whole-body, while animals were free to move around in the cage. InhSMF-exposure was shown earlier not to introduce significant changes in the locomotor activity or anxiety behavior of animals (**Locomotor activity and anxiety behavior in healthy mice**). With the double sized cages, 3 comparison options aourse: (i) Between the SMF and sham side within the double-sized cage, (ii) between the SMF side in the double-sized cage and identical SMF in the single-sized cage, and (iii) between the sham side in the double-sized cage and the sham side in the single-sized cage.

The vertical components of the magnetic induction vector were probed at planes 3, 10, and 15 mm from the topmost surface of the magnet(s) in the lower matrix. These planes would intersect the body of a mouse moving in the cage approximately at its feet, its lower back, and its head. These magnetic induction values for inhSMF and hSMF were shown already in Table **3.4**. Since both kinds of magnetic materials were magnetized in the vertical direction, all horizontal components were regarded as stray field components.

Other Conditions

The lighting conditions inside the cage were again basically independent of the location of the mouse within the cage. A light gradient only occurred between the front (transparent) and the back (opaque) side of the cage. The arrangement was illuminated with fluorescent lights from above during the experiments. The shaded area in the back was always bigger than 94×140 mm or 94×280 mm during the experiments. The fluorescent lamps generated a scattered light in the shaded area of the cage with intensity between 5.7 and 15.5 mW/m^2. The fluorescent light sources emit light over many wavelengths with peaks at 403, 435, 475, 550, 580, 610, and 710 nm. The calculated light intensity maximum corresponds to 3.9×10^{16} photons/ s/m^2 (integral), which is below the intensity threshold for eliminating the *AE* in mice in magnetic field-shielded environments measured by Prato *et al.* [227].

Background noise never exceeded 52 dBC in the animal laboratory throughout the experiments. No site difference was found between the left and right sides of the different cage configurations used. The temperature during the exposure was identical to the housing temperature of mice (20±2°C). We did not observe any temperature gradients inside the exposure cage.

Monitoring Locomotion

Locomotion was monitored in the case of inhSMF&sham by measuring the duration of stay in one or in the other (sham or inhSMF) side of the cage. The total durations were then compared. Two animals were in the cage at the same time, one of which received *i.p.* acetic acid according to the writhing test. One of the animals was marked in a randomized order in a series. The inhSMF and sham side of the inhSMF&sham chamber were also swapped between experiments in a randomized order because of the potential but not verified lateral differences in lighting and noise amplitudes.

Statistical Analysis

We defined the *AE* of a treatment; when calculating the measure (or merit) of effectiveness (*ME*) in a similar form, the examined quantities were time periods (in s) spent in the unmagnetized $<x>$ or magnetized $<y>$ side of the double-sized cage. We estimated the F value, the critical value of F (F_{crit}), the probability value (p), and the size effect value (η^2) by one-way ANOVA. In an expression, these appear as $F_a=b$, $a=F_{crit}$, and $b=F$. We accepted statistical significance at the 95% confidence level if $p<0.05$; two groups were compared at one time. One-way ANOVA is not sensitive to a slight unbalance in group sizes; Microsoft Excel works properly; and confounded data do not alter the statistical consequences. We used pooling only if the F test between data sets provided similar variances.

Approximation of B(x;y;z)

Reminding the Reader to **Constraints, solutions** we concluded that we can approximate the measured values of the periodic inhomogeneous SMF distribution (type 2) along the x axis (our statements hold for the y axis as well, for symmetry reasons). We can fit normal (Gaussian) probability density functions to the individual peaks, where the contribution of the kth peak to the distribution was $\pm\frac{1}{\sigma\sqrt{2\pi}}e^{-\frac{[x-(k-1)\lambda]^2}{2\sigma^2}}$ with $k=1,2,3,\ldots$ (σ is considered equal for all peaks), λ equal in both (x and y) directions. This simple 2D approach is widely used for finding the spatial resolution in laterally or vertically periodic systems [228]. $B(x,y)$ can then be approximated by the linear combination of the periodic functions for x and y, *c.f.*, the Error Function Superposition Approximation (EFSA) introduced by Marton *et al.* [229]:

$$B(x,y)=B_x\frac{1}{\sigma\sqrt{2\pi}}\sum_{k=1}^{m}e^{-\frac{[x-(k-1)\lambda]^2}{2\sigma^2}}+B_y\frac{1}{\sigma\sqrt{2\pi}}\sum_{k=1}^{m}e^{-\frac{[y-(k-1)\lambda]^2}{2\sigma^2}}\quad \text{for } k=1,2,3,... \tag{1}$$

with B_x and B_y inductions in the x and y directions, respectively. In the present model $B_x=B_y=B_0$ and we further approximate $B(x,y)$ with:

$$B(x,y)\approx\frac{B_0}{\sigma\sqrt{2\pi}}\sum_{k=1}^{m}e^{-\frac{\left(\frac{M\lambda}{2}+1-k\right)^2\lambda^2}{2\sigma^2}}\left\{\boldsymbol{sin}\left[\pi\left(\frac{x}{M\lambda}-1\right)\right]+\boldsymbol{sin}\left[\pi\left(\frac{y}{M\lambda}-1\right)\right]\right\} \tag{2}$$

where M is the partitioning number. The limit of this approximation is the finitude of the resolution, namely the following condition for the resultant derivative of $B(x)$ (as well as for $B(y)$) in the range $0\leq x\leq M\lambda$ (and $0\leq y\leq M\lambda$) must hold:

$$\frac{\partial B(x)}{\partial x}=B_0\frac{(k-1)\lambda-x}{\sigma^3\sqrt{2\pi}}\sum_{k=1}^{m}e^{-\frac{[x-(k-1)\lambda]^2}{2\sigma^2}}\begin{cases}=0, \text{ if } x=\dfrac{M\lambda}{2}\\ \neq 0 \quad \text{elsewhere}\end{cases} \tag{3}$$

and similarly for $\partial B(y)/\partial y$. This gives a non-analytic solution for the $\sigma(\lambda)$ function (and thus for the resolution, $\Delta z=2\sigma$) with the geometrical constraint $\lambda\geq d$.

In the z direction of the arrangement perpendicular to the cylindrical magnets' surface along the axis, SMF is z-dependent only

$$B(z)=\frac{B_r}{2}\left\{\frac{h+z}{\left[R^2+(h+z)^2\right]^{1/2}}-\frac{z}{\left(R^2+z^2\right)^{1/2}}+\frac{h+D-z}{\left[R^2+(h+D-z)^2\right]^{1/2}}-\frac{D-z}{\left[R^2+(D-z)^2\right]^{1/2}}\right\} \tag{4}$$

and its gradient:

$$\frac{\partial B_z}{\partial z}=\frac{B_r R^2}{2}\left\{\frac{1}{\left[R^2+(h+z)^2\right]^{3/2}}-\frac{1}{\left(R^2+z^2\right)^{3/2}}+\frac{1}{\left[R^2+(D-z)^2\right]^{3/2}}-\frac{1}{\left[R^2+(h+D-z)^2\right]}\right. \quad \textbf{(5)}$$

can be expressed in analytic form. In this approximation we take into account 2 (lower and upper) magnets along their common axis (in-axis) in a distance of D=46 mm from each other. More specifically at z=20 mm, this value must well estimate the measured vertical average value obtained in a first-neighbor approximation (∇B). Inductions as well as their gradients have horizontal components, but they were a minimum of 2 orders of magnitude below the vertical components at any position in-axis and therefore, were neglected as fringe field components. Similarly, the off-axis vertical components were neglected for the same reasons. We also introduced N, the number of gradients per distance as the number of inflection points of the vertical magnetic induction component per average linear ambulation distance (L).

If SMF is also inhomogeneous laterally, mice sense a time-dependent magnetic flux (φ) by crossing the field lines during their ambulation in the cage. We estimated the induced current density in the mouse.

Ambulation Model, Approximation of Mouse Motion

Linear Model

Our first assumption is that the mouse moves in a 2D plane always along a straight line with constant speed (v) as long as it reaches a boundary/wall at $0 \leq x \leq a$ and $0 \leq y \leq b$, then changes direction semi-randomly (in a degree of α pointing into the cage) and continues its movement (Fig. **5.24**). (This simple model can be justified by the fact that the length of the mouse's body is only about 3-4 times smaller than the longer side length of the cage size $a \times b$.) The iterative equations of motion of the ith linear section are as follows:

$$\begin{aligned} x_i &= \Delta t \,|v|\, \boldsymbol{cos}(a_i)+x_{i-1} \\ y_i &= \Delta t \,|v|\, \boldsymbol{sin}(a_i)+y_{i-1} \end{aligned} \quad \textbf{(6.1)}$$

where Δt is an equidistant time step. Since $x=x(t)$ and $y=y(t)$, $B(x,y)=B(t)$ as if the

SMF would be time-dependent.

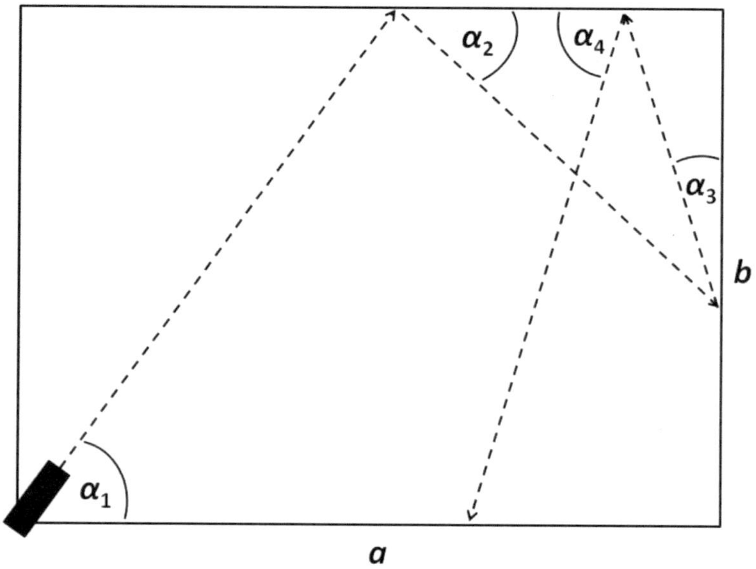

Fig. (5.24). Linear model of mouse ambulation in cage of size a×b according to Eq. (6.1).

Random Model with Identical Probabilities

The $a \times b$ cage is here divided into cells. There is a finite probability that the mouse gets into a cell on its way. We assume that this probability is independent of the cell coordinates. (We shall refine this assumption in the next point.) The ambulation is mapped to a random 2D motion with the only exception that backward locomotion was forbidden, the incidence of which is much lower than marching ahead. We also keep the speed constant; it is one step per unit time. We also allow for obstacle(s) in the cage that can be at rest or can move like another mouse. In case of potential confrontation (more than one mouse entering the same cell), one or both of the mice shrink from collision. Matlab was used for this model, a mouse was represented by a 2×1 cell rectangle, and the cage was 8×8 cells. In Fig. (**5.25**) the flash of the ambulation of 3 mice can be seen.

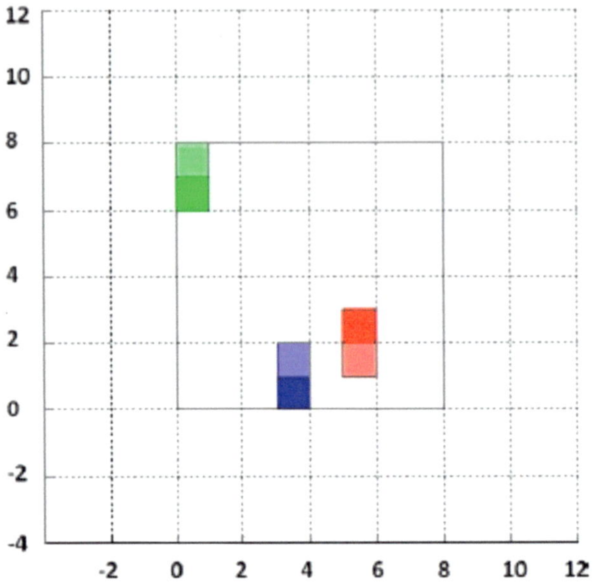

Fig. (5.25). Random ambulation model of the simultaneous ambulation of 3 mice.

Mice started from different corners. A cell position at a certain time point of *i* is given with its integer coordinates *j* and *k,* thus real space coordinates are

$$x_i(j,k)=j*a/n$$
$$y_i(j,k)=k*b/m \qquad \textbf{(6.2)}$$

with *n* and *m* number of partitions in the *x* and *y* directions, respectively. The trajectory of a mouse is then

$$x_i(j,k)=f*x_{i-1}(j\pm1,k)$$
$$y_i(j,k)=f*y_{i-1}(j,k\pm1) \qquad \textbf{(6.3)}$$

due to the fact that the mouse moves continuously. Here $f\equiv1$ is the uniform and time-independent probability of changing position. The choice of direction then goes by a random selection between next available 2-4 cells taking into account the boundary conditions

$$
\begin{aligned}
&x_i(1,k)=f^*x_{i-1}(2,k)\\
&y_i(1,k)=f^*y_{i-1}(1,k\pm1)\\
&x_i(n,k)=f^*x_{i-1}(n-1,k)\\
&y_i(n,k)=f^*y_{i-1}(n,k\pm1)\\
&x_i(j,1)=f^*x_{i-1}(j\pm1,1)\\
&y_i(j,1)=f^*y_{i-1}(j,2)\\
&x_i(j,m)=f^*x_{i-1}(j\pm1,m)\\
&y_i(j,m)=f^*y_{i-1}(j,m-1)
\end{aligned} \quad \textbf{(6.4)}
$$

Random Model According to Measured Probabilities

This model is based on the previous one; the probability of a mouse entering a cell is still time-independent, but it is not uniform ($f<1$). For weighing the probabilities we used ambulation data obtained by the system described in **HEALTHY ANIMALS Locomotor activity and anxiety behavior in healthy mice** and Fig. (**5.8**). Amulation data of 48 mice monitored for 30 min suggested that rodents prefer the sides of the cage to the center (one sample trajectory can be seen in Fig. **5.26**). On the basis of these observations we attributed a higher probability of occurrence to the cells along the walls. The weights of probabilities were proportional to the ratio of average time spent in cells at the walls and in the center (Fig. **5.27**).

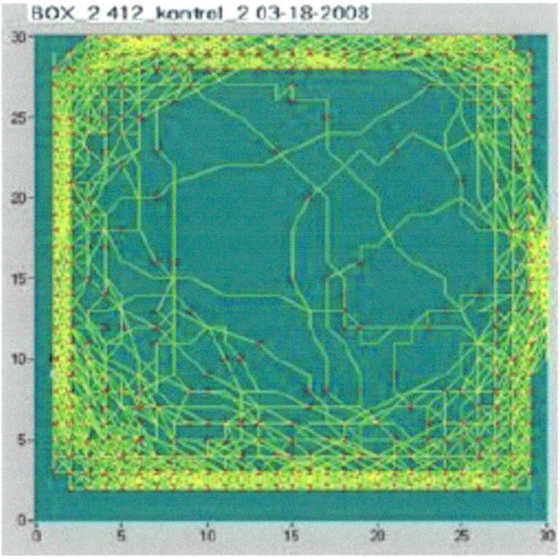

Fig. (5.26). Ambulation path of a single mouse in the Conducta System box.

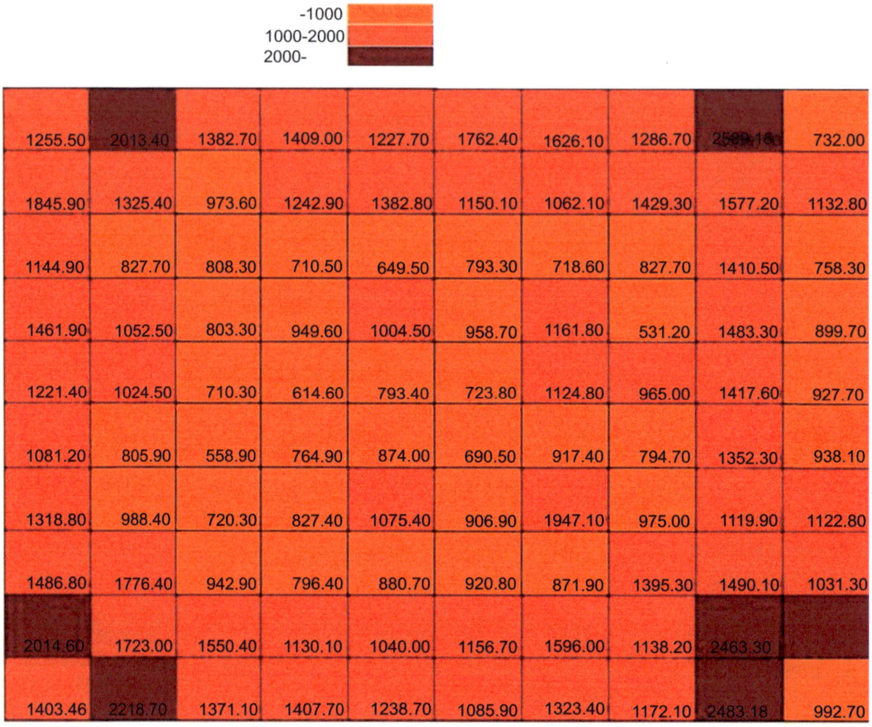

Fig. (5.27). Average times (s) mice spent in different cells of the box as measured in the Conducta System. Different shading denotes different ranges of times.

In this model Eq. (6.3) still holds, but all $f(j,k)<1$. Actually, f values generate a matrix $\overline{\overline{F}}$ based on the values cited in Fig. (**5.27**). $\overline{\overline{F}}$ is a sparse matrix, since cell transfer is still restricted to first available neighbors. Eq. (6.3) becomes an underdetermined system of linear equations. In order to reduce the number of unknowns, transfer to neighboring cells can be optimized in a way that the distribution of transfers is the "smoothest". Those elements of $\overline{\overline{F}}$ that are non-zero should be minimized by the least square method allowing for a positive transfer probability to the next neighbor cells. If $\vec{F}$ is the vector of non-zero elements of $\overline{\overline{F}}$, by keeping $f > 0$, we must solve the min $(\vec{F} * \vec{F})$ linear optimization task. This method creates the weights to f. The results of this calculation are presented in Fig. (**5.28**). The similar shading of Fig. (**5.27**) and Fig. (**5.28**) confirms the applicability of the method.

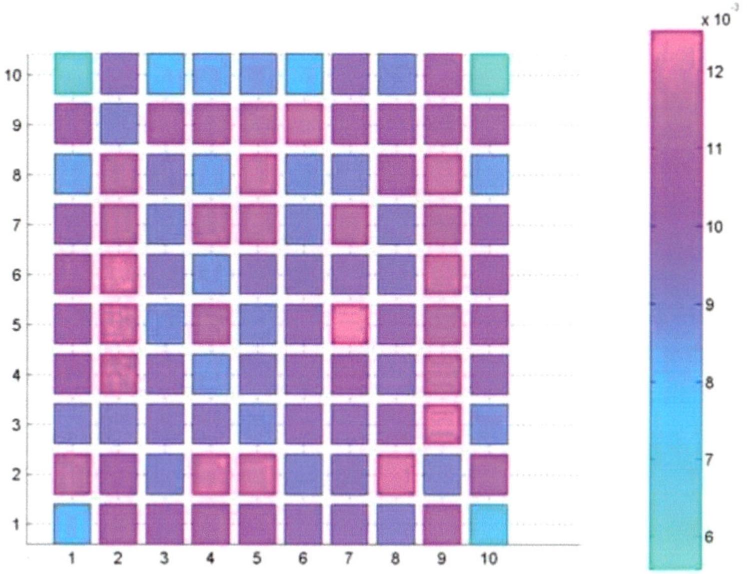

Fig. (5.28). The calculated $\overline{\overline{\boldsymbol{F}}}$ matrix with the probability ranges for the first neighbor cell transfer of a mouse.

Approximation of Induced Electric Current Density

As described by Maxwell's 4th (Faraday's) law, the induced electromotive force (εmf) in the mouse is:

$$\varepsilon mf = \oint_l \vec{E}d\vec{l} = -\frac{d\varphi}{dt} = -\frac{d}{dt}\int_A \vec{B}d\vec{A} \tag{7}$$

where $\vec{E}$ is the induced electrostatic field in the mouse and $d\vec{l}$ is an infinitesimal section of the circumference (l) of the mouse's area $(\vec{A})$ exposed to SMF. We assume that the surface of a mouse perpendicular to the magnetic induction vector is A (with the assumption $\vec{B}\|d\vec{A}$), $|\vec{B}|$ can be regarded as constant on A, and the homogeneous specific electric resistivity of the mouse is constant (ρ). Then the induced current density is:

$$j_i = -\frac{1}{\rho l}\frac{dB}{dt} \tag{8}$$

Using Eq. (6.1), the induced current density of the *i*th section can be expressed as:

$$j_i = -\frac{2\pi|v|B_0}{\rho l\lambda}\left\{cos(\alpha_i)cos\left[\frac{2\pi}{\lambda}(\Delta t|v|cos(\alpha_i)+x_{i-1})\right]+sin(\alpha_i)cos\left[\frac{2\pi}{\lambda}(\Delta t|v|sin(\alpha_i)+y_{i-1})\right]\right\} \quad \textbf{(9)}$$

In case of the model of ambulation with measured probabilities (Eq. (6.3)) we can estimate the magnetic induction gradient per a single step from one cell to another.

Data used for the estimate were: $|v|\approx 1$ m/s (average speed after [214, 215]), $\rho\approx 1.82\times 10^{11}$ $\Omega mm^2/m$ [216], $l\approx 100$ mm, $B_0=0.5$ T (after fitting to the actual dosimetric values), $\lambda=10$ mm, $k=20\pi$ mm^{-1}, $x_i\leq min(a;b)\approx 140$ mm, $y_i\leq min(a;b)\approx 140$ mm).

Results

<u>Effect of SMF-exposure and Cage Size on AE (%) of Acute Peritoneal Pain in Mice</u>

<u>Writhing Number Comparison Between inhSMF/hSMF- and Sham-exposed Groups (Group 1s vs 1i, Group 2s vs 2h, and Group 3s vs 3h)</u>

Table **5.6** shows the detailed results for all situations in this section. To analyze the side preference and possible pain induced locomotion of animals between sham- and inhSMF- or hSMF-exposure, a daily control arrangement was also provided in order to testify and validate the previously described *AE* of inhSMF- (generator 11) or hSMF-exposure (generator 16 in **Optimization of SMF parameters**). When applying inhSMF (Group 1s *vs* 1i), the difference in the writhing numbers between unexposed and inhSMF-exposed groups was statistically significant. The average writhing numbers decreased from 6±1.53, 36±2.08, 21±1.73, and 63±5.13 to 1.67±0.88, 10.33±1.20, 11.67±1.45, and 23.67±1.20 in the 0-5, 6-20, 21-30, and 0-30 min time periods, respectively. This represents AE_{inh}=62% for the total 30 min period of time (see case A in Fig. **5.29**).

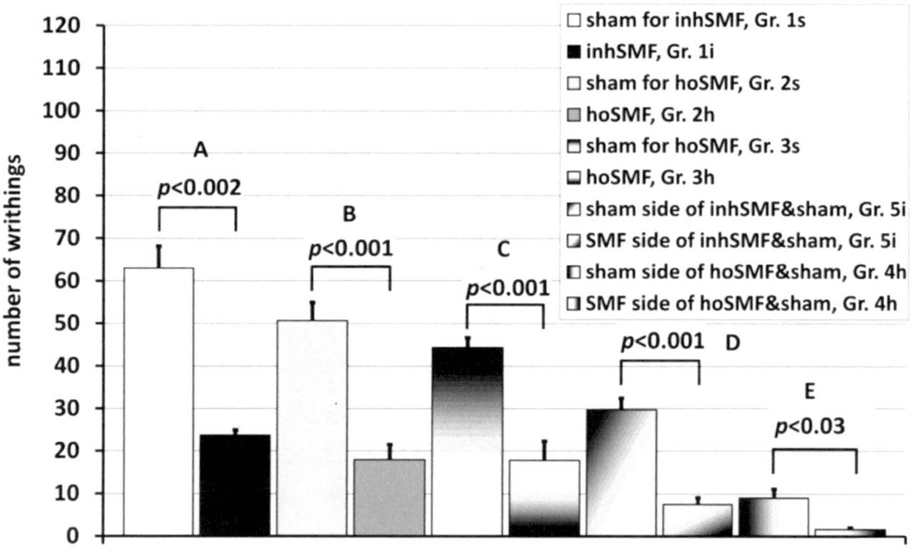

Fig. (5.29). Number of writhings in the 30 min long writhing test in challenged mice exposed to either sham field or SMF. Statistical significance relates to the corresponding sham-exposed control group. Positive error bars represent SEM. A and B refer to exposure in Cage 1; C refers to exposure in Cage 2.

Furthermore, in the hSMF-exposure situation in the single-sized cage (Group 2s *vs* 2h), AE_{ho}=64%, and in double-sized cage (Group 3s *vs* 3h), *AE*=60% (see Table **5.6** and cases B and C in Fig. **5.29**).

Writhing Number Comparison Between inhSMF/hSMF and Sham Sides of the Double-sized Cage (Cage 2, Group 4h, and Group 5i)

The double sized cage was suitable to look for differences in the writhing numbers between the sham and SMF, inhSMF&sham, and hSMF&sham sides. Group 5i (inhSMF) showed AE_{inh}=75%. For hSMF-exposure, Group 4h resulted in AE_{ho}=81% (see cases D and E in Fig. **5.29**).

Effect of Cage Size on Writhing Numbers (Group 1s vs 6s and Group 2h vs 3h)

If we compared the writhing numbers of challenged mice (Group 1s *vs* 6s) in the sham cages (single-sized cage *vs* sham side of double-sized cage), we found no significant difference (*AE*=9%; see case A in Fig. (**5.30**)). The same holds for challenged mice exposed to hSMF (Group 2h *vs* 3h, *AE*=1%; see case B in Fig. (**5.30**)).

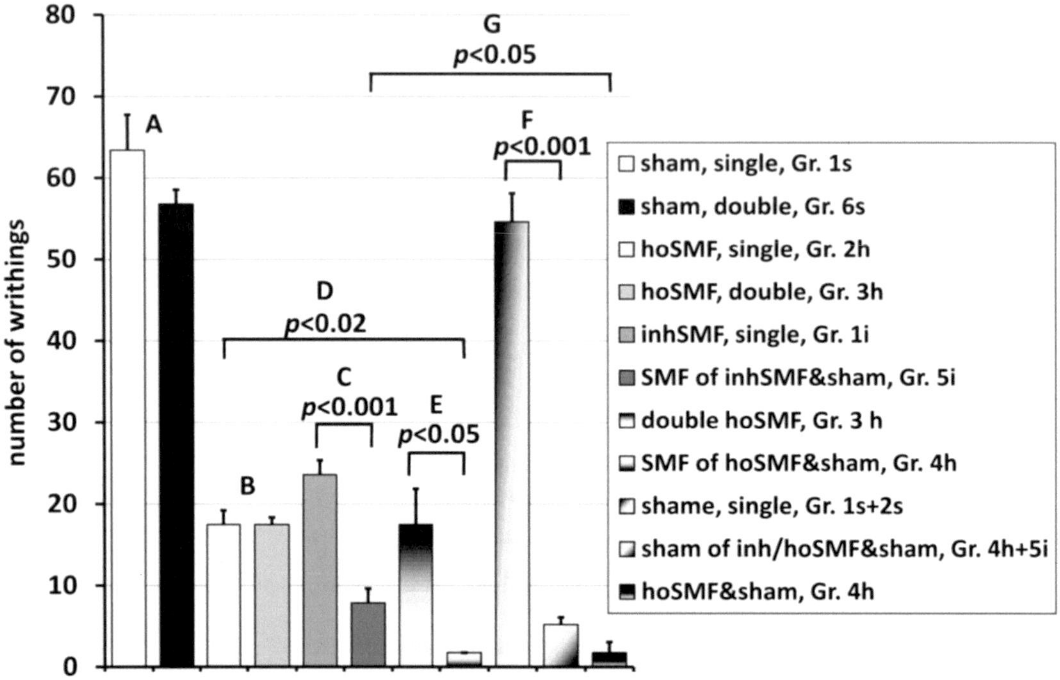

Fig. (5.30). Number of writhings in the 30 min long writhing test in challenged mice exposed to either sham field or SMF. Statistical significance relates to the corresponding sham-exposed control group. Positive error bars represent SEM. "Single" refers to Cage 1; "double" refers to Cage 2. A-C: Effect of cage size; D-F: Exclusive effects of SMF gradients; G: Homogeneous *vs* inhomogeneous SMF-exposure.

Exclusive Effect of Magnetic Field Gradients (Group 1i vs 5i, Group 2h vs 4h, Group 3h vs 4h, and pooled Group 4h and 5i vs pooled Group 1s and 2s)

Animals in the magnetic side of inhSMF&sham (Group 5i) showed significantly fewer pain syndromes than those in the single-sized cage under inhSMF-exposure (Group 1i). This effect was demonstrated by AE_{inh}=68% (see Table **5.6** and case C in Fig. (**5.30**)). The situation is similar under hSMF-exposure (Group 2h *vs* 4h); the effect is AE_{ho}=91% (Group 4h), shown by case D in Fig. (**5.30**). However, in this case we can also compare Group 3h to 4h: AE_{ho}=91% (represented by case E in Fig. (**5.30**)).

When we compared the writhing numbers of sham exposed mice in the single-sized cage (Group 1s and 2s pooled) with those in the sham side of the double-sized cage (Group 5i and 4h pooled), we found that mice in the double-sized cage showed fewer pain responses, represented by AE=90% (case F in Fig. (**5.30**)).

hSMF- vs inhSMF-exposure (Group 4h vs 5i)

When we compare writhing numbers of Group 5i (inhomogeneous SFM side of double-sized Cage 2) with 4h (homogeneous SFM side of double-sized Cage 2), we can see the effects of the difference in the homogeneity of the SMF. The inhibition of hSMF-exposure (Group 4h, SMF *vs* sham side) was undefined in the first 5 min (all 6 writhing numbers were zero), and changed to 83% between 6 and 20 min, 78% between 21 and 30 min, and 81% for the whole period; while it was 67%, 64%, 64%, and 64% in Group 5i in the 0-5, 6-20, 21-30, and 0-30 min periods, respectively. The inhSMF-exposure condition was more beneficial in inhibiting pain (than the homogeneous AE_{inh}=78%; see case G in Fig. (**5.30**)).

Measure of Effectiveness of SMF-exposure on Locomotion and Social Behavior in Mice with Acute Peritoneal Pain (Control Group vs Challenged Animals Exposed to inhSMF&sham)

Table **5.7** shows the results concerning locomotion in inhSMF&sham with the double-sized cage (control *vs* challenged animals exposed to inhSMF&sham). No significant differences between the groups could be identified. In the control group, 5 out of 9 mice spent more time in the inhSMF side of the inhSMF&sham arrangement than in the sham side. In the acetic acid-challenged group, the results were opposite; 5 out of 9 mice spent more time in the sham side. The difference was not significant. Unchallenged mice crossed the boundary between the 2 sides 632 times while challenged mice did this 551 times. This difference is also not significant.

We then looked for the differences at every 10 min interval. In the first 10 min, when mice make exploratory ambulation in general, the challenged mice spent significantly more time in the sham side than in the other (ME_{inh}=-27%, $p<0.01$). In the second 10 min, when mice started to adapt to their new environment, unchallenged mice spent significantly more time in the inhSMF side than in the other (ME_{inh}=42%, $p<0.005$). Comparing the 10 min intervals to each other, we realized that the first 10 min made the difference. Excluding this exploratory 10 min period from the estimate, we found that the only significant difference was that unchallenged mice spent somewhat more time in the inhSMF side than in the other (ME=24%, p<0.05).

Table 5.7. Statistical characteristics of time periods (s) Mice spent in the SMF or Sham side of the animal cage penetrating into the SMF-exposure chamber.

	time (s) unchallenged mice (n=9) spent on the		time (s) mice challenged with acetic acid (n=9) spent on the	
	SMF side (t_{SMF})	sham side (t_{sham})	SMF side (t_{SMF})	sham side (t_{sham})
average	996.25	804.30	859.98	940.30
S.E.M.	99.65	99.57	160.43	160.37
ratio	55%	45%	48%	52%
ME	19.27%		-9.34%	

We can confirm the fact that mice are socially sensitive since mice spent considerably longer times together; that is, in the same side of Cage 2 than separately (control *vs* challenged animals exposed to inhSMF&sham). Almost 19 out of 30 min mice spent time together representing ME_{inh}=38%, $F_{4.49}$=12.51, p<0.003, and η^2=44%.

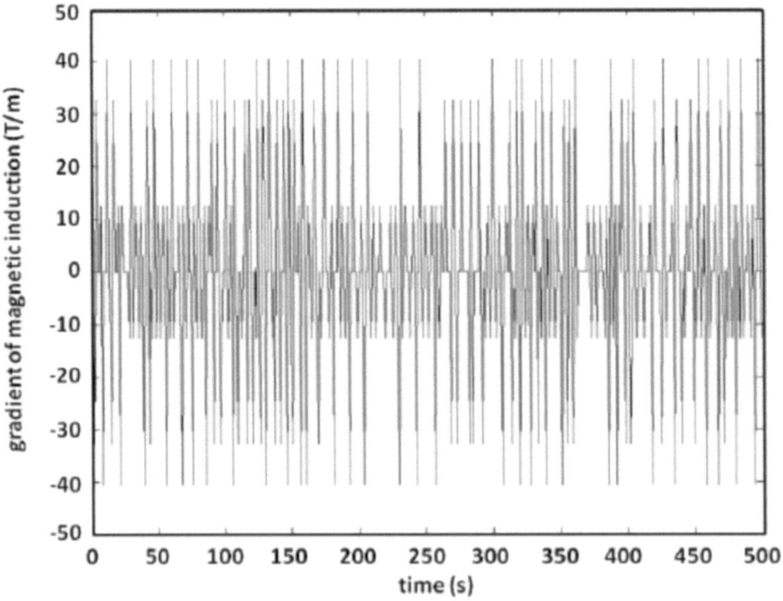

Fig. (5.31). Simulated magnetic field induction gradients in the course of mouse locomotion for 500 s.

Using Eq. (6.3) and the simulation in the random model with measured probabilities result in $\left|\Delta\vec{B}\right| \leq 40$ mT between neighboring cells simply due to the animal crossing "SMF lines" as shown in Fig. (**5.31**).

The Effect of Partitions of SMF on Acetic Acid Induced Abdominal Pain in Mice

Table **5.6** and Fig. (**5.32**) show the average number of writhings of mice exposed to type 2 SMF (*M*=1, 2, 3, 4, 5, and 6) for a total of 30 min exposure time. The corresponding *AE* values are listed in Table **5.7**. *p* values were always below 0.05. We note here that case *M*=1 is a replication of our results with generator 11 (**Optimization of SMF parameters**).

We also simulated *MEWR* and *MESR* in the *M*-SMF system. Table **5.7** presents how dosimetric data and data from the ambulation model correlate with the pain assay results.

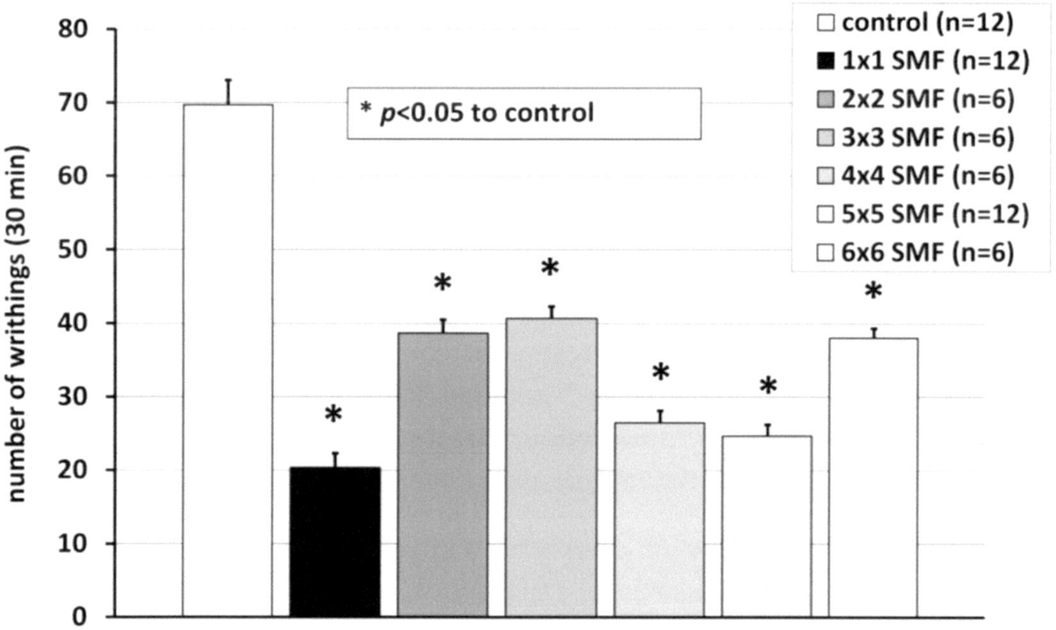

Fig. (5.32). The average number of writhings and SEM in the writhing test in mice for 30 min exposure to SMF with different partitionings (M=1, 2, 3, 4, 5, and 6). * denotes $p<0.05$ significant difference to control assessed by one-way ANOVA.

Discussion, Conclusions

Locomotion

Reminding the Reader to our special section on locomotion of healthy mice under SMF-exposure in **HEALTHY ANIMALS Locomotor activity and anxiety behavior in healthy mice**, mice in the present series were partly free to move in the double-sized cage penetrating into the SMF-exposure chamber allowing them to choose their resting place on their own and partly, were challenged with acetic acid. In contrast to rats exposed to 7 T magnetic induction [66], mice in our experiments showed no behavioral signs of aversion to SMF. A possible physiological mechanism behind circling and the development of taste aversion in rats subsequent to SMF-exposure could be the vestibular activation [230]. The proper characterization of advantageous or eventually harmful biological effects of the applied SMF has become an important issue since the widespread utilization of magnetic resonance (MR) devices. Magnetic induction typically varies between 0.5 and 3 T for human diagnostic MRI devices; for research and experimental purposes it can be up to or even over 10 T. According to guidelines of, for example, the US Food and Drug Administration (Silver Spring, MD, USA), 8 T is the highest magnetic induction without significant risk to human health [231]. This value is also accepted in the EU. Even if there were vestibular excitation involved in our experiments, it might not have been necessarily aversive for the mice. More specifically, a mammal in an SMF without self-motion is unlikely to become subject to SMF induced Faraday induction or perceptible flow potentials, if we disregard the potentials exerted by the dynamics of the fluid motion within the body. These potentials may not rise to a level of excitation below 8 T magnetic induction. The time mice spent in the cages was mostly resting time (beyond the first 10 min of exploratory motion).

Constant but increased induction compared to the geomagnetic field also exhibits several molecular- and cellular-level effects including nitric oxide signalization and vasodepressive tendency in rat hypertension models [232]. In contrast to rats however, short-term SMF-exposure of humans does not result in a significant reduction in either BP or heart rate [233]. Based on our findings it is highly probable that the moderate inhSMF or hSMF arrangements in our experiments did not result in significant vestibular excitation. Unchallenged animals spent significantly more time in the inhSMF/hSMF side of Cage 2 ($p<0.04$), supporting that neither type of SMF-exposure was aversive.

Subsequent to the verification of SMF-exposure not being aversive; our next goal was to test whether the exposure was preferentially chosen by the challenged mice. In our visceral pain assay, challenged mice spent approximately the same time in the inhSMF/hSMF and sham side of Cage 2; there was no significant site preference for the challenged animals. During the total 30 min duration of a single exposure to inhSMF/hSMF, it is unlikely that conditioned learning had arisen as several hours are required to develop conditional taste aversion in mice [136]. Mice in our measurements failed to recognize the beneficial effects of inhSMF/hSMF within the 30 min time limit of the experiments; the challenged group did not prefer either the SMF or the sham side of the cage.

When introduced to a new environment animals started to explore their new cage. This exploratory activity usually takes several minutes and can be quantified based on the number of exploratory rearings [234]. This occurrence of this activity of both challenged and unchallenged mice is supported by our observations. The analysis of separate 10 min intervals (0-10, 11-20, and 21-30 min) revealed that the behavior of the animals during the first 10 min of the experiment is mainly governed by random exploratory motion. No significant difference was found when cumulative 0-20 min data were compared with cumulative 0-30 min data on time spent in the inhSMF/hSMF and sham side. A possible explanation for the lack of inhSMF/hSMF preference of challenged mice was that crossing the boundary (with a strong lateral gradient of inhSMF/hSMF) caused enough pain inhibition. Staying or moving within the inhSMF/hSMF side did not provide excess analgesia.

Effect of Cage Size

According to our measurement data, behavioral pattern and pain response (number of writhings) of challenged animals in the single- and double-sized cage did not differ significantly when hSMF or inhSMF was applied. Stress and aggression is not only dependent on the area per animal but also on the number of animals in the same cage. Other authors reported an increased number of agonistic encounters below 125 cm^2 area per mouse when 3 to 8 mice were accommodated in the same cage [235]. In our experiments, the area per mouse in the double-sized cage varied between 130 and 196 cm^2 with 2 or 3 animals simultaneously in the cage. Agonistic encounters did not occur during the 30 min experiments. This observation, together with the similar number of writhings, excludes the stressor role of even the single-sized cage.

Effect of Social Behavior

Social cooperation rather than agonistic encounters was recorded between both unchallenged and challenged mice in the double-sized cage. Mice spent almost 2/3 of the total experimental period together (either in the sham or inhSMF/hSMF side of double-sized cage), which is supported by other observations applying the same 0.9% acetic acid induced visceral pain assay [44]. As a proof of empathy based on visual perception, cage mates recognize the pain behavior of each other mutually. If both mates were challenged with similar noxious stimuli, the behavioral response of one animal tended to imitate that of the other. Because only one mouse was challenged inside the cage at a time in our experiments, the only applicable measure of cooperative behavior was the time spent together. Unchallenged mice did not perform writhing behavior and most likely did not influence the response of the challenged ones.

Cross Interactions

As previously concluded, mice did not recognize the *AE* of inhSMF/hSMF; they did not prefer to spend more time exposed to inhSMF/hSMF. For this reason, the effectiveness of inhSMF/hSMF was analyzed comparing the number of writhings as being more objective signs of pain response. Significantly fewer pain syndromes were observed in mice in either the hSMF or inhSMF side of the double-sized cage compared to the sham side. This is in agreement with previous data where pain responses were monitored only in Cage 1, either entirely expsosed to inhSMF/hSMF or under sham conditions (**Optimization of SMF parameters**).

Exclusive Effect of SMF Gradients

A critical analysis on how pain inhibition in the writhing test depended on different parameters of SMF was provided in **Optimization of SMF parameters** already. The most prominent relationship occurred between inhibition and the vertical component of the magnetic induction measured at 3 mm from the magnet surface. The *AE* also strongly correlated with the polarity of the magnet arrangement. Since "unidirectional" magnet arrangements modeling a uniform SMF achieved far less antinociception than "bidirectional" arrangements modeling a strongly inhomogeneous SMF, the correlation with the SMF gradient was also suggested even if a quantitative relationship could not be established. In order to understand whether inhSMF/hSMF themselves or the spatial gradients of the inhSMF/hSMF play a more important role in the *AE* in visceral pain, we performed a deeper statistical analysis of the raw writhing data. Keeping in mind that cage size had no effect on visceral pain responses, animals in the double-sized cage were free to cross the sham inhSMF boundary in the inhSMF&sham arrangement and the sham-hSMF boundary in the hSMF&sham setup. Comparing the number of writhings in the sham side of the double-sized cage to those in the single-sized cage under sham conditions, and the writhing in the inhSMF side of the double-sized cage to those observed in the inhSMF with the single sized cage, significantly fewer pain responses were found in the double-sized cage. A plausible explanation for this is that it was not the SMF itself but its gradient that was more crucial in analgesia. The same stands for the experiments in the hSMF if we compare the analgesic action (*AE*) of mice in the single-sized cage exposed to hSMF to mice in the double-sized cage exposed to hSMF&-sham. Furthermore, cross-checking pain reactions in the double-sized cage with hSMF&sham and double hSMF (where the hSMF covers the entire cage area), the results were identical. The *AE* was more prominent when only half of the cage was exposed to the hSMF and mice were not restricted in motion. Crossing over the inhSMF/hSMF boundary elicits similar physical effects to an extremely low frequency (ELF) magnetic field on a static object (*c.f.*, in **Clinical MRI**). ELF fields, where the frequency of magnetic induction variation is typically several Hz, possess contradictory physiological effects in animals; they can induce opioid-peptide-mediated analgesia in land snails [74, 169] and mice [83], for instance.

Both an aversive thermal response and morphine induced analgesia were attenuated in snails [74, 236]; also the antioxidant enzyme capacity in rat brains decreased [237]. However, these conclusions have to be taken with a grain of salt due to the small number of animals involved in the experiments.

hSMF Versus inhSMF-Exposure

Previous results on optimizing SMF for analgesic therapy (**Optimization of SMF parameters**) suggest that application of an inhSMF is preferable to hSMF for analgesia. Our data analysis supports this hypothesis; the inhSMF-exposure condition resulted in stronger pain inhibition.

Aversiveness to Moderate SMF-exposure

Short-term (5-30 min) exposure to strong SMF instantaneously triggers taste aversion in rats [66]. The underlying behavioral and molecular processes are the focus of scientific interest with many parameters being currently still unclear. In several brainstem regions of rats exposed to such SMF, c-Fos induction occurred parallel to the taste aversion [127] underlining its possible role as a mediator. Experiments in deer mice revealed that the conditional taste aversion though existent, is not instantaneous [165]. Sexual steroids are also thought to play a role in the long-term persistence of taste aversion. In ovariectomized rats, taste aversion was found to be more prominent; however, estrogen replacement eliminated the aversive behavior. Male rats acquired a stronger initial aversion but it extinguished faster than in females [238]. Repeated exposure to SMF attenuates this biological response possibly due to habituation to vestibular perturbation subsequent to the exposure [239]. The aversive response is abolished by labyrinthectomy, which further supports the possibility of a vestibular stimulus upon SMF-exposure [230]. Mice were similarly treated with high SMF, resulting in similar aversive responses to those of rats [136]. One main goal of the present study was to analyze the aversiveness of the applied moderate type 1 inhSMF/hSMF in contrast to previous measurements which were performed under steady inhSMF/hSMF- or sham-exposure without the free choice of resting location for the animals (sections **Optimization of SMF parameters** and **Clinical MRI**). In the case of a prompt vestibular activation, aversive behavior and sham site preference would have been expected provided that the animals had been able to move freely across the inhSMF/hSMF- and sham-exposed sides of cages, which they are indeed able to do in the present experiment. This aversiveness might compete with the *AE* of the inhSMF/hSMF, but the cognitive performance of mice can prevent the rapid realization of this beneficial effect of inhSMF/hSMF. Another possibility that explains the absence of aversiveness might be due to the complex stimulation of the brain, resulting in either a sedative or anxiogenic activity. An anxiogenic effect of chronic exposure to ELF was observed in rats [240], but was not found in healthy mice as reported in **HEALTHY ANIMALS Locomotor activity and anxiety behavior in healthy mice**.

When a mouse crosses a boundary between type 2 SMF partitions, it undergoes a change of the magnetic induction in a short time. From the physical point of view this effect is identical to either, when

i. a living object is moved into the bore of a high field MR apparatus from practically stray field, or
ii. the MR proceeds gradient switching on a static living object inside its bore.

Applying the ambulation model for the motion induced current densities (Eq. (9)), two conclusions could be drawn.

1. Its long-time average in the mouse moving in a periodic SMF is zero, since the trigonometric terms result in zero in the integration. This fact can be generalized for every rectilinear motion in a laterally periodic SMF supposing that the typical "wavelength" of the periodicity is not bigger than the typical linear ambulation distance of the animal. If so, the resolution obeys the rule defined in Eq. (3), and the decay time of PNS is much shorter than the time it takes for an animal to cross a boundary with strong SMF induction gradient. The partitioned SMF are periodic with wavelengths λ=10, 20, 30, and 40 mm. The periodicity in case of M=5 and 6 is questionable. The boundary widths are shorter than the typical linear ambulation distances in the cage (140 mm) with the exception of M=5 and 6. Thus, the discrepancy of the *AE* results for these cases may be due to the failure of the 2D model assumptions. According to models of electric signal propagation along the axon (Chapter 3 in the book of

Malmivuo and Plonsey [241]), we estimate that an impulse strong enough to stimulate a peripheral nerve would decay at a certain location in less than 2 ms, meanwhile a mouse needs 10-60 ms to intersect a boundary.

2. For a single linear path the time dependence of the motion induced current density can be non-zero. Can this non-zero induced current density contribute to inhibition (*AE*)?

As has been mentioned in the Discussion part of **Clinical MRI** already, the threshold of the motion induced current density for PNS was first estimated to be at 0.01 mA/m^2 [214], later 0.48 A/m^2 was proposed for human nerves [215]. Now the threshold values are accepted to be at 1-10 mA/m^2 [216]. The size-corrected value for mice is 0.16-1.6 mA/m^2. In our ambulation model the absolute value of the motion induced current density remains below 1.8 mA/m^2, not excluding an effect. We must assume that the pain inhibitory effect of SMF-exposure based on the endogenous μ-opioid receptors (as shown in **Clinical MRI**) is either more effective and/or has a preventive manner as compared to the nerve stimulatory effect leading to pain sensation.

The clinically determined PNS threshold for the MR's switching rate is between 50 [221] and 60 T/s [224]. The mean PNS threshold is at 90 T/s and the mean cardiac stimulation threshold is by 2 orders of magnitude higher [224]. In our experiments *MEWR* lay between 46 and 164 mT/s, 2 orders of magnitude below threshold. Switching rates were shown not to contribute to pain inhibition in clinical studies; rather the contrary was found [125]. On the other hand, Table **5.8** illustrates a strong correlation between *AE* and *MEWR*. We may resolve this contradiction remembering that the inhomogeneity of SMF was demonstrated earlier in **Clinical MRI** not to be necessary to achieve *AE*; the homogeneous SMF of a 3 T clinical MR apparatus was also able to exert 69% *AE* in the writhing test in mice. Although the *P-P* amplitude of the magnetic induction does not have a strong correlation with *AE* directly (Table **5.8**), it may have through its gradient though.

We may interpret these facts as *AE* not being exclusively related to the inhomogeneity of SMF. The 1D single axis slew rates of clinical MR devices are typically 20 T/m/s and above. *MESR* calculated in our model for case (i) above remains well below threshold, at *cca.* 1 T/m/s for a clinical MR. The estimated *MESR* values in Table **5.8** are in fact, all below typical slew rates. From the correlations of the *M*-SMF induced inhibition to the *MESR* (Table **5.8**), we may conclude for case (ii) that the higher the *MESR*, the more expressed the inhibition.

Table 5.8. Correlation of the inhibition (AE in %) to the measured values of the *P-P* amplitudes of the magnetic induction, to their gradients (∇B), to the numbers of gradient per distance (N), to the MR-equivalent switching and slew rate (both MEWR and MESR data estimated *via* the ambulation model) in the M-SMF. Vertical dosimetric data measured at *z*=20 mm are shown with the assumption that this is the average target distance from the magnets' surface, where AE takes place in the mouse. The absolute values of induction gradient are averaged values in first-neighbor approximation. N reflects numbers of inflection points of the vertical magnetic induction component per average linear ambulation distance (140 mm). For *v*=1 m/s average ambulation speed MEWR are equal in their numerical value to the magnetic induction gradients.

partitioning number, *M*	*M*-SMF dosimetry			ambulation model	SMF-induced analgesic effect (*AE* %)
	P-P amplitude of the magnetic induction *B*) at *z*=20 mm (mT)	absolute value of induction gradient (*MEWR*) at *z*=20 mm (mT/m)	numbers of gradient (*ñB* per distance	MR-equivalent slew rate (*MESR*) at *z*=20 mm (T/m/s)	
1	1.6	162	19	16.2	71
2	17.7	46	9	2.3	44
3	64.9	90	6	3.0	42
4	133.8	140	3	3.5	62
5	191.2	164	3	3.3	65
6	212.5	154	2	2.6	45
correlation to *AE* (%)	**-53.1**	**17.2**	**66.5**	**67.0**	
correlation to *AE* excluding *M*=5 (%)	**-85.8**	**3.9**	**78.8**	**87.5**	

For the simulation model it is easy to estimate, on the basis of Fig. (**5.31**), that the magnetic induction gradient per a single 10 mm step from one cell to another was always below 40 mT, indicating that PNS might not disturb either the motion, or any other response of the animal for that matter.

Present data do indeed confirm that neither inhomogeneous, nor homogeneous SMF-exposure in the applied magnetic induction range is aversive to mice. We determined that the exposure to the spatial SMF gradient might have been responsible for the pain inhibition in the writhing test rather than the exposure to the SMF itself. We also verified that mice are socially sensitive based on the observation that couplets preferred to spend more time together on the same side of the cage. We concluded that the conditioning of mice with the applied short-term SMF-exposure is not possible; the cognitive perception of analgesia and either inhomogeneous, or homogeneous SMF site preference was not developed. Let us now turn to the pharmacological analysis of *AE* in the writhing test model in mice.

PHARMACOLOGICAL ANALYSIS

Pharmacological Analysis of Static Magnetic Field-Induced Antinociceptive Action in the Mouse

Goals

The aim of this study was to analyze the following questions:

Does SMF-exposure inhibit pain responses evoked by the Epsom salt challenge?
2. What mechanisms are involved in the *AE* due to SMF-exposure?
3. Does SMF-exposure affect morphine induced analgesia?

Materials and Methods

Magnetic Exposure Conditions, Drugs

SMF was produced by generator 11 (**Generators 1-16**). Naltrindole, naloxone, and norbinaltor-phimine were purchased from Sigma-Aldrich, and β-funaltrexamine from Tocris. The drugs were given either *s.c.* or intracerebroventricularly (*i.c.v.*) in a volume of 20 ml/kg or 10 μl/mouse, respectively. Morphine (Sigma-Aldrich) was given *s.c.* in an amount of 10 mg/kg, 20 min preceding the acetic acid challenge. Had we used the same dose of morphine in the pain assay as in the behavioral tests (**HEALTHY ANIMALS Locomotor activity and anxiety behavior in healthy mice**), we would have completely suppressed the possible effect of SMF-exposure.

Statistical Analysis

All the results are expressed as mean±SEM. The statistical analysis of the data was executed by one-way ANOVA for repeated measures followed by the Newman-Keuls test for *post hoc* analysis. A probability of $p<0.05$ was considered statistically significant.

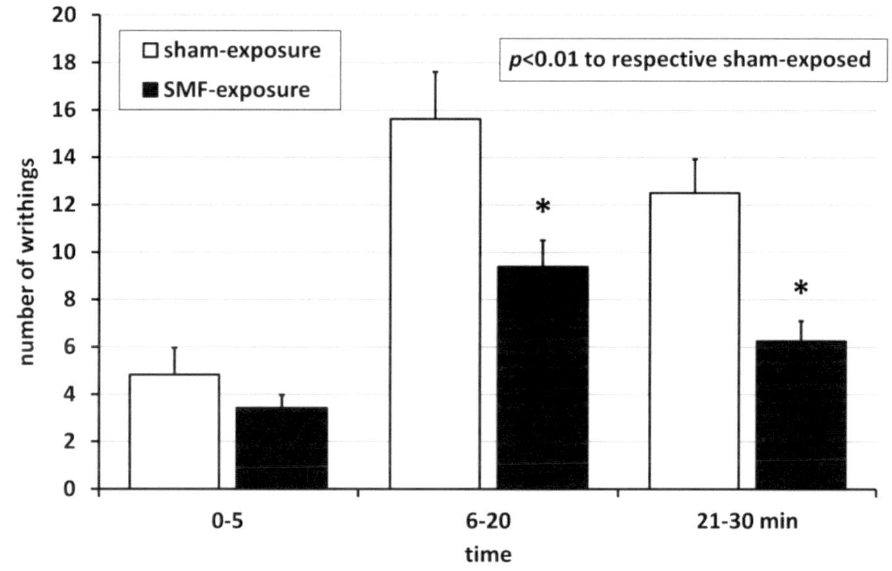

Fig. (5.33). Inhibitory effect of SMF-exposure on abdominal contractions (writhing movements) induced by i.p. injection of 2% Epsom salt. Mice were placed into the SMF or sham cage 5 min before the injection of the irritating agent and stayed there during the whole experimental period. Results are shown as means with SEM of n=6-12 animals/group. * p<0.01 SMF- *vs* sham-exposure (Bonferroni's modified Dunnett's test).

Results

The Effect of SMF-exposure on Epsom Salt Induced Abdominal Pain

In control mice intraperitoneal injection of 2% Epsom salt elicited 4.8±1.2, 15.7±2.0, and 12.7±1.4 writhing movements in the 0-5, 6-20, and 21-30 min intervals, respectively. Exposure of mice to SMF resulted in 26%, 39%, and 52%

decrease of Epsom salt-evoked nocifensive behaviors. Although the inhibitory effects in the 2nd and 3rd examination periods proved to be statistically significant, the degree of inhibition was smaller than for acetic acid (89%, 80%, and 89%, respectively as compared Fig. (**5.33**) with generator 11 in Table **5.3**).

The Effect of Naloxone, β-funaltrexamine, Naltrindole and Norbinaltorphimine Given Peripherally on SMF Induced AE

Naloxone in the dose of 1 and 0.2 mg/kg *s.c.* resulted in a significant inhibition of *AE* induced by SMF applied for 30 min after the acetic acid challenge (Fig. **5.34**). The μ-opioid receptor selective irreversible antagonist β-funaltrexamine (20 mg/kg *s.c.*) also inhibited the SMF induced *AE*. Naltrindole (0.5 mg/kg *s.c.*) decreased in a significant manner the SMF induced *AE* as well, but the inhibition of the action was not complete. In contrast, norbinaltorphimine (20 mg/kg *s.c.*) failed to affect SMF-induced *AE* in any way (Fig. **5.35A-C**).

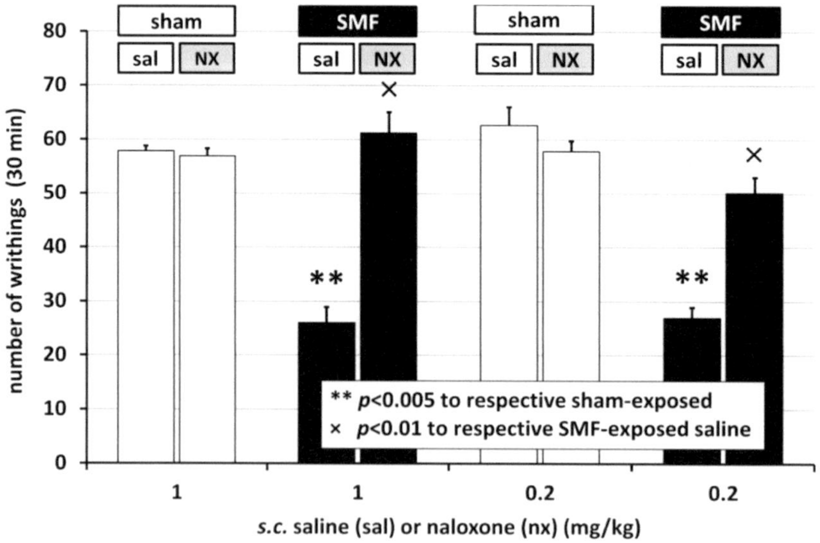

Fig. (5.34). The effect of 1.0 and 0.2 mg/kg of naloxone (NX) given s.c. on SMF induced AE on writhing syndrome in mice. Open columns: Control animals injected with saline (sal) unexposed to SMF. Dark columns: Mice exposed to SMF. Each column represents the mean±SEM of 12 mice (summation of 2 experiments, 6 mice/group/experiment). ** $p<0.005$ compared to control groups (columns 1 and 5, respectively). × $p<0.01$ compared to SMF-saline group assessed by Bonferroni's modified Dunnett's test.

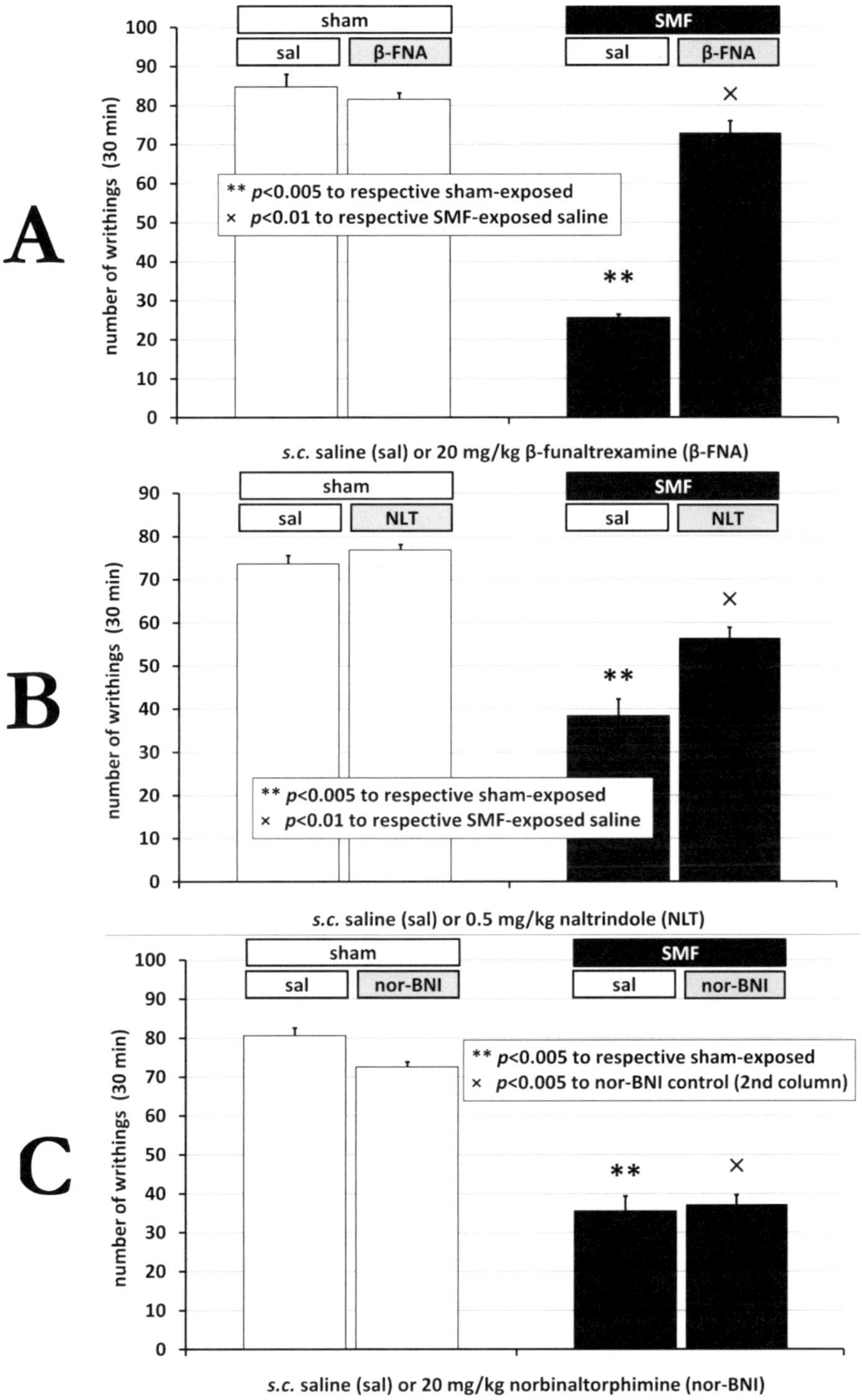
A
sham
SMF
sal
β-FNA
sal
β-FNA
number of writhings (30 min)
100
90
80
70
60
50
40
30
20
10
0
** p<0.005 to respective sham-exposed
× p<0.01 to respective SMF-exposed saline
**
×
s.c. saline (sal) or 20 mg/kg β-funaltrexamine (β-FNA)
B
sham
SMF
sal
NLT
sal
NLT
number of writhings (30 min)
90
80
70
60
50
40
30
20
10
0
**
×
** p<0.005 to respective sham-exposed
× p<0.01 to respective SMF-exposed saline
s.c. saline (sal) or 0.5 mg/kg naltrindole (NLT)
C
sham
SMF
sal
nor-BNI
sal
nor-BNI
number of writhings (30 min)
100
90
80
70
60
50
40
30
20
10
0
** p<0.005 to respective sham-exposed
× p<0.005 to nor-BNI control (2nd column)
**
×
s.c. saline (sal) or 20 mg/kg norbinaltorphimine (nor-BNI)

Fig. (5.35). The effect of **A)** β -funaltrexamine (β -FNA) (20 mg/kg s.c.), **B)** naltrindole (0.5 mg/kg s.c.) **C)** norbinaltorphimine (nor-BNI) (20 mg/kg *s.c.*) on SMF induced AE on writhing syndrome in mice. Open columns: Control animals unexposed to SMF. Dark columns: Mice exposed to SMF. Each column represents the mean±SEM of 6 mice. ** $p<0.005$ compared to saline-control groups (column 1). In panel (A) and (B) × $p<0.01$ compared to β-funaltrexamine- or naltrindole-control group (column 2). In panel (C) × $p<0.005$ compared to norbinaltorphimine-control group (column 2). All p values were assessed by Bonferroni's modified Dunnett's test.

The Effect of Naloxone on SMF Induced AE Given i.c.v.

Exposure of mice to SMF resulted in more than 50% inhibition of acetic acid induced pain reaction. On the other hand, Naloxone given *i.c.v.* (10 mg/mouse) failed to affect the SMF induced *AE* (Fig. **5.36**).

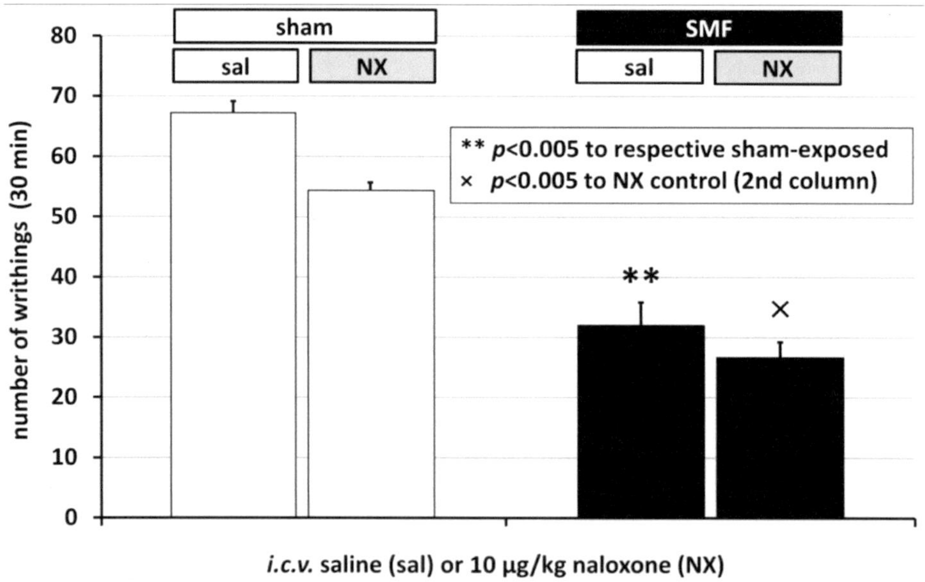

Fig. (5.36). The effect of naloxone given i.c.v. (10 µg/mouse) on SMF induced AE on writhing syndrome in mice. Open columns: Control animals. Dark columns: Mice exposed to SMF. Each column represents the mean±SEM of 12 mice (summation of 2 experiments, 6 mice/group/experiment). ** $p<0.005$ compared to saline-control group. × $p<0.005$ compared to naloxone-control group assessed by Bonferroni's modified Dunnett's test.

The Effect of an Inhomogeneous SMF on Morphine Induced AE

Fig. (**5.37**) demonstrates the average number of writhings±SEM of mice that were exposed to the SMF for 30 min. Morphine in the dose of 0.5 mg/kg induced a 43% inhibition of pain reaction; SMF-treatment elicited 66% reduction of abdominal pain. Similarly, 67% inhibition developed, when SMF was applied in morphine-treated mice. 2 mg/kg MO plus SMF-exposure caused a maximum average number of writhings below 2 and therefore, is not shown in Fig. (**5.37**). The number of animals was 6 in each group, except for morphine treatment in an amount of 2 mg/kg, where n=3.

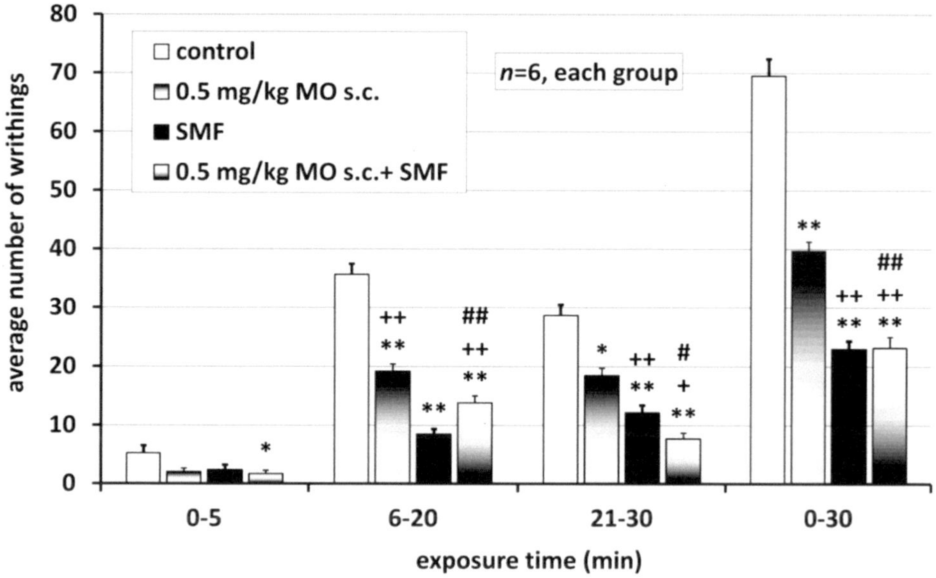

Fig. (5.37). The effect of inhomogeneous SMF-exposure applied for 30 min on the number of writhings (± SEM) of mice per se or in combination with morphine (MO, 0.5 mg/kg s.c.). The number of animals was 6/group. * $p<0.05$, ** $p<0.001$ compared to control group, + and ++ denote $p<0.05$ and $p<0.001$ compared to SMF-treated group, respectively, # and ## mean $p<0.05$ and $p<0.001$ compared to morphine-treated group, respectively. Statistical significance was estimated by one-way ANOVA followed by Dunnett's post hoc test.

Discussion, Conclusions

It was shown that SMF-exposure can modify analgesic responses; for example, stress induced analgesia in mice was inhibited by hypogeomagnetic environment [242] as well as by exposure to an artificial SMF, and this analgesia was likely to involve a light-dependent mechanism [243]. Furthermore, nociceptive sensitivity in mice was enhanced by exposure to pulsed magnetic field [130]; a rotating magnetic field significantly reduced the analgesic and locomotor effects of morphine in mice [153]. The inhibitory effect of extremely low frequency magnetic field on opioid analgesia induced by enkephalinase inhibitor was also observed in land snails [244]. Furthermore, daily repeated SMF shielding was shown to effectuate analgesia in mice [27].

The present data demonstrated first that SMF exerted *AE* against visceral pain elicited by Epsom salt. The SMF induced inhibition was more pronounced on the abdominal writhing response evoked by acetic acid than by Epsom salt. This difference might be explained by distinct pain-producing mechanisms of these chemicals: The nocifensive response elicited by Epsom salt may be due to the direct stimulation of visceral chemonociceptors, while an acute inflammatory reaction is likely to be involved in the acetic acid induced behavior [182]. *AE* in the writhing test was fully reversed by naloxone (1 mg/kg) indicating that an opioid component is likely to be involved in the action. This was already shown in the land snail, *Helix pomatia* (**Experiments on invertebrates *in vivo***) and also in mice in the bore of an MRI (**Clinical MRI**). Interestingly, [27] found that *AE* induced by repeated daily exposure to SMF shielded environment was also reversed by naloxone in hot plate test in the mouse.

The existence of 3 distinct opioid receptors: μ, δ and *x* was suggested by Martin *et al.* [245]. The question was raised which opioid receptor may play a role in *AE* of SMF. Since naloxone (0.2 mg/kg) as well as the μ-opioid receptor selective irreversible antagonist β-funaltrexamine inhibited *AE* of SMF, the involvement of μ-opioid receptors in *AE* may be suggested. The *δ*-opioid receptor antagonist naltrindole also highly reduced the effect of SMF. On the contrary, *x*-opioid receptor antagonist norbinaltorphimine failed to affect *AE*. These results indicate that activation of μ-, as well as δ-, but not *x*-opioid receptors may play a role in the SMF induced *AE* in the mouse. Our results are consistent with the findings of Thomas *et al.* [77], who suggested that *x*-opioid receptors may not be involved in *AE* of SMF in land snail against thermal nociception.

Several endogenous ligands for opioid receptors have been described, such as leu- and met-enkephalins, β-endorphin, dynorphins, and the recently discovered pair: Endomorphin-1 and endomorphin-2 [246]. Enkephalins have higher affinity for δ-opioid receptor than for μ-opioid receptors, β-endorphin shows slightly higher binding affinity to μ- than to δ-opioid receptors, dynorphin is an endogenous ligand of *x*-opioid receptors [150], whereas endomorphins exhibit the highest affinity and specificity for μ-receptors of any endogenous compound found so far in mammalian nervous system [246]. Thus, it might be speculated that the release of either the μ-opioid receptor selective agonist endomorphins and/or the δ- and μ-opioid receptor agonist β-endorphin may be responsible for *AE* of SMF in the mouse.

The potential role of opioid peptides in SMF-exposure induced biological responses is supported by the findings that increased concentration of β-endorphin (and substance P) was observed in the hypothalamus following repeated exposure of rats to extremely low frequency magnetic field [169].

The potential site of action of SMF induced *AE* has also been studied. I.c.v. administration of naloxone failed to affect *AE* of SMF-exposure indicating that the site of action is not likely to be at the supraspinal level. However, spinal mechanism in the SMF induced *AE* can also be raised. Specifically, acetic acid induced pain reaction was suggested to involve inflammatory components [182], which can result in a prolonged afferent input and the concomitant physiological changes. For example, repetitive small afferent input leads to release of active factors in dorsal horn neurons, initiating a spontaneous afferent traffic [64]. Endomorphin-2 is present in the primary afferent fibers and in the spinal cord [247 - 249] and endomorphin-2 released from fibers may function to modify pain sensations from the visceral organs [247]. Furthermore, β-endorphin was also identified in the spinal cord [250]. Consequently, it may be speculated that *AE* of SMF may be due to the release of either β-endorphin or endomorphin-2 in the spinal cord.

Since naloxone antagonized the SMF induced analgesic response given peripherally but not centrally, the role of the peripheral opioid system is likely to be dominant. β-endorphin [251] and endomorphin [252] were identified in immune cell subpopulation as well as in inflamed and non-inflamed lymph nodes. Inflammation increases the expression of opioid peptides both *in vivo* and *in vitro* [253, 254]. In addition, opioid peptides can be found in circulating granulocytes [255]. It is to be determined whether SMF-exposure can induce the release of opioid peptides from these cellular elements.

Further studies are needed to clarify, whether other mechanisms also contribute to

AE of SMF against abdominal pain reaction. For example, it was raised that the cAMP-dependent protein kinase (PKA) signal transduction cascade contributes to nociceptive processing at the spinal cord level and intrathecal infusion of PKA inhibitor, H89 partially reversed the visceral pain induced effects elicited by intracolonic injection of mustard oil. Although the 2 pain models are different, it is to be analyzed, if SMF-exposure might affect the PKA signal transduction pathway [256].

Moreover, further studies are needed to determine, whether SMF-exposure affects the voltage-gated sodium channel, since its blockade may also result in the inhibition of spinal neurotransmission [257].

The reason is unclear, why SMF-exposure results in a "morphine-like" *AE*, but does not mimic the effect of MO on locomotion (*c.f.*, **Locomotor activity and anxiety behavior in healthy mice**). One of the possibilities might be that the role of the various opioid receptors and endogenous opioid systems is dissimilar in these 2 functions [150]. However, the role of other factors, for example various, not yet deorphanised orphan G-protein coupled receptors [258] in the effect of SMF-exposure cannot be excluded.

In the next section, we make an attempt to reveal whether SMF-exposure can affect visceral inflammation in a murine model.

CHRONIC MODELS

Peripheral action

Neuropathic pain

Exposure to Static Magnetic Field Ceases Mechanical Allodynia in Neuropathic Pain

Preliminaries

Nearly 1/3 of the human population experience severe chronic pain in some point in life. For many patients, pain continues to produce severe distress, dominating, and disrupting the quality of their lives. Much of currently available clinical treatment is only partially effective and may be accompanied by distressing side effects or have abuse potential [259]. As mentioned already in the previous **Visceral action** for PTB, the search for reliable, safe, and effective treatments for neuropathic pain also remains a major challenge and patients continuously explore alternative approaches. Among a number of other treatment strategies, magnetic therapy is increasingly used to alleviate pain. Magnetic field therapy as a self-care intervention has led to the conduct of more than 50 randomized controlled human trials (reviewed by Colbert *et al.* [43]). Results obtained from studies that tested *AE* of SMF therapy in chronic pain are inconsistent. Some authors demonstrated a positive effect of SMF-exposure on achieving anesthesia in neuropathic, inflammatory, musculoskeletal, fibromyalgia, rheumatic, and postsurgical pain [40, 260 - 268]. Others claimed that SMF-exposure had no advantage over sham-exposure in reducing pain intensity in patients with diabetic polyneuropathy, chronic low back pain, or carpal tunnel syndrome [269 - 274]. Sporadic studies in animals have not provided more consistent results either. There are reports showing that rodents exposed to SMF exhibited strong analgesia to various painful stimuli [27, 153, 275]. On the other hand, increased pain sensitivity has also been shown to occur after exposure to SMF [130, 242, 276]. However, since the parameters of the applied magnetic fields were poorly defined and the pain models that were supposed to be treated varied from investigation to investigation, the interpretation of the results obtained from these studies is quite ambiguous.

Goals

To avoid the obvious problems in the interpretation of the results of earlier studies, here we utilized an experimental approach, in which both the parameters of the applied SMF and the pain model supposed to be treated were carefully standardized. Firstly, for the generation of an inhomogeneous SMF we used an apparatus the parameters of which has been carefully tested and adjusted to small experimental animals (sections **Optimization of SMF parameters** and **Clinical MRI**). Secondly, we tested the effectiveness of SMF-exposure on a well established animal model of chronic neuropathic pain (Seltzer model) which makes our results controllable and reproducible.

Materials and Methods

Animals and Surgical Procedure

Experiments were carried out on 30 male mice (BALB/c, 20-25 g, Gödöllő, Hungary). Animals were divided into 5 experimental groups with 6 animals/ group. Animals in the different experimental groups went through the following procedures:

Group 1: No surgical procedure was carried out on these animals; they were not exposed to SMF.
Group 2: The animals were deeply anesthetized with sodium pentobarbital (3.5 mg/100 g body mass; *i.p.*). Following an incision at the level of the mid thigh, the left sciatic nerve was exposed by blunt dissection. Without making any further surgical intervention the incision was sutured and the animals were allowed to recover. Animals were not exposed to SMF.
Groups 3-5: The animals were deeply anesthetized with sodium pentobarbital. Following blunt dissection a suture was passed through the dorsal third of the nerve and tied tightly according to Seltzer *et al.* [277]. The incision on the skin was then sutured and the animals were allowed to recover.
Group 3: Animals were not exposed to SMF.
Group 4: Animals were exposed to SMF repetitively, once a day on post-operative days 1 to 14.
Group 5: Animals were exposed to SMF repetitively, once a day on post-operative days 15 to 28

Magnetic Exposure Conditions

Generator 11 was used to generate SMF in this series of experiments. For SMF-exposure, animals were put into the Plexiglas cage one at a time and then the cage with the animal was inserted into the SMF-exposure chamber for 30 min. The behavioral test on the days of SMF-exposure was performed within 20 min after the exposure as SMF-exposure was shown to have a prolonged *AE* in an acute pain model (**Optimization of SMF parameters**).

Behavioral Test

All mice were tested for withdrawal responses to noxious mechanical stimuli using a dynamic plantar aesthesiometer (Ugo Basile) similarly to that described in **Peripheral action**. Animals were placed upon a network platform and covered with a Perspex enclosure that rendered the animal unrestrained for the duration of the experiment. The hind paw of the animal was positioned above a von Frey-type filament with a tip diameter of about 1 mm. The filament exerted an increasing pressure to the plantar surface until the animal removed its paw. At this point the measurement was terminated and the actual force at which paw withdrawal occurred was recorded. The measurement was repeated 5 times in each case. The mechanical withdrawal threshold (MWT) for both hind paws was determined before surgery (day 0) and the test was repeated on postoperative days 1, 4, 6, 8, 11, 13, 15, 18, 20, 22, 25, 27, 29, 36, and 40.

Table 5.9. Mechanical withdrawal threshold values for the right hind paws measured before surgery (day 0) and on postoperative days 1, 4, 6, 8, 11, 13, 15, 18, 20, 22, 25, 27, 29, 36 and 40. The responsiveness of the right hind paw to mechanical stimulation was similar in all animals in all experimental groups throughout the entire length of the experiment. Thus, here we calculated the average values and SEM of data obtained from all experimental animals (5 experimental group, 6 animal in each group, 5 measurements in each animal).

Mechanical withdrawal threshold	**days**															
	0	**1**	**4**	**6**	**8**	**11**	**13**	**15**	**18**	**20**	**22**	**25**	**27**	**29**	**36**	**40**
average	4.70	4.73	4.62	4.74	4.75	4.62	4.70	4.75	4.69	4.87	4.81	4.85	4.85	4.87	4.84	4.83
SEM	0.05	0.05	0.06	0.05	0.04	0.05	0.05	0.05	0.05	0.04	0.04	0.04	0.04	0.04	0.04	0.04

Statistical Analysis

All numerical values presented in the text and figures were calculated from 30 experimental data (6 animals in each experimental group, 5 measurements on each animal). Results indicate mean values±SEM. Statistical differences between multiple experimental groups were assessed by one-way ANOVA completed with Dunnett's *post hoc* test for the comparison between pairs of data series. Equal numbers of data were compared. Probabilities (*p*) of less than 0.05 were considered to be statistically significant.

Results

MWT of the non-operated right hind paw was very similar in all animals in all experimental groups throughout the entire duration of the experiment (Table **5.9**). It varied between 4.62±0.05 g and 4.87±0.04 g with an average of 4.76±0.02 g. Thus, our further description will focus exclusively on the findings that were obtained on the operated left hind paws.

The Effect of Sham Operation on the Mechanical Withdrawal Threshold

MWT in the untreated control animals (group 1) varied randomly between 4.61±0.14 g and 4.91±0.04 g during the experiment (Fig. **5.38**). The sham operation (group 2) caused a transient but significant drop in MWT. On postoperative day 1, MWT of sham operated animals decreased to the value of 3.99±0.29 g. After this however, animals showed a rapid spontaneous recovery. MWT figures continuously increased day by day and reached the control values on postoperative day 11 (4.66±0.15 g).

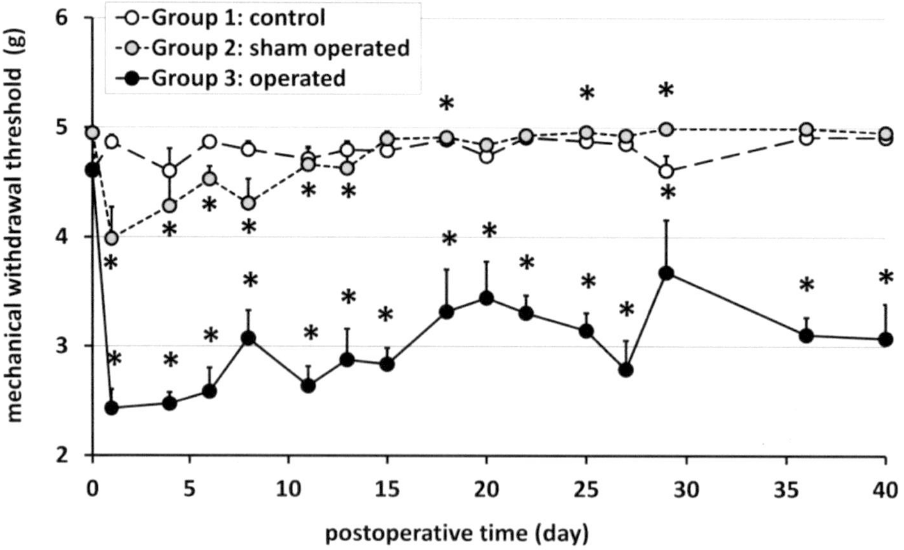

Fig. (5.38). Development of MWT of control (group 1), sham operated (group 2), and operated animals with partial nerve ligation of the left sciatic nerve (group 3). None of the animals in groups 1, 2, or 3 were exposed to SMF. Threshold values are represented as means; the vertical bars at measurement points represent SEM. Asterisks along the histogram curves of groups 2 and 3 label measurement points that are significantly different ($p<0.05$) from corresponding control values as estimated with Dunnett's post hoc test.

The Effect of Partial Nerve Ligation on the Mechanical Withdrawal Threshold

The partial ligation of the sciatic nerve resulted in a sudden and dramatic drop in MWT. On postoperative day 1, MWT values decreased to 2.43±0.18 g, 2.63±0.17 g 2.49 ±0.24 g in animals within groups 3, 4, and 5, respectively (Fig. **5.38**, Fig. **5.39**, and Fig. **5.40**). Without SMF-exposure this condition did not improve within the 40 days long experimental period. Although MWT value showed a slight elevation with time, it was still at the level of 3.07±0.31 g at postoperative day 40 in group 3 animals (Fig. **5.38**).

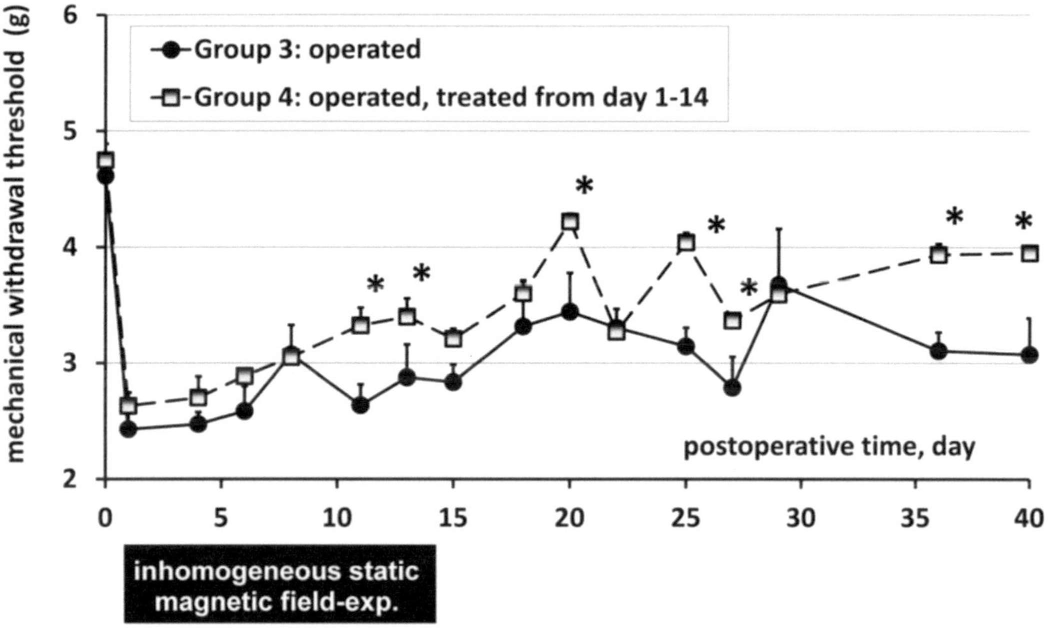

Fig. (5.39). Development of MWT of 2 groups of animals with partial nerve ligation of the left sciatic nerve (groups 3 and 4). Animals in group 4 were exposed to SMF once a day on postoperative days 1 to 14. Asterisks along the histogram curve of group 4 label measurement points that are significantly different ($p<0.05$) from corresponding values obtained from group 3 animals as estimated with Dunnett's post hoc test.

The Effect of Magnetic Exposure on the Mechanical Withdrawal Threshold in Animals With Partial Nerve Ligation

Daily exposure to SMF during the first postoperative week did not inhibit the decrease of MWT values in animals with partial nerve ligation. By postoperative day 8, MWT of animals in group 4 elevated to 3.05±0.21 g, whereas it remained

3.07±0.25 g and 2.93±0.17 g for animals in groups 3 and 5, respectively that did not receive SMF-exposure (Fig. **5.39** and Fig. **5.40**). However, by the end of the 2 week long SMF treatment, MWT values of animals that were and were not exposed to SMF showed a modest but significant difference (Table **5.10**). On postoperative day 13, MWT was 3.40±0.16 g for animals in group 4, 2.88±0.28 g and 2.91±0.52 g for animals in groups 3 and 5, respectively (Fig. **5.39** and Fig. **5.40**). In addition, with transient drops during the 3rd and 4th weeks, MWT kept rising even after the termination of SMF-exposure and reached the value of 3.95±0.16 g by postoperative day 40, whereas the MWT of nerve-ligated animals without SMF-exposure (group 3) was only 3.07±0.31 g (Fig. **5.39**).

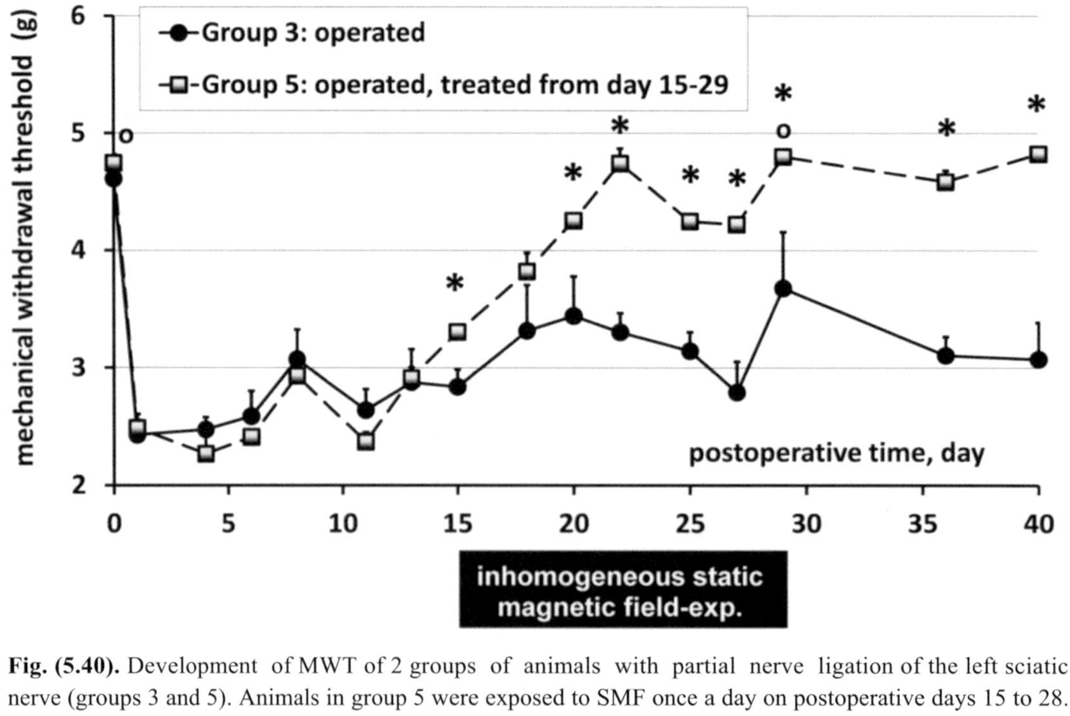

Fig. (5.40). Development of MWT of 2 groups of animals with partial nerve ligation of the left sciatic nerve (groups 3 and 5). Animals in group 5 were exposed to SMF once a day on postoperative days 15 to 28. Asterisks along the histogram curve of group 5 label measurement points that are significantly different ($p<0.05$) from corresponding values obtained from group 3 animals. The 2 open circles along the histogram curve of group 5 mark measurement points that are not significantly different ($p>0.05$) from corresponding values obtained from control (group 1) animals as estimated with Dunnett's post hoc test.

The effectiveness of exposure to SMF was much more prominent when it was applied between postoperative days 15 and 28. MWT was noticeably elevated right after the first treatment (Fig. **5.40**). On postoperative day 15, animals in group 5 showed an elevated MWT (3.31±0.11 g) that was significantly higher than MWT of animals in group 3 (2.84±0.15 g; Table **5.10**). During the experiment MWT showed a remarkable continuous increase and by the end of the 2 week long repetitive exposure period it reached the control value. On postoperative day 29, MWT for animals in group 5 was 4.80±0.11 g. On top of this, this value was maintained even after the cessation of the treatment as far as postoperative day 40 (the end of the experiment), when MWT was still 4.82±0.05 g for these animals.

Table 5.10. Statistical differences between experimental groups computed by using Dunnett's post hoc test for the comparison between pairs of data series. Equal numbers of MWT for the right hind paws measured before surgery (day 0) and on postoperative days 1, 4, 6, 8, 11, 13, 15, 18, 20, 22, 25, 27, 29, 36, and 40 were compared. Probabilities (p) of less than 0.05 were considered to be statistically significant and marked with asterisks in the table.

groups of animals		2 and 1		3 and 1		4 and 3		5 and 3	
days	**0**	0.119		0.964		0.309		0.329	
	1	<0.001	*	<0.001	*	0.278		0.770	
	4	<0.001	*	<0.001	*	0.187		0.219	
	6	<0.001	*	<0.001	*	0.108		0.388	
	8	<0.001	*	<0.001	*	0.922		0.565	
	11	0.001	*	<0.001	*	0.004	*	0.249	
	13	<0.001	*	<0.001	*	0.010	*	0.907	
	15	0.165		<0.001	*	0.102		0.040	*
	18	0.011	*	<0.001	*	0.319		0.093	
	20	0.616		<0.001	*	0.002	*	0.001	*
	22	0.668		<0.001	*	0.894		<0.001	*
	25	0.031	*	<0.001	*	<0.001	*	<0.001	*
	27	0.976		<0.001	*	0.015	*	<0.001	*
	29	<0.001	*	<0.001	*	0.715		<0.001	*
	36	0.602		<0.001	*	<0.001	*	<0.001	*
	40	0.084		<0.001	*	<0.001	*	<0.001	*

Discussion, Conclusions

Magnetic therapy has been used for treating painful injuries for centuries (for a review see [278]), and is still used to alleviate pain. The beneficial effect of SMF-exposure in treating pain has also been demonstrated in controlled experimental conditions. Some authors reported positive effects of SMF-exposure on achieving anesthesia in patients suffering from various neuropathic and inflammatory pain conditions [40, 261 - 268]. Rodents exposed to SMF also exhibited strong analgesia to various painful stimuli [27, 153, 275].

However, results obtained from studies that tested the analgesic efficacy of SMF therapy in chronic pain are inconsistent. For example, the latest systematic review of 29 reports [42] that assessed the efficacy of magnetic therapy for pain reduction concluded that the evidence did not support the use of magnets for pain relief. We argue that this conclusion is unwarranted if the parameters of the SMF and the dosage applied were inappropriate for the clinical condition treated. Actually, it is highly probable that this was the case in the majority, if not all earlier clinical trials, since the most effective dose or dosing regimen have not been defined for any clinical conditions yet. Thus, it is imperative that dosing conditions be optimized before attempting to test the efficacy of SMF therapy. To reach any reliable conclusion on the usefulness of SMF therapy on alleviating pain of different origin, authors are urged to describe the parameters of their applied technique and exposure system as precisely and rigorously as possible as proposed by Colbert *et al.* [29] to allow others to replicate the experiments, and to permit correct interpretation of the reported results.

The exposure system that has been designed and carefully tested as shown in **Optimization of SMF parameters** and has been shown to generate an inhomogeneous SMF in a well-defined strength appears to be useful for attenuating responses evoked by noxious chemical irritation of the peritoneum or the hind paw (sections **Optimization of SMF parameters** and **Clinical MRI**). In addition, here we demonstrated that its application is also beneficial in neuropathic pain. If applied appropriately, the inhomogeneous SMF generated by this apparatus can diminish mechanical allodynia evoked by partial ligation of the sciatic nerve in mice.

It has been demonstrated that exposure to SMF greater than about 1 T induces flow potentials around the heart and major blood vessels [218]. The physiological significance of these potentials however, is likely to be negligible, since several hour long exposures at the thoracic part of the body with inductions of up to 8 T did not result in any measurable cardiovascular effects in pigs [225]. The maximum *P-P* magnetic induction generated by the apparatus that we used in our experiments was below 0.5 T. Thus, it is unlikely that the exposure to SMF might have caused any substantial change in the cardiovascular system of the experimental animals, and could thus bias our results.

It has been generally accepted that currents are generated in the body of animals when they move in an external SMF [124]. This topic has been discussed already in **Clinical MRI**. In principle, these motion induced currents may stimulate peripheral nerves if the time derivative of the induction is larger than 40 T/s [16, 210, 221 - 223]. Taking the measured physical parameters of the device into account and calculating with the estimated value of 0.5 m/s for the motion velocity of the animals within the cage (according to the rigorously precise measurements of Yang *et al.* [279] the normal walking speed of a mouse is around 0.03 m/s), the time derivative of the induction for our SMF apparatus cannot be larger than 24 T/s. If we then continue this calculation by using the value of maximum induced current estimated for a human phantom [212] with a size conversion from human to mouse according to the inverse-square law [213], it turns out that the maximum induced current in a mouse in our SMF can be around 0.04 mA/m^2. This is far below the values of 480 mA/m^2 for humans and 1.6 mA/m^2 for mice that are now accepted as threshold values for the induction of currents [15, 217, 220]. Thus, it appears unlikely that motion induced currents could achieve PNS in our animals and could cause a misinterpretation of the experimental data.

In case of whole-body SMF-exposure that we utilized in the present study the SMF may influence all levels of this complex information processing neural apparatus from peripheral receptors to cortical microcircuits as already mentioned in **Peripheral action**. Thus, at the present state of our investigations it is impossible to define which parts of the pain processing apparatus responded to

SMF-exposure in a way that resulted in the normalization of the mechanical withdrawal threshold.

Although at the moment, we cannot identify the mechanisms and sites of action, it is unlikely that the effect of inhomogeneous SMF-exposure on nociceptive receptors and primary afferents in the peripheral nervous system might have played a substantial role in diminishing the increased sensitivity to mechanical stimuli. We found that the exposure to SMF on the first postoperative week, when the activity evoked chemical reorganization of nociceptive receptors and primary afferents (known as peripheral sensitization) occur in the early phase of chronic pain generation [156, 280, 281], did not prevent the development of mechanical allodynia. Thus, it appears that the SMF-exposure could not exert a substantial influence on neural events that lead to the development of peripheral sensitization.

However, the effectiveness of daily exposure to SMF was slightly more effective during the second postoperative week and was remarkably prominent when it was applied between postoperative days 15 and 28. It has been widely documented that just after the sensitization of nociceptive receptors and primary afferents long-lasting painful events like partial nerve ligation evokes a dramatic chemical reorganization also in the central pain processing apparatus that leads to the development of central sensitization of pain processing neural microcircuits in the central nervous system [156, 280, 281]. Most of these neural events that result in the development of central sensitization and consecutive chronic pain occur during the 1st and 2nd week after the commencement of pathologic processes such as nerve injury. Thus, it appears to be likely that SMF-exposure may have an influence on the chemical reorganization mechanisms of pain processing neural circuits and can effectively act on the pain processing apparatus after the development of central sensitization. The site of action may be multiple as suggested in **Pharmacological analysis**, but further pioneer studies also suggest, among many other possible targets, endogenous opioid systems may also be sensitive to SMF-exposure [27, 281].

We found that exposure to inhomogeneous SMF did not prevent the development of mechanical allodynia following partial nerve ligation. However, a 30 min long daily repetitive SMF-exposure that started just after the nerve ligation elevated

MWT by the end of the 2nd week to a modest but significant extent. More interestingly, first in the literature we also demonstrated that the effectiveness of a daily exposure to SMF was much more prominent when it was applied between postoperative days 15 and 28. In this case, MWT was already noticeably increased after the 1st treatment and it practically reached the control values by the end of a fortnight long period. The results suggest that exposure to SMF cannot prevent the development of mechanical allodynia, but can inhibit processes that maintain the increased sensitivity to mechanical stimuli in neuropathic pain. If neuropathy is induced by diabetes rather than direct nerve injury, would SMF-exposure influence the symptoms?

NEUROPATHIA DIABETICA

Exposure to Static Magnetic Field Reduces Symptoms of Neuropathia Diabetica

Preliminaries

As mentioned in **Exposure to static magnetic field ceases mechanical allodynia in neuropathic pain** already, neuropathic pain, and especially neuropathia diabetica is an illness that causes severe persistent pain in some point in the life of hundreds of million people worldwide. The search for reliable, safe, and effective treatments for neuropathic pain remains a major challenge [282].

If MRI is used for diagnostic goals in diabetic patients [283, 284], its SMF component may have an unexpected physiological effect as suggested in **Exposure to static magnetic field ceases mechanical allodynia in neuropathic pain**. Electromagnetic fields were shown to induce an effect, which was analgesia [285], vulnerability of diabetic rats [286], decrease of neurological deficit and required insulin daily dose, nerve conduction velocity increase, increase of the muscle compound action potentials (muscle power), and peripheral outflow [287].

Results obtained from studies that tested *AE* of SMF therapy in chronic pain are inconsistent. SMF treatment lowered the blood glucose levels and improved eye conditions in diabetes [288]. Magnetic insoles were found to have a positive effect [289]. Another clinical trial showed that permanent magnets applied in a sole reduced the numbness, burning pain, and tingling of the feet as effectively like gabapentine, tramadol, or lamotrigine treatment [267]. In this human trial the existence of sensory and motor diabetic peripheral neuropathy were required as an inclusion criterion. Others claimed that SMF-exposure had no advantage over sham-exposure in reducing pain intensity in patients with chronic lower back pain [269] or diabetic polyneuropathy [274]. More than 40 randomized, double-blind, placebo-controlled clinical trials of SMF therapy were collected and analyzed [43], also dosimetric considerations were completed [29].

Sporadic studies in animals have not provided more consistent results either. There are reports showing that rodents in a magnetically shielded environment showed strong analgesia [27]. On the other hand, increased pain sensitivity has also been shown to occur after exposure to a SMF environment [130, 242, 276]. However, since the parameters of the applied magnetic fields and models varied, most results are not intercomparable.

Goals

To avoid the obvious problems in the interpretation of the results of earlier studies, here

i. we used an apparatus for the generation of an inhomogeneous SMF, the parameters of which have been carefully tested and adjusted to small experimental animals (**Acute models**).
ii. The effectiveness of SMF on a well established model of neuropathic pain, neuropathia diabetica in mice was tested. We used a model of diabetes according to Khan *et al.* [290].

Our goal in the present examination was not only to prove or drop the assumption that the 30 min repetitive, daily exposure to SMF has an effect on mice with neuropathia diabetica, but also to compare our previous results obtained in the Seltzer model of neuropathic pain, but with the same SMF generator (previous **Exposure to static magnetic field ceases mechanical allodynia in neuropathic pain**).

Materials and Methods

Magnetic Exposure Conditions, Chemical Treatment

For SMF-exposure in generator 11 (**Generators 1-16**), two-three animals were put into the Plexiglas cage at a time keeping in mind that mice are socially sensitive [44], then the cage with the animals was inserted into the exposure chamber for 30 min per day for a period of time animals were alive (minimum of 6 weeks). The treatment was whole-body exposure, while animals were free to move in the cage. The magnetic exposure created with this magnetic exposure system did not cause any change in the anxiety behavior and locomotor activity of animals (**Locomotor activity and anxiety behavior in healthy mice**). Blinding was provided by keeping 2-3 control animals (not exposed to SMF, sham) at a time in identical Plexiglas cages for 30 min daily.

Streptozocin (STZ, provided by Tocris) was administered *i.p.* in some animals in different doses (100, 150, or 200 mg/kg) to induce diabetes.

Increasing-temperature Hot Plate Test

The increasing-temperature hot plate test [291] was used in the experiments. The plate (in contact with the paws) is slowly warmed from body temperature and the threshold temperature producing the first nocifensive behavior (*e.g.* paw licking) is recorded. By contrast, in the conventional, constant-temperature hot plate test, the plate is maintained at a noxious (52°C) temperature and the latency of paw licking nocifensive response is measured. The effect of even weak analgesics can be well assessed with the increasing-temperature hot plate method, because of its higher sensitivity and thus higher relevance than standard hot plate assay that is insensitive to such compounds [291, 292]. This method excludes the possibility of conditional reflex development and mice do not show paw licking behavior before the placement onto the plate. Since the temperature is increased only gradually into the noxious range, stress associated with the testing procedure is minimized, and thus the results obtained can more convincingly be thought of as reflecting true thermonociceptive thresholds.

The increasing-temperature hot plate test equipment was produced by Supertech.

The heated surface dimensions were 110×80 mm surrounded by 350 mm high transparent Plexiglas walls. The commanding computer program was set to produce a 3°C/min temperature increase of the plate. When hind paw licking or flinching were observed the threshold temperature was recorded. The measurement was terminated, when the plate temperature reached 50°C to avoid tissue damage [292].

Diabetes Induction by Single Dose of Streptozotocin Administration

Mice were rendered diabetic by a single dose of *i.p.* administered STZ in 100, 150, or 200 mg/kg body mass [290, 293]. STZ was prepared freshly by dissolving in 0.9% sterile physiological saline. Aside the 200 mg/kg dose, the 2 lower doses of STZ were set up for modeling the illness with reduced severity. All of the STZ-treated animals were included irrespective of their blood glucose level, because the SMF-exposure sequence was commenced 1 day after the STZ challenge.

Animals and Groups

Forty two CD-1 as well as 12 CFLP mice were kept at 22±3°C; the relative humidity was 30-70%, and the light/dark cycle was 12/12 h. They were maintained on a standard rodent pellet diet with tap water available *ad libitum.*

Animals were randomly divided into the following experimental groups.

Group 1: Animal number was 3. These animals did not get STZ at all. This was the non-treated group (negative control, sham, no STZ).
Group 2, 3, and 4: Animal number was 6/group, STZ was administered in an amount of 100, 150, and 200 mg/kg, respectively.

Animals in Groups 1-4 were not exposed to SMF (sham-exposure). Animals in Groups 5-8 were exposed to 30 min/day inhomogeneous SMF from day 1 until death.

Group 5: Animal number was 3. These animals did not get STZ at all. This was the SMF-exposure without STZ treatment group (SMF, no STZ).
Group 6, 7, and 8: Animal number was 6/group, STZ was administered in an amount of 100, 150, and 200 mg/kg, respectively.

Ethics

Altogether 54 naïve mice participated in 10 series of experiment. 36 animals got *i.p.* STZ, 27 animals were exposed to SMF.

Statistical Analysis

Single-factor ANOVA was used to test significant differences among multiple data sets. Statistical differences between binary experimental groups were estimated by Dunnett's *post hoc* test. Unequal sized data sets were compared using the Bonferroni's correction. Data series were considered significantly different, if their mean values differed with a probability (p) less than 0.05. The following statistical values are provided numerically in the text: F number for (between-group variability)/(between-group variability), F_{crit} critical value of F determining, whether the null hypothesis should be accepted or rejected, η^2 ratio of variance explained in the dependent variable by a predictor, while controlling for all other predictors ($SS_{treatment}/SS_{total}$, where SS stands for sum of squares).

Results

Although the experimental series was designed for 11 weeks, the 200 mg/kg STZ-administered animals died irrespective of the SMF treatment in the 6th week.

Effect of 30 min/day Inhomogeneous SMF-exposure on the Body Mass of Mice

Fig. (**5.41**) demonstrates the time evolution of the body mass in g averaged for the animals in the group (SEM is designated as positive error bars) for control and diabetic (200 mg/kg STZ) animals (Group 5 *vs* 1, and Group 8 *vs* 4).

Fig. (**5.41**) suggested that there might be a body mass effect of SMF-exposure for non-diabetic mice. In order to check this assumption, we introduced an additional set of experiments with 6 CFLP mice/group (Fig. **5.42**). Here we also registered water and rodent pellet consumption. We found no significant difference between body mass, water, or pellet consumption of SMF-treated and control mice in a 30 day long examination period. The slight difference in body mass following the first fortnight was due to a single mouse in the untreated and another in the treated group. The results of the ANOVA of the average body mass, water, and rodent pellet consumption values are collected in Table **5.11**. *p* stands for probability, two sets of data are statistically significantly different at the 95% confidence level, if $p<0.05$. Since we used different strains of mice, the results in Fig. (**5.42**) cannot be regarded as clear reproductions of those in Fig. (**5.41**). We think that the additional experimental series is reproducible.

Table 5.11. Statistical evaluation of the effect of 30 min/day SMF-exposure on the body mass, water, and rodent pellet consumption of non-diabetic mice. The table shows the probability of significance (p) at 95% confidence level and the corresponding p, F, F_{crit}, and η^2 values as obtained from single factor ANOVA estimation.

SMF- *vs* sham-exposed (*n*=6/group)	single factor ANOVA			
	P	*F*	F_{crit}	η^2(%)
Body mass	>0.05	0.19	4.10	0.49
Water consumption	>0.05	0.02	4.11	0.06
Rodent pellet consumption	>0.05	0.04	4.11	0.10

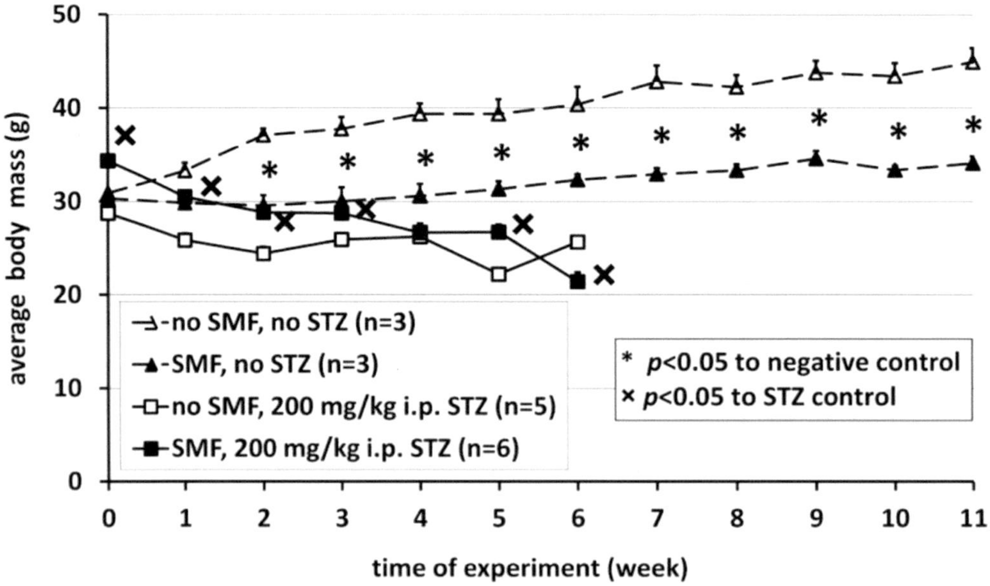

Fig. (5.41). Time evolution of the changes in the body mass (g) of non-diabetic, diabetic CD-1 mice with or without 30 min/day SMF-exposure starting with day 1 (before the STZ challenge). Note that diabetic mice died in the 6th week. Markers and error bars indicate mean values and SEM, respectively. * and × denote the probability of significant difference at the 95% confidence level between SMF- and sham-exposed groups for no STZ and 200 mg/kg STZ animals, respectively. Straight lines between markers guide the eye only.

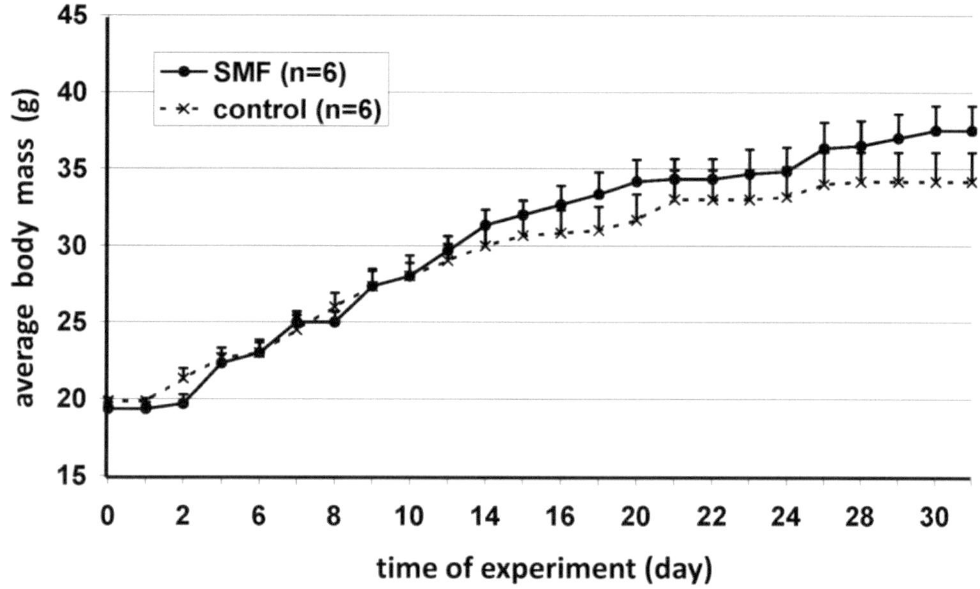

Fig. (5.42). Time evolution of the changes in the body mass (g) of non-diabetic CFLP mice with and without 30 min/day SMF-exposure. Markers and error bars indicate mean values and SEM, respectively. The time axis is not equidistant. The figure is no reproduction of Fig. (**5.41**).

Fig. (**5.43**) presents the dose dependence of the body mass in g averaged for the animals in a certain group and for the time period of the experiment (SEM is designated as positive error bar) in a column diagram. Animal numbers (*n*), time of the experiment (*t*) in weeks, and probability of significant difference at the 95% confidence level are also shown for Group 5 *vs* 1 (no STZ), Group 6 *vs* 2 (100 mg/kg STZ), Group 7 *vs* 3 (150 mg/kg STZ), and Group 8 *vs* 4 (full diabetes: 200 mg/kg STZ). Table **5.12** contains the results of the ANOVA analysis.

Table 5.12. Statistical evaluation of the effect of 30 min/day SMF-exposure on the body mass of diabetic and control mice. The table shows the probability of significance (p) at 95% confidence level and the corresponding p, F, F_{crit} and η^2 values as obtained from single factor ANOVA estimation.

SMF- *vs* sham-exposed (*n*=6/group)	condition (STZ)	single factor ANOVA			
		P	*F*	F_{crit}	η^2(%)
Group 6 *vs* 2	100 mg/kg	>0.05	0.59	3.91	0.41
Group 7 *vs* 3	150 mg/kg	<0.001*	40.58	3.91	22.22
Group 8 *vs* 4	200 mg/kg	<0.001*	15.76	3.97	16.99

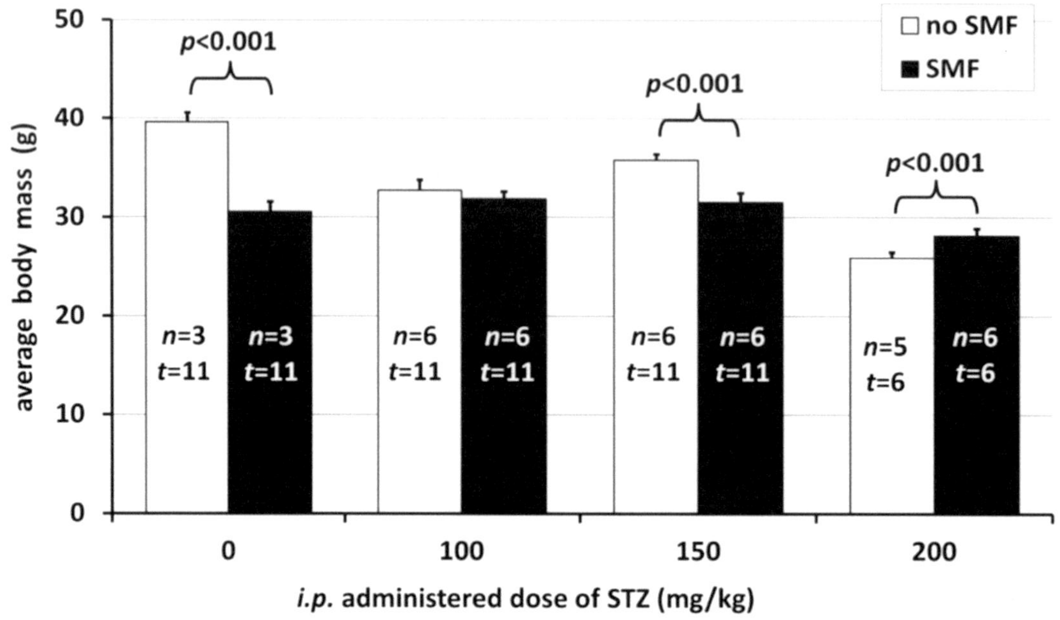

Fig. (5.43). Effect of 30 min/day SMF-exposure on the body mass (g) in diabetic CD-1 mice treated with i.p. STZ in an amount of 100, 150, or 200 mg/kg. The columns and error bars represent mean and SEM values, respectively. Open columns: Control (sham-exposed). Dark columns: SMF-exposed. The number of animals (n), testing time in weeks (t), and the significance level (p) between the corresponding data sets are indicated in or on top of the columns assessed by Dunnett's post hoc test.

Effect of 30 min/day Inhomogeneous SMF-exposure on the Blood Glucose Level of Mice

Fig. (**5.44**) demonstrates the time evolution of the blood glucose level in mM/l averaged for the animals in a certain group for control and diabetic (200 mg/kg STZ) animals (Group 5 *vs* 1, and Group 8 *vs* 4). * and × denote the probability of significant difference at the 95% confidence level between SMF- and sham-exposed groups for no STZ and 200 mg/kg STZ animals, respectively. The difference between SMF-treated and untreated animals was rarely significant; this happened on 2 days only and probably does not suggest any biological difference between the groups. For non-diabetic mice, there is no observable effect of SMF treatment. For diabetic mice, SMF treatment decreases average blood glucose level between 6.44% and 40.36%, by 22.83% on average.

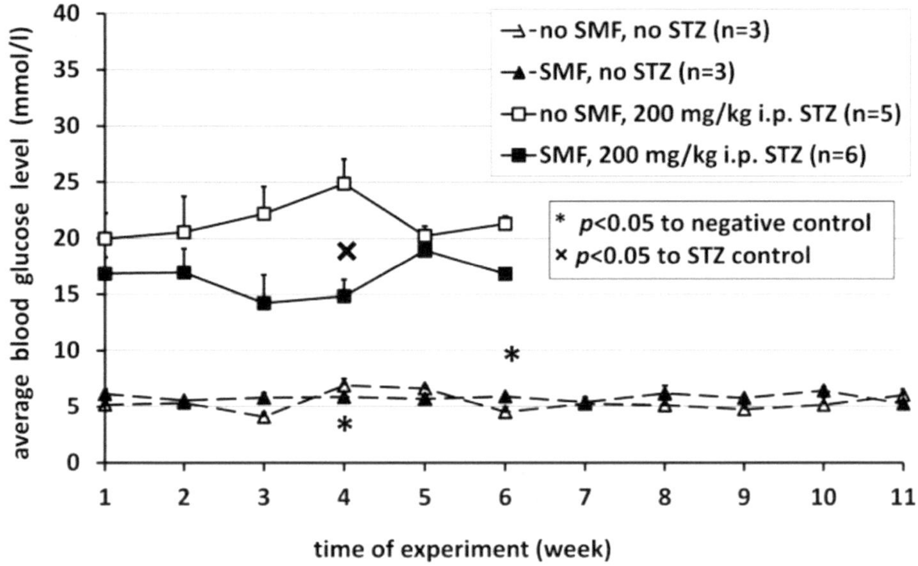

Fig. (5.44). Time evolution of the changes in blood glucose level (mM/l) in non-diabetic, diabetic CD-1 mice with or without 30 min/day SMF-exposure starting with day 1 (following the STZ challenge). Note that diabetic mice died in the 6th week. Markers and error bars indicate mean values and SEM, respectively. * and × denote the probability of significant difference at the 95% confidence level between SMF- and sham-exposed groups for no STZ and 200 mg/kg STZ animals, respectively. Straight lines between markers guide the eye only.

Fig. (**5.45**) presents the dose dependence of the blood glucose level in mM/l averaged for the animals in a certain group and for the time period of the experiment in a column diagram. Animal numbers (*n*), time of the experiment (*t*) in weeks, and probability of significant difference at the 95% confidence level are also shown for Group 5 *vs* 1 (no STZ), Group 6 *vs* 2 (100 mg/kg *i.p.* STZ), Group 7 *vs* 3 (150 mg/kg *i.p.* STZ), and Group 8 *vs* 4 (full diabetes: 200 mg/kg *i.p.* STZ). Table **5.13** contains the results of the ANOVA analysis.

Table 5.13. Statistical evaluation of the effect of 30 min/day SMF-exposure on the blood glucose level (mM/l) in diabetic and control mice. The table shows the probability of significance (*p*) at 95% confidence level and the corresponding p, F, F_{crit} and η^2 values as obtained from single factor ANOVA estimation.

SMF- *vs* sham-exposed (*n*)	condition (STZ)	single factor ANOVA			
		p	*F*	F_{crit}	η^2(%)
Group 5 (3) *vs* 1 (3)	-	<0.05*	4.56	3.99	6.65

(Table 5.13) contd.....

SMF- *vs* sham-exposed (*n*)	condition (STZ)	single factor ANOVA			
		p	*F*	F_{crit}	η^2(%)
Group 6 (6) *vs* 2 (6)	100 mg/kg	>0.05	1.22	3.93	1.12
Group 7 (6) *vs* 3 (6)	150 mg/kg	>0.05	1.83	3.92	1.51
Group 8 (6) *vs* 4 (5)	200 mg/kg	<0.001*	16.41	4.01	22.66

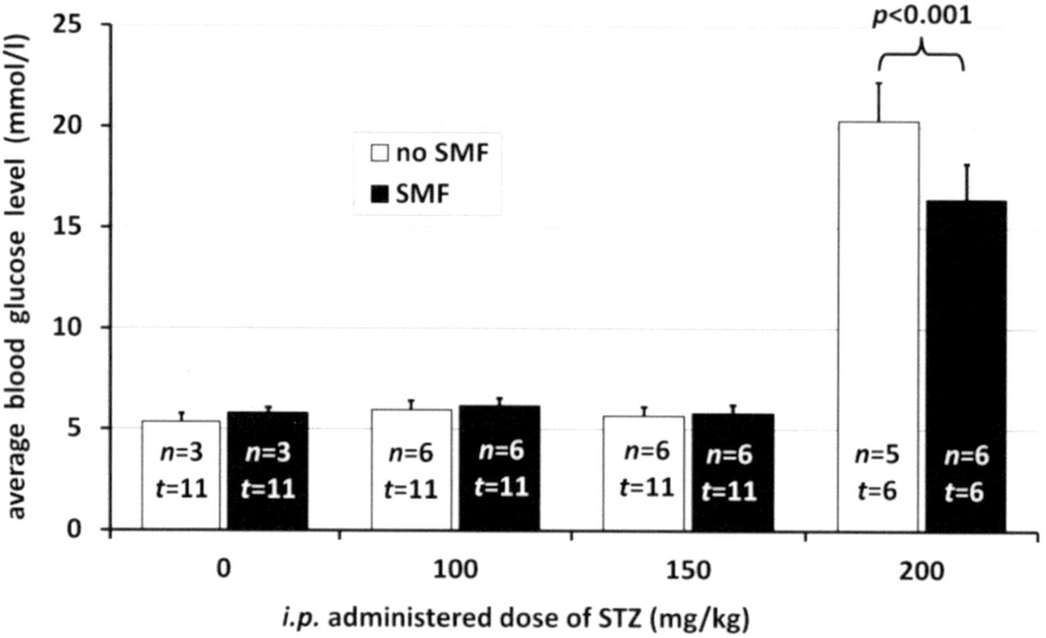

Fig. (5.45). Effect of 30 min/day SMF-exposure on blood glucose level (mM/l) in diabetic CD-1 mice treated with i.p. STZ in an amount of 0, 100, 150, or 200 mg/kg. The columns and error bars represent mean and SEM values, respectively. Open columns: Control (sham-exposed). Dark columns: SMF-exposed. The number of animals (n), testing time in weeks (t), and the significance level (p) between the corresponding data sets are indicated in or on top of the columns. Time evolution of the changes in nociceptive temperature threshold (°C) measured by increasing-temperature hot plate assay at non-diabetic, diabetic CD-1 mice with or without 30 min/day SMF-exposure starting with day 1 (following STZ challenge). Note that diabetic mice died in the 6th week. Markers and error bars indicate mean values and SEM, respectively. Straight lines between markers guide the eye only.

Effect of 30 min/day Inhomogeneous SMF-exposure on the Nociceptive Temperature Threshold of Mice in the Hot Plate Test

Fig. (**5.46**) demonstrates the time evolution of the thermonociceptive threshold temperatures in °C averaged for the animals in a certain group for control and diabetic (200 mg/kg STZ) animals (Group 5 *vs* 1, and Group 8 *vs* 4). * and ×

denote the probability of significant difference at the 95% confidence level between SMF- and sham-exposed groups for no STZ and 200 mg/kg STZ animals, respectively. No effect of the SMF treatment is observable for either non-diabetic or diabetic mice.

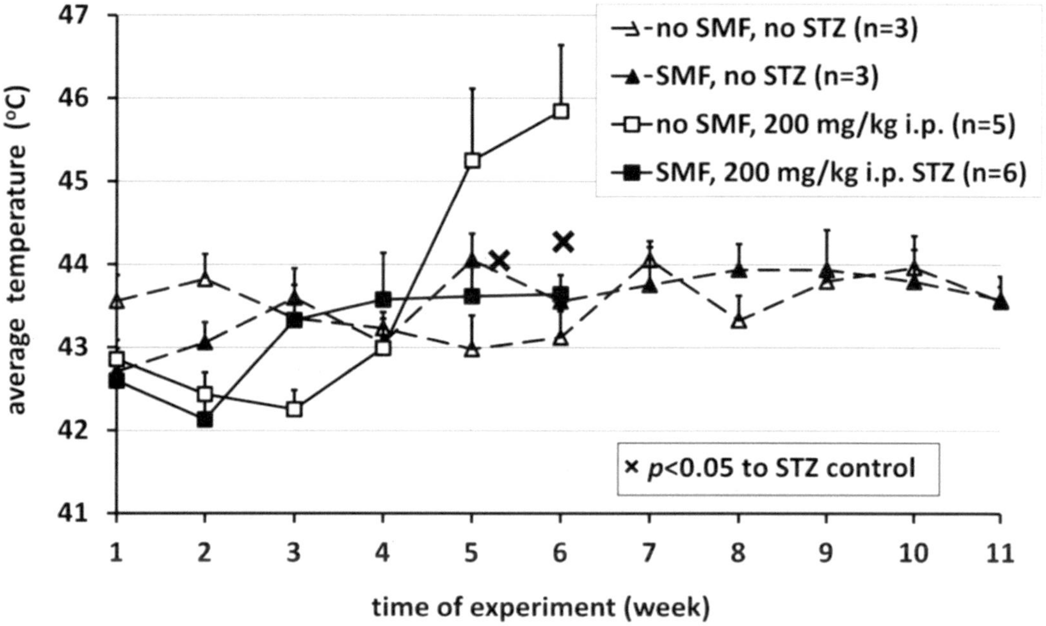

Fig. (5.46). Time evolution of the changes in nociceptive temperature threshold (°C) measured by increasing-temperature hot plate assay at non-diabetic, diabetic CD-1 mice with or without 30 min/day SMF-exposure starting with day 1 (following STZ challenge). Note that diabetic mice died in the 6th week. Markers and error bars indicate mean values and SEM, respectively. Straight lines between markers guide the eye only.

Fig. (**5.47**) presents the dose dependence of the thermonociceptive threshold temperatures in °C averaged for the animals in a certain group and for the time period of the experiment in a column diagram. Animal numbers (*n*), time of the experiment (*t*) in weeks, and probability of significant difference at the 95% confidence level are also shown for Group 5 *vs* 1 (no STZ), Group 6 *vs* 2 (100 mg/kg STZ), Group 7 *vs* 3 (150 mg/kg STZ), and Group 8 *vs* 4 (full diabetes: 200 mg/kg STZ). Due to the consistency of data and accordingly very small standard deviation (0.09 and 0.11), Group 6 and 2 were statistically slightly significantly different (p=0.043), even though no biological difference could be attributed to this fact (averages 43.54°C and 43.26°C, respectively). For the diabetic mice (Group 8 and 4) the nociceptive temperature threshold was significantly higher without SMF treatment, but the biological relevance is again questionable (averages 44.22°C and 43.15°C, respectively). Table **5.14** contains the results of the ANOVA analysis.

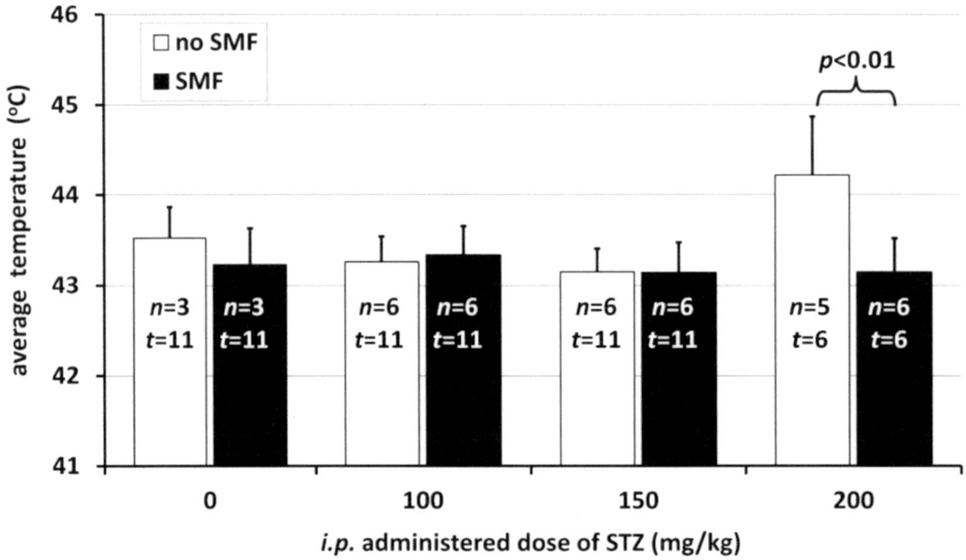

Fig. (5.47). Effect of 30 min/day SMF-exposure on temperature threshold (°C) measured by increasing-temperature hot plate assay in diabetic CD-1 mice treated with i.p. STZ in an amount of 0, 100, 150, or 200 mg/kg. The columns and error bars represent mean and SEM values, respectively. Open columns: Control (sham exposed). Dark columns: SMF-exposed. The number of animals (n), testing time in weeks (t), and the significance level (p) between the corresponding data sets are indicated in or on top of the columns.

Table 5.14. Statistical evaluation of the effect of 30 min/day SMF-exposure on the temperature threshold level measured by increasing-temperature hot plate assay at diabetic and control mice. The table shows the probability of significance (p) at 95% confidence level and the corresponding p, F, F_{crit} and η^2 values as obtained from single factor ANOVA estimation.

SMF- *vs* sham-exposed (*n*)	condition (STZ)	single factor ANOVA			
		p	F	F_{crit}	η^2(%)
Group 5 (3) *vs* 1 (3)	-	>0.05	2.17	3.99	3.28
Group 6 (6) *vs* 2 (6)	100 mg/kg	<0.05*	4.18	3.91	3.11
Group 7 (6) *vs* 3 (6)	150 mg/kg	>0.05	1.16	3.92	0.92
Group 8 (6) *vs* 4 (5)	200 mg/kg	<0.01*	7.99	4.02	12.69

Discussion, Conclusions

Effect on Body Mass

Several studies demonstrated that SMF-exposure has no significant effect on body mass. Developmental effects were studied in pregnant albino-mice after exposures to homogeneous 1 T SMF on days 7, 10, or 13 post conception [294]. No postnatal effects were observed in exposed mice as compared to unexposed control. Yan *et al.* [295] investigated the effects of SMF on bone formation of rat femurs evaluated using tapered rods made of magnetized and unmagnetized samarium cobalt of the same size. Authors failed to find any specific changes in the body mass of animals with either magnetized or unmagnetized rods. The potential adverse biologic effects of subchronic (cumulatively 10 weeks) exposure to a high SMF (9.4 T) were evaluated in young adult male and female Fischer rats as well as in their progeny in the study of High *et al.* [195]. Authors reported biologic end points including birth and also monitored body masses weekly. Findings from this study did not show any adverse biologic effects in male and female adult rats or their progeny that could be attributed to the exposure to SMF. Tablado *et al.* [296] examined the influence of *in utero* exposure to SMF in mice. Females were exposed to 0.5-0.7 T SMF from day 7 of gestation to the day of birth. No significant differences were found between exposed and sham-exposed animals with respect to body mass during the gestational period, body mass of male pups at the day of birth, and body mass gain of pups from birth to day 35.

Two studies suggested the contrary. In the study of Tsuji *et al.* [135] the effects of 5 T SMF-exposure on food and water intake in BALB/c mice were examined. The authors examined body mass changes resulting from changes in food and water intake. They concluded that exposure to 5 T SMF for 48 h suppresses eating and drinking behavior and supposed that the decreased body mass after exposure were due to body fluid loss resulting from decreased food and water intake. Hashish *et al.* [297] have more recently investigated the effects of continuous whole-body exposure to either SMF or 50 Hz electromagnetic field for 30 days on the body mass of mice. SMF-exposure resulted in a gradual mass loss. This was coupled with a significant decrease in the level of blood glucose.

In our experiments the animal model included STZ administration in different doses resulting in latent or severe diabetes. 150 and 200 mg/kg STZ led to opposite effects in the body mass, while no change was observed compared to control, when STZ was injected in a dose of 100 mg/kg. These results suggest that whole-body SMF treatment is controversial and depends on the diabetic state. Daily SMF-exposure was double-checked in CFLP mice so as not to cause a significant body mass change between non-treated and SMF-exposure without STZ-treatment groups. Neither have we experienced any difference in the food, nor in the water intake between exposed and unexposed animals.

Effect on Serum Glucose Levels

70 mg/kg STZ-hyperglycemic rats were shown to predispose the eye to produce high levels of IL-1β cytokines [298]. Large animal models with toxin-mediated pancreatic damage have been used extensively in research with respect to diabetes mellitus and cardiovascular diabetic complications. Lu *et al.* [299] used a Chinese Guizhou minipig model with 125 mg/kg STZ induced diabetes. They observed a significant elevation in the serum glucose levels 1 month and 6 months after STZ induction. Western blot analysis demonstrated a significant elevation of IL-1β as revealed by RT-PCR (reverse transcription-polymerase chain reaction). The NPI (neonatal porcine islets) are a potentially useful source of beta cells for transplantation to treat type 1 diabetes mellitus. Acute oxidative stress causing STZ, a nitric oxide-generating beta cell cytotoxin was able to impair *in vitro* NPI beta cell insulin release, whereas human pro-inflammatory cytokines (*e.g.* IL-1β) did not affect the secretory response, nor were they cytotoxic *in vitro*. Pro-inflammatory cytokines were shown though, to be cytotoxic to B cells, in part through the generation of nitric oxide [300]. High-fat diet and low dose (40 mg/kg) STZ induced diabetic rats were given NPH (Neutral Protamine Hagedorn) insulin or gliclazide for 3 weeks, initiated at the 3rd day after STZ injection as early treatment and NPH for 3 weeks at 1 month for late treatment. A decreased level of interleukin IL-1β in the liver was observed [301]. Ehses *et al.* [302] concluded that elevated islet IL-1β activity in Goto-Kakizaki rats promoted cytokine and chemokine expression leading to the recruitment of innate immune cells. Rather than being directly cytotoxic, IL-1β may be the driving force behind tissue inflammation that impacts both B cell functional mass and insulin sensitivity in

type 2 diabetes.

Pregnant rats were exposed to 128 mT SMF for 1 h/day from day 6 to day 19 of pregnancy. At 25°C, the exposure of rats for 13 consecutive days to SMF significantly induced an increase in hematocrit level by 6%, hemoglobin concentration by 12%, and LDH (lactate dehydrogenase) levels by 67% suggesting a hypoxia-like state. Moreover, exposure to SMF increased blood glucose and decreased insulin release leading to a diabetic-like state in pregnant rats [303]. The effect of SMF-exposure on the survival rate of LPS (*lipopoly*saccharide) induced male BALB/cByJ mice was tested [304]. Mice were exposed to 0.25 T SMF for 2 h before LPS injection. Additionally, the effect of a 2 h SMF treatment on the production of anti-inflammatory cytokines was examined. No significant changes in inflammatory cytokines including IL-1α, IL-6 in plasma were found following the exposure. The results showed that the plasma levels of IL-1ra (interleukin-1 receptor antagonist) were higher in the SMF-exposed group than in the sham group. The authors suggested that the exposure to SMF increased the plasma levels of IL-1ra.

Our experiments showed that 200 mg/kg STZ significantly elevated blood glucose level by about 4 times. This level could be significantly reduced by approximately 25% *via* SMF treatment on a daily basis.

In sum, we can hypothesize that the effect of 30 min/day whole-body SMF-exposure for several weeks can evoke an effect resembling the IL-1β receptor antagonist. Its effect may be equivalent to insulin intake in the sense that it reduces the malign influence of STZ, decreases oxidative stress, lowers IL-1β level, assists insulin release, discourages the recruitment of innate immune cells, and thus diminishes blood glucose level.

Effect on Peripheral Nociception

Sensory symptoms of 180 mg/kg STZ induced diabetic neuropathy were shown to be able to manifest as positive (painful), negative (insensate), or both [305]. Responses of diabetic mice in the cited experiments were significantly reduced during the 2nd phase of the formalin test beginning 3 weeks post-STZ. These results demonstrated that the reduced sensation occurring from progressive peripheral axon loss results in functional deficits in spinal cord activation. We presented similar results as the conclusion of SMF-exposure already in **Exposure to static magnetic field ceases mechanical allodynia in neuropathic pain**. Kamei *et al.* [306] showed that in the course of diabetic neuropathy development STZ treated mice show an allodynia phase in the first 3-4 weeks after STZ administration; hypoesthesia develops gradually afterwards. A similar effect may be seen in our present results; however, not for SMF-exposed mice. This suggests that a homeostatic defense mechanism may have been activated when SMF was applied. When comparing the present results to those of our previously discussed study (**Exposure to static magnetic field ceases mechanical allodynia in neuropathic pain**), we realized that the present results were far less convincing from the point of view of the beneficial effect of SMF-exposure in the treatment of neuropathic pain.

In the case of *in vivo* experiments with mammals, Xu *et al.* [307] made efforts to explore the role of SMF-exposure on modulating the muscle capillary microcirculation in pentobarbital-anesthetized mice under whole-body exposure to SMF. They found that the peak blood velocity significantly increased at SMF induction above 1 mT. Ichioka *et al.* [308] tested whether the skin temperature of rats in high induction (8 T) SMF decreased, but found no convincing evidence. Okano *et al.* [309] showed in a series of investigations that there was a relationship between the spatial gradients of SMF and the suppression of BP elevation in rats. They observed that under hypertensive conditions, the whole-body exposure to non-uniform SMF with peak magnetic gradient in the carotid sinus baroreceptor significantly attenuated the vasoconstriction and suppressed the elevation of BP. Del Seppia *et al.* [130] investigated the effect of exposure of low frequency electromagnetic fields on open field behavior and nociceptive responses in mice. They concluded that exposure to altered magnetic fields induced a more rapid habituation to a novel environment. McLean *et al.* [310] carried out experiments to find a potential supplement or alternative to the pharmacological treatment of epilepsy. They studied how SMF could modulate the severity of audiogenic seizures and anticonvulsant effects of phenytoin in DBA/2 mice and found that SMF pretreatment potentiated the effect of phenytoin. Shupak *et al.* [131] used a low frequency magnetic field to induce *AE* in mice.

Their experimental results suggested that pulsed magnetic fields could induce *AE* in mice without the side effects often associated with opiates like morphine. Veliks *et al.* [311] were interested in how SMF-exposure influenced the brain function of rats. They found that the predominant effects were bradycardia and the disappearance of respiratory sinus arrhythmia. The mechanism of pain relief of SMF-exposure in arthritic rats involves an increased blood circulation caused by the rise in the tail surface temperature [312]. These phenomena can interfere with the temperature threshold of pain sensation in our experiments as well. Nonetheless, the biphasic development of hyper- and hyposensitivity in temperature induced pain threshold is completely abolished by the daily SMF-exposure. Following an initial decrease in the temperature threshold the weekly measured values were not significantly different from the control. This might imply that it was the spontaneous repair mechanism of the injured nerve indeed that was assisted by the exposure as suggested in **Exposure to static magnetic field ceases mechanical allodynia in neuropathic pain** and not the improvement of the diabetic state.

The present results show that a 30 min/day whole-body SMF-exposure for several weeks failed to significantly affect the peripheral thermonociceptive pain threshold measured by increasing-temperature hot plate assay in STZ treated diabetic mice. The fact that animals died after 6 weeks in the SMF and STZ (200 mg/kg) treated group (Group 8) and after the 7th week in the STZ (200 mg/kg) treated group (Group 4) leads us to the conclusion that, in contrast to the improvement in the blood glucose level and temperature threshold, the severity of diabetes may have been higher compared to the animals treated with only STZ. Thus, the SMF treatment influences the survival of severe diabetic mice insignificantly. Among the physiological parameters measured in series week by week, no signs of agony were observed. Exposure to strong SMF can cause disturbances and can cause death among immune cells; however, non-dividing cells are not affected [313]. As STZ can cause B cell death *via* the mechanism of DNA damage precipitating poly(ADP-ribose (adenosine diphosphate-ribose)) synthetase activation followed by lethal nicotinamide adenine dinucleotide depletion [314] and free radical formation, which leads to DNA strand breaks. These breaks induce DNA repair involving the activation of poly(ADP-ribose) polymerase [315]. For this reason we hypothesize that SMF-exposure reduces the repair machinery as it disturbs the dividing cells.

Although many questions remain unanswered, the present study provides evidence that 30 min/day, whole-body exposure to inhomogeneous SMF significantly diminishes plasma glucose level as compared to control in diabetic mice. A parallel increase of the survival rate could not be observed. Water and food intake together with body mass and peripheral thermonociceptive threshold seemed to remain unaffected by the SMF-exposure. The next question that was deemed necessary to look into was whether SMF-exposure had an effect on a neurodegenerative disease of CNS.

VISCERAL ACTION

Exposure to Static Magnetic Field Delays Induced Preterm Birth Occurrence in Mice

Preliminaries

Despite intensive research, preterm birth (PTB) remains a central problem in modern perinatal medicine. PTB occurs in 5-10% of all pregnancies. Clinical, epidemiological, and experimental studies indicate that urogenital tract infections play a critical role in the pathogenesis of PTB. Moreover, intrauterine infections are often associated with the development of organ system diseases, such as cerebral palsy, asphyxia, or chronic lung disease. They significantly increase perinatal morbidity and mortality [316]. Ascending infection occurs, if pathogenic bacteria pass the cervical barrier. They can cause decidual and chorioamnial inflammation characterized by the bacterial infection of the amniotic fluid. The presence of bacteria induces the release of pro-inflammatory cytokines, *i.e.* interleukin 1 (IL-1) and tumor necrosis factor (TNF) by macrophages, amnion, deciduas, and myometrium. These pathophysiological mechanisms are leading to the induction of labor and dilation of the cervix [317]; moreover, cytokines are essential in balancing between neurotrophism and neurotoxicity [316].

The wide spectrum of reasons leading to PTB has not been clarified yet. In the past decades treatment and management of PTB have not improved much, the rate of PTB occurrence did not change significantly. It has been known for long that infections in mothers raise the risk of complications arising during delivery. Several risk factors of PTB have been identified: Intrauterine infection, inflammation, vascular pathophysiological conditions, uteroplacental ischemia, intrauterine bleeding, and over tension of the uterus. Genetic polymorphisms enhancing the intensity and/or the duration of the inflammatory reaction may also increase the risk of PTB [318].

Several of the well known risk factors of PTB increase inflammatory disposition [319]. It is well-known that inflammatory processes trigger a wide range of uterotonic factors, *e.g.* the influx of inflammatory cells into the uterus. Also elevated levels of pro-inflammatory cytokines (IL-1β, IL-6, IL-8, TNF-α) and prostaglandins were observed in the human amnion during parturition [320]. Pro-inflammatory cytokines can induce preterm spasms of the pregnant uterus by synthesizing prostaglandins among others [321]. The physiological activation of the decidua is responsible for the induction of uterine contractions. Latent inflammation in the uterus can activate the decidua well before term, which may lead to preterm contractions and to PTB [317]. The risk of PTB under autoimmune conditions is high [322] suggesting the participation of inflammatory processes mediated by the immune system in the commencement of preterm spasms of the uterus.

In the present experiments we used a murine model to explore the relation of inflammation of the uterus and PTB. Either local or systemic exposure to microbial products leads to PTB in several experimental models. LPS plays a key role in eliciting an inflammatory response that includes the activation of the immune cells and the release of enzymes involved in remodeling of the extracellular matrix leading to PTB [323]. LPS is recognized by a protein of the innate immune system including Toll-like receptor 4 (TLR4) [324]. Types of TLR4 serve as sentinels of uterine immunity in terms of the response to pathogens [325]. The connection between PTB and bacterial inflammation is proven by the effective antibiotics therapy in women at risk of PTB (see the review [326]).

There are reports of experimental studies showing that rodents exposed to SMF exhibited strong analgesia to various painful stimuli [27, 153, 275]. SMF-exposure was also demonstrated to deaden the pain originating from the inflamed peritoneum in the mouse (**Visceral action: The writhing test**).

The direct effect of SMF-exposure on inflammatory conditions was studied by Morris and Skalak [166]. Localized inflammation was induced *via* injection of inflammatory agents λ-carrageenan or histamine into rat hind paws, alone or in conjunction with pharmacological agents. Application of a 10 or 70 mT, but not 400 mT SMF for 15 or 30 min immediately following histamine induced edema resulted in a significant, 20-50% reduction in edema formation. A 2 h, 70 mT SMF-exposure to λ-carrageenan induced edema also resulted in significant (33- 37 %) edema reduction. We also showed in **Peripheral action** that inhomogeneous SMF-exposure significantly diminished the duration of formalin-evoked paw lickings and liftings in both phase I (acute somatic nociception) and phase II (acute inflammatory nociception). Selective inactivation of capsaicin-sensitive sensory fibers by high dose resiniferatoxin pretreatment decreased nocifensive behaviors in phase II of the formalin test indicating that pro-inflammatory neuropeptides, such as substance P and calcitonin gene-related peptide (CGRP) released from these fibers are involved in this inflammatory reaction.

Human experiences with local SMF-exposure on the pelvic domain are scarce. Holcomb *et al.* [263] studied 2 patients diagnosed with intervertebral disk disease at spinal cord levels that could be responsible for their chronic pain in the abdomen and genitals. The authors found a surprisingly rapid relief in both cases upon continuous local SMF-exposure with a quadrupolar arrangement of 4 permanent magnets B_r=1.2 T); not to mention that the effect was sustained for over 2 years. Brown *et al.* [266] performed a randomized, double-blind, placebo-controlled trial with 32 patients at a gynecology clinic. They confirmed a significant effect in Pain Disability Index, Clinical Global Impressions-Severity, and Clinical Global Impressions-Improvement scores in the group treated with continuous local exposure with 50 mT compared to the group receiving sham-exposure. They admitted, though, that it was likely that patients could identify the type of treatment they received.

Goals

The main initiatives to perform our experiments were:

i. To potentially broaden the treatment options of pregnant women with pain and inflammation. Many of the currently available clinical treatments of the inflammatory state have limited effectiveness and their action is often accompanied by distressing side effects. The search for reliable, safe, and effective treatments for inflammation remains a major medical problem, and not surprisingly, patients have continuously been exploring complementary or alternative approaches (for a the review see *e.g.* [327]). Among a number of other treatment strategies, magnetic therapy is increasingly used to alleviate pain and shorten the period of healing. Magnets appeal to patients because they promise a simple solution for pain relief; they are relatively safe, drug free, durable, and non-invasive [328].

ii. The proliferation of high field Magnetic Resonance Imaging (MRI) equipments makes it necessary to tackle any possible (beneficial or adverse) effects of SMF-exposure, gradient magnetic field, and radio-frequency electromagnetic radiation that may be exerted on living tissues [329], with special emphasis on pregnant women [330]. We decided to test the effectiveness of SMF-exposure in inflammation induced PTB first in the literature. Inflammation was produced by *i.p.* administered bacterial lipopolysaccharide (LPS) in mice. The rationale was to explore the effect of an inhomogeneous SMF-exposure on inflammation induced PTB in a widely used experimental rodent model under easily reproducible experimental circumstances and with an SMF optimized for pain inhibition, and validated for rodent experiments. We also planned to make dose dependence.

Materials and Methods

Magnetic Exposure Conditions, Animals

Inhomogeneous SMF was produced by generator 11 (*c.f.*, **Generators 1-16**). The time period of SMF-exposure, 40 min was chosen in order to obtain results comparable with those in the writhing test (**Visceral action: The writhing test**). The idea of the frequency of SMF-exposure was confirmed; robust results could be achieved with the same magnetic treatment under different, induced pathological conditions. SMF-exposure created with this specific magnetic exposure system was shown not to introduce significant changes in the anxiety behavior and locomotor activity of the animals (**HEALTHY ANIMALS Locomotor activity and anxiety behavior in healthy mice**).

E. coli LPS (serotype 0111:B4, Sigma-Aldrich) was dissolved in phosphate buffer solution (PBS). LPS was administered *i.p.* in mice in an amount of 25 μg/mouse (~1 mg/kg) on a single occasion on day 15 of gestation. According to the literature this dose induces PTB within 17 h following the challenge [331].

Timed-pregnant C57BL/6 mice were used in the experiment. Gestation age was determined with the help of a vaginal plug (day 0 of gestation). The conventional timing of gestation was used, where pregnancy begins with the maternal recognition of the embryo around the time of implantation (day 5 of gestation).

Thirty four female mice were randomly divided into the following 5 experimental groups:

Group 1: Intact (untreated) gravid animals (n=6). This was negative control group.
Group 2: Gravid animals exposed to 40 min/day whole-body SMF-exposure starting on day 14 of gestation, cumulated exposure time *cca.* 6×40 min, n=6.

In Group 1 and 2 the expected delivery was on day 19 of gestation. In Groups 3-5 gravid animals were treated with *i.p.* LPS to induce PTB.

Group 3: Gravid animals not exposed to SMF (n=7). This group served as positive control group.
Group 4: Gravid animals exposed to 40 min/day whole-body SMF-exposure starting on day 14 of gestation until delivery, cumulated exposure time 3×40 min, n=7.
Group 5: Gravid animals exposed to 40 min/day whole-body SMF-exposure starting on day 1 of gestation until delivery, cumulated exposure time 17×40 min, n=8.

One male mouse was randomly allocated to each group of females. These male mice were utilized to impregnate all the females in their specific groups and were then separated from the females. Male mice did not participate in the experiment otherwise; neither were they injected with LPS, nor were they exposed to SMF.

Control animals (both negative and positive) were kept in identical perforated Plexiglas cages for 40 min/day. For all treatments (sham and SMF) 2 animals were put into the Plexiglas cage at a time keeping in mind that mice are socially sensitive creatures [44], then the cage with the animals was either inserted into the exposure chamber (SMF) or left alone (sham) for 40 min every day of the treatment.

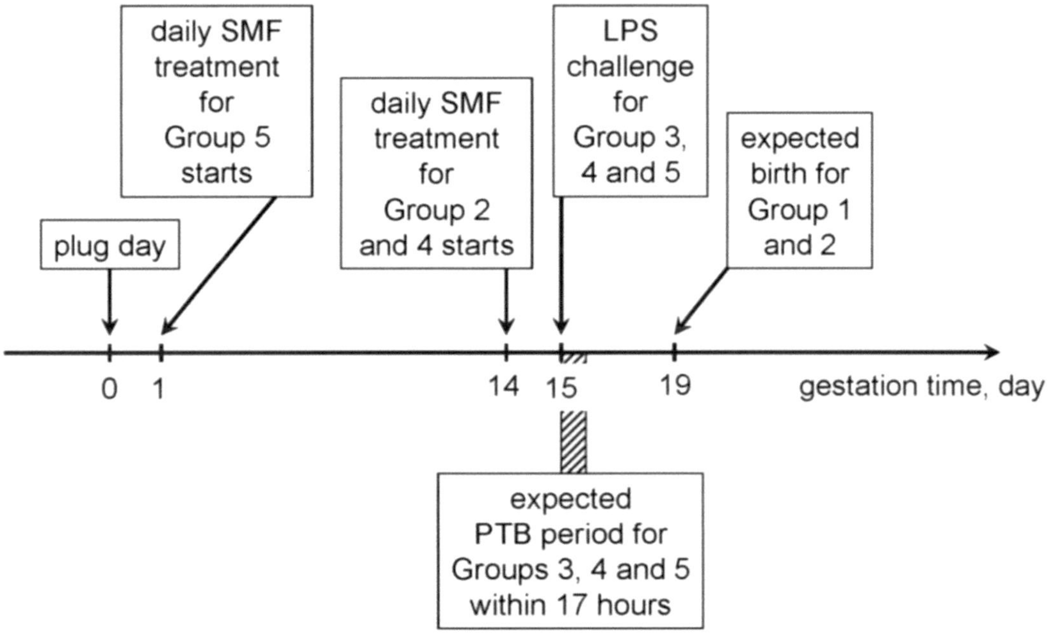

Fig. (5.48). Flow diagram of the series of experiments. LPS designates 25 μg/mouse intraperitoneal (i.p.) lipopolysaccharide challenge, SMF stands for 40 min/day whole-body inhomogeneous static magnetic field-exposure starting on day 1 (Group 5) or day 14 (Group 2 and 4) of gestation. Plug day is by definition day 0 of gestation.

The treatment of animals in Group 2 and 4 started on gestation day 14 only, because previous experimental results suggested that the SMF-exposure of healthy animals may not have any physiological effects [166], **HEALTHY ANIMALS Locomotor activity and anxiety behavior in healthy mice** in this book. However, we intended to test this assumption by introducing Group 5. We presumed that data of Group 4 and 5 could be pooled, supposed their averages do not significantly differ from each other. The flow diagram of the experimental series can be seen in Fig. (**5.48**).

C57BL/6 mice were kept at 22±3°C; the relative humidity was 30-70%, the light/dark cycle was 12/12 h. They were maintained on a standard rodent pellet diet with water *ad libitum*. Care was taken to treat animals (SMF-treated as well as controls) during the same time of the day preventing the circadian cycle of mice disturb the measurements.

The Plexiglas cage was illuminated with halogen lights from above during the experiments. The shaded area was always bigger than 94×140 (×46) mm during the experiments similarly to the circumstances described in **Clinical MRI**. The lamps generated a scattered light in the shaded area of the cage between 3.9-20.6 lx. Background noise in the laboratories remained below 50 dBC. Lighting and noise stimuli were identical for control and treated animals.

Since the results showed only minimal inter-animal variations within the experimental groups and because of the bioethical necessity of minimizing animal suffering by keeping the number of experimental animals as low as possible, we did not involve more animals than absolutely necessary to achieve statistically adequate sample sizes. Altogether 34 naïve female mice participated in 5 types of experiment. 22 animals got *i.p.* LPS injection, 21 animals were exposed to SMF.

Statistical Analysis

In general, we applied 2-contrasts testing. We carried out a dose-effect evaluation with 2 doses plus control. Our null hypothesis was that in Group 4 and 5 the times of delivery would be bigger than in Group 1 (effect test). We also presumed that the values will be bigger in Group 5 than in Group 4 (dose test). In order to evaluate the effect, we pooled Group 4 and 5 and compared this data series to that of Group 1 using a one sided Dunnett's test. Another one sided Dunnett's test proved the dose effect between Group 4 and 5. For multiple group analysis we used one-way ANOVA, F, F_{crit}, and p are shown in the text.

Results

Gestation time in days was compared between Group 1 (negative control) and Group 2 (6×40 min cumulative SMF-exposure starting on day 14) animals. The average values (±SEM) were not significantly different (19.33±0.21 *vs* 19.00±0.26), one-way ANOVA resulted in F=1.00, F_{crit}=4.96, and p=0.17. The expected value based on the literature is 19 days (from gestation day 0). No birth occurred during exposure.

The pups born after the SMF-exposure did not show any major changes in outlook or behavior compared to their unexposed mates.

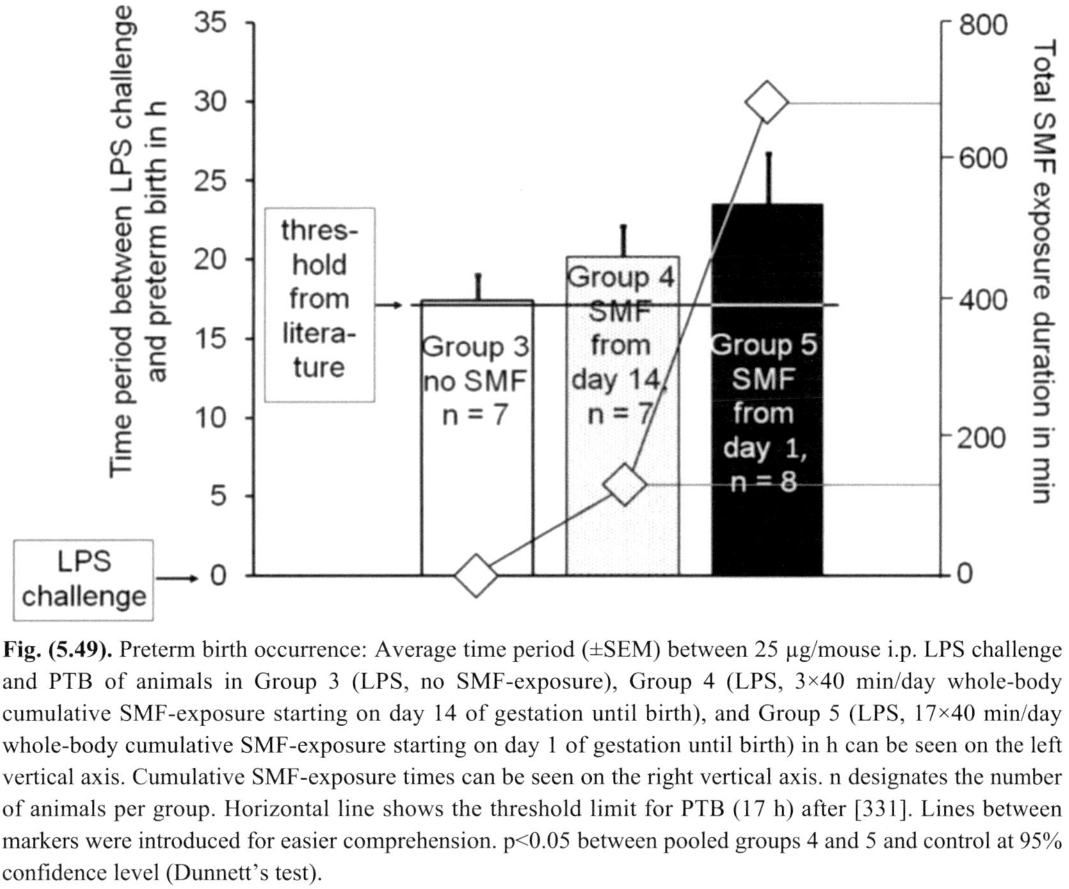

Fig. (5.49). Preterm birth occurrence: Average time period (±SEM) between 25 µg/mouse i.p. LPS challenge and PTB of animals in Group 3 (LPS, no SMF-exposure), Group 4 (LPS, 3×40 min/day whole-body cumulative SMF-exposure starting on day 14 of gestation until birth), and Group 5 (LPS, 17×40 min/day whole-body cumulative SMF-exposure starting on day 1 of gestation until birth) in h can be seen on the left vertical axis. Cumulative SMF-exposure times can be seen on the right vertical axis. n designates the number of animals per group. Horizontal line shows the threshold limit for PTB (17 h) after [331]. Lines between markers were introduced for easier comprehension. p<0.05 between pooled groups 4 and 5 and control at 95% confidence level (Dunnett's test).

The length of time between LPS challenge and PTB was compared between Group 3 (positive control or sham), Group 4 (3×40 min/day cumulative SMF-exposure starting on day 14), and Group 5 (17×40 min/day cumulative SMF-exposure starting on day 1). The average values (±SEM) were not significantly different (17.43±1.59, 20.14±1.96, and 23.50±3.20, respectively), one-way ANOVA resulted in F=1.57, F_{crit}=3.52, and p=0.23. The data can be seen in Fig. (**5.49**) completed with a function of cumulative SMF-exposure time in min.

Although the statistical analysis could not reveal significant differences between data series, the observed PTB times show an interesting phenomenon: They increase by about 20% with increasing SMF-exposure time from 17 to 20 h and then to 23 h for 0, 3×40, and 17×40 min total SMF-exposure, respectively. The correlation between the cumulated SMF-exposure time and the time period between LPS challenge and PTB occurrence is 96%. This manifests a dose-dependence at fixed magnetic induction. The dose effect was not significant, times of delivery in Group 4 and 5 did not differ from each other significantly. The effect test was positive, the difference between sham-exposed (Group 1) and SMF-exposed groups (Group 4 and 5 pooled) was statistically significant (p=0.043).

Discussion, Conclusions

<u>General Consequences</u>

In **Optimization of SMF parameters**, it was demonstrated that a single SMF-exposure of 30 min duration could achieve an antinociception over 80% in the writhing test (based on an acute visceral inflammation in the peritoneum) in mice.The results of **Pharmacological analysis** suggest that acute exposure of mice to SMF results in an opioid-mediated analgesic action in the writhing test. This *AE* is likely to be mediated by μ-opioid receptors. It was also speculated that *AE* of SMF may be due to the release of either β-endorphin or endomorphin-2 in the spinal cord. Pain sensation in women on the other hand, is often related to visceral inflammation [332]. On the basis of these observations we may have predicted that exposure of animals to SMF evoked changes in the pain processing apparatus of the nervous system and reduce inflammation. Placing mice under

SMF-exposure for 30 min was shown in **Peripheral action** not to affect their rotarod performance; conclusively, the impairment of motor function cannot be considered as a factor influencing labor.

The effect of 0.25 T homogeneous SMF on the production of IL-1 receptor antagonist has recently been studied *in vivo* in BALB/cByJ male mice that were exposed to SMF for 2 h before the *i.p.* injection of 50 mg/kg LPS [304]. Authors found that both the survival rate and the plasma IL-1ra level in the SMF-exposed group were higher by almost 100% than in the sham-exposed group. The authors proposed that the possible mechanism by which SMF-exposure prevents the development of disseminated intravascular coagulation is *via* the up regulation of IL-1ra rather than *via* the down regulation of pro-inflammatory cytokines. In other words, the changes in this marker suggest that SMF-exposure exerts an anti-inflammatory effect by stimulating the binding of IL-1ra to IL-1 receptors, thereby rendering IL-1 incapable of inducing an inflammatory response [333].

In a number of pathologic situations leading to PTB (cervical insufficiency, uterine stress, fetal-placental hypoxia, *etc.*) no relationship has been established to inflammatory conditions, to the release of pro-inflammatory cytokines. Studies of such situations under SMF-exposure are missing in the literature. We are aware of one single study [303] that was devoted to the effect of 1 h/day exposure of female rats to 128 mT SMF from gestation day 6 through day 19 on hematopoiesis and biochemical parameters. SMF-exposure was found to, thought slightly, but significantly increase the hematocrit level and the hemoglobin concentration, and strongly and significantly increase the lactate dehydrogenase, indicating a hypoxia-like state. Exposure also increased blood glucose level and decreased insulin release, leading to a diabetic-like state in pregnant rats.

The similarity between results of Group 1 and 2 suggested a week long, daily 40 min SMF-exposure for one week affected neither the timing of the implantation, nor the occurrence of birth. Because of prostaglandin release and cytokine up regulation term labor itself shows inflammatory-like pathology. We know that prostaglandin plays an important role in bone formation. SMF-exposure was shown to promote osteoblast differentiation *in vitro* and increase bone formation *in vivo* and in clinical studies. A study [334] reported that 10 T with no gradient had no effect either on prostaglandin E(2) (PGE(2)) secretion from a mouse osteoblastic cell line, MC3T3-E1, or PGE(2)-synthesizing enzyme, cyclo-oxygenase 2 (COX-2), and translocation of the transcription factor nuclear factor xB (NF-xB), which is involved in the induction of COX-2 expression. PGE(2) secretion was about 50%, COX-2 expression 100%, and NF-xB translocation by 100-200% higher under 6 T and maximal 41.7 T/m SMF-exposure than under sham conditions. (We must add that Breunig *et al.* [335] did not find any effect of PGE(2) release due to 85-120 mT continuous exposure for 72 h.) If we put all these facts together, we may conclude that an inhomogeneous SMF-exposure may be able to affect even term labor, but the expected effect lies probably within the error limit of the present measurement.

We checked the health condition of the newborn pups, since it was shown that even a short period of exposure of pregnant mice to a strong, homogeneous (400 mT) SMF in a dorso-ventral (DV) direction had teratogenic effects on the developing fetuses Saito *et al.* [336]. The authors observed various malformations of fetuses, which were exposed to the SMF *in utero* for 60 min/day from days 7.5 to 14.5 of pregnancy. Yip *et al.* [337] reported that a combined exposure of 1.5 T SMF, 64 MHz radio-frequency electromagnetic wave and a switched gradient field mimicking an MRI sequence was applied on chicken eggs for 6 h. Exposed embryos after 6 day incubation showed a trend toward higher abnormality and mortality rates than controls. In our experiment the applied inhomogeneous SMF had magnetic induction components in the DV direction; however, the processing and outcome of pregnancy were normal and the pups of animals not treated with LPS although, exposed to SMF-exposure from day 14 of gestation were born alive, and they looked, and behaved healthily.

The difference of almost 4 h in PTB occurrence between SMF-exposed and unexposed mice is not only statistically significant, but the results extrapolated to humans may be of clinical importance.

Limitations of the Present Study, Alternative Interpretations of the Results

As discussed earlier in **Lateral gradients**, the body of freely moving rodents in a SMF is subject to magnetic fluxes and consequently, induced electric currents.

The study design could not reveal differences between direct action of the exposure and indirect action through motion induced magnetic induction. The significant effect of daily SMF-exposure on PTB occurrence may or may not be due to electric currents in the body of the moving mice.

A 40 min daily SMF-exposure statistically significantly prolonged the duration of time between LPS challenge and PTB. This result suggests that exposure to SMF does not affect the timing of nidation or the length of pregnancy in intact animals, but may delay delivery in mice with *i.p.* infection. It appears plausible to hypothesize that 40 min/day exposure to inhomogeneous SMF delays the onset of PTB. Although this method may be quite new to the Reader, but especially obstetricians and gynecologists should be aware of the (patho)physiological effects involved, when their patients get exposed to the strong SMF in MRI devices. The applicability of the method, if proven to be effective in human therapy, relies also on MRI, where whole-body exposure can be the easiest realized, supposed the effect is directly due to the exposure. A potential limitation to clinical relevance is the repetitive, daily SMF-exposure starting 1 to 14 days before the LPS challenge for Group 4 or Group 5, respectively. Comparison between pre- and post-challenge exposure in the writhing test (**Optimization of SMF parameters**) showed however, that post-challenge application is more effective; the effect of pre-challenge exposure may be due to the prolonged effect of the exposure.

High field MRI devices are often reported to cause vertigo, nausea, metallic taste, magnetophosphenes, headache (see the review [338]). However, these symptoms seem to be reversible. No other significant side effects have been found so far. Further studies are needed to analyze the background mechanisms in detail and determine the value of the present technique in human therapy.

Having collected a series of strong experimental evidence about the effect of SMF-exposure in different animal models we may as well take a look at whether SMF-exposure was found similarly effective in measurements including human cells or humans as subjects.

CHAPTER 6

Human Investigations

Keywords: γ-ray irradiation, Cytokines, Dental, DNA repair, Human cell, Human subjects, Lymphocytes, Macrophages, Osteoporotic, Stomatological, TPT, VAS pain rating.

Table **6.1** summarizes the subjects with the disease (if any) and methods of testing we shall focus in the present chapter.

Table 6.1. Subjects with disease (if any) and methods of testing.

	Healthy volunteers	Patients with erosive gastritis	Patients with vertebral deformity	Patients with alveolitis	Patients with oral aphta	Patients with temporo-mandibular disorder	Patients with caries	Patients in preparation of prosthetics
Laboratory			×					
Numerical rating scale							×	×
Thermal pain threshold	×							
Tolerance threshold measurement							×	×
Visual analogue scale		×	×	×	×	×		

The WHO [12] in a Research Agenda encouraged the following in terms of human studies: "Cognitive and behavioral effects of static magnetic fields with the rationale: The cognitive and behavioral effects due to exposure to static magnetic fields should be investigated further. However, the available data do not suggest particular risks to specific aspects of cognition nor do they suggest which

János F. László

parameters should be tested in the laboratory. In the absence of a clear direction, a possible approach would be to investigate the effects of exposure on the performance of a battery of cognitive tasks that encompass standard tests of attention, reaction time and memory, if only to act as an initial screen pending more focused work. The initial work could be done with volunteers as part of experimental studies."

Taking up the challenge and following Galen's indication, who advocated the application of magnetic therapy for curing scars that are caused by infectious materials [339], interesting human experiments have been carried out during the past 2 decades concentrating on the applicability of SMF-exposure and low frequency (<1 Hz) electromagnetic field irradiation in medicine as a non-contact, non-invasive, and cheap physiotherapeutic method. An increasing amount of evidence indicates that SMF or low frequency electromagnetic fields can induce *AE* in humans, mostly with regard to chronic pain. The beneficial effect of SMF in curtailing the inflammatory period was also observed [340]. Among the participants of published trials were patients with pain in the abdomen and genitals (see Holcomb *et al.* [263]), with musculoskeletal disorders due to prolonged sitting (see Capodaglio and Vicenzi [341]), with fibromyalgia (see Alfano *et al.* [264]), with foot disorders (see Suomi *et al.* [342] and Simoncini *et al.* [343]), with chronic pelvic pain (see Brown *et al.* [266]), with chronic knee pain (see Hinman *et al.* [233]), with osteoarthritis [344], spine disorders [345], with myofascial pain syndrome (see Smania *et al.* [346]), or even diabetic neuropathic pain [267]. In these studies, the beneficial effect of SMF-exposure in the form of either *AE* or the shortening of the inflammatory period was observed and reported. Engström *et al.* [347] conducted an experiment on how exposure to strongly inhomogeneous SMF influenced myosin phosphorylation and found that the magnitude of magnetic induction alone could not be responsible for the effect. Gmitrov and Ohkubo [9] suggested the use of local SMF-exposure to moderate sympathetic activation and baroreceptor dysfunction. Salvatore *et al.* [348] showed how SMF could be fruitfully combined with chemotherapy in patients with advanced malignancy. Others found no effect of SMF on nociceptive transmission and pain symptoms in humans [272, 349]. Yet other studies dealt with the effects caused by SMF-exposure in humans, such as Mayrovitz *et al.*

[350] who found no change in the resting skin blood flow in humans under the influence of 85 mT SMF measured by laser-Doppler.

Precise evaluation of the efficacy of several differently applied magnetic therapies has led to conflicting conclusions in meta-analysis; SMF therapy showed no benefits compared to placebo controls [42]. These contradictory results are mainly due to human factors that are inevitable. Many clinical studies are limited either because of subject awareness of the control group (lack of magnetic properties of sham devices is easily detectable); because of an incorrect or incomplete characterization of the applied SMF [351],or because there is high variability in the biological response to pain [352]. Colbert *et al.* [29] fortunately enumerated a 10point list of conditions for the standardized description of SMF-exposure in a trial. In the long-run this list will foster intercomparability of measured results.

MATERIALS

Chemicals were purchased from (in alphabetical order) Abbott (Chicago, IL, US A), ALK-Abello (Hørsholm, Denmark), Beckman Coulter (Brea, CA, USA), Cambrex BioScience (Verviers, Belgium), Roche Diagnostics (Mannheim, Germany), DiaSorin (Stillwater, OK, USA), GIBCO (Carlsbad, CA, USA), ICN Biomedicals (Irvine, CA, USA), Merck (Whitehouse Station, NJ, USA), Reanal (Budapest, Hungary), Sanofi (Paris, France), Sigma-Aldrich (St. Louis, MO, US A). Kits and devices were provided by (in alphabetical order) Denjoy Dental (Changsha, Hunan, China), Iwaki (Tokyo, Japan),Kinetic Imaging (Bromborough, UK), Lincoln Diagnostics (Decatur, IL, USA), GE Healthcare (Little Chalfont, Bucks, UK), Metripond Plus (Hódmezővásárhely, Hungary), Nikon (Kawasaki, Kanagawa, Japan), OMRON Electronics (Budapest, Hungary), Pharmacia Biotech (Stockholm, Sweden), Roche Diagnostics (Basel, Switzerland), Siemens (Munich, Germany), and Spektrum-3D (Debrecen, Hungary).

IN VITRO EXPERIMENTS

DNA Damage

Static magnetic field-exposure fails to affect repair of DNA damage damage

Preliminaries

The proliferation of magnetic resonance imaging (MRI) as a diagnostic device has evoked a range of experiments where the potential adverse effect of static magnetic field (SMF) and electromagnetic radiation was studied. In many of these experiments, the focus was on genotoxicity. The subjects were healthy or pathologic human cells, and the method was *in vitro*: Chromosome aberration, sister chromatid exchange, micronucleus formation, assays for mutagenesis or tests for the DNA damage. The results are contradictory even within one single publication; authors reveal positive as well as negative effects. The reports published by WHO [12] and by Scientific Committee on Emerging and Newly Identified Health Risks of the EU [13] give a fair summary of the literature.

Pacini *et al.* [353] exposed human skin fibroblasts to 0.2 T SMF in an MR. They studied cell morphology after 1 h exposure and found a decrease of thymidine incorporation and of 2nd messenger formation. Takashima *et al.* [354] also assessed the possibility that exposure to strong SMF caused DNA damage and mutation. The exposure to 2, 5, or 14 T SMF for 24 h caused a statistically significant enhancement in somatic recombination frequency in the post-replication repair-deficient *Drosophila melanogaster*. Salerno *et al.* [355] investigated the release of cytokines, expression of surface markers, cell proliferation, and levels of cytosolic free calcium in human $CD4^+$ T-cell lines in a 0.5 T MR with 2 h exposure time. Their results showed that SMF gave rise to transient biological effects on T lymphocytes. Ghibelli *et al.* [356] demonstrated a strong (1.8-2.5 fold) increase of damage induced apoptosis by 1 T SMF-exposure in human tumor cells of hematopoietic origin. Tenuzzo *et al.* [357] observed that the effect of the exposure to 0.6 mT SMF for 24-48 h exposure durations on the apoptosis of human lymphocytes, mice thymocytes, and cultures of 3DO, U937, HeLa, HepG2, and FRTL-5 cells served as the promotion of apoptosis and mitosis, but not of necrosis or modifications of the cell shape. In their study, Schwenzer *et al.* [358] used a 3 T MR to study the clonogenic ability, proliferation, and cell cycle in embryonic human lung cell lines. They found no effect attributable to SMF-exposure. Amara *et al.* [359] examined the effect of SMF-exposure on the DNA damage in THP cells with exposures of 250 mT for 1, 2, or 3 h. They could not identify any change in the DNA damage.

There were examinations devoted to the effect of exposure to inhomogeneous SMF as well. Okano *et al.* [360] studied the effects of a moderate intensity, inhomogeneous SMF in the early stage development of endothelial capillary tubule formation using co-cultured human umbilical vein endothelial cells and human diploid fibroblasts. The co-cultured cells within a well were exposed to SMF of an induction up to 120 mT with the maximum spatial gradient being 21 T/m. Their findings suggested that the application of SMF to intact or VEGF-A stimulated vascular endothelial cells lead mainly to promote or enhance arteriogenesis in the peripheral part of the wells, where the spatial gradient increased relative to the central part. Hashish *et al.* [297] dealt with the effect of continuous SMF-exposure for 30 days on some liver and blood parameters in mice. Their dosimetric value for the induction was ±2.9 μT. A significant decrease in the counts of monocytes, platelets, peripheral lymphocytes as well as splenic total, T and B lymphocyte levels was observed.

Goals

The present study aims at studying the effect of homogeneous and different inhomogeneous SMF-exposure on the repair of radiation-induced DNA damage. We tested the effects of homogeneous SMF and, for the first time in the literature, 3 different inhomogeneous SMF, 8 different exposure times, as well as before and after γ-irradiation in human blood cells.

Materials and Methods

Magnetic Exposure Conditions

Two separate exposure chambers (generator 16 and 11, see in **Generators 1-16**) were used for homogeneous and inhomogeneous magnetic exposures, respectively similarly to the conditions described in Chapter 4 (***In Vitro* Experiments on Microorganisms**), Where the Subjects Were microorganisms. The *in vitro* samples could be positioned in these chambers too. Human blood samples were placed in Petri dishes with an internal diameter of 35 mm, then in the inhomogeneous SMF-exposure chamber. Three Petri dishes were stacked upon each other. A positioning mould made of plastic was used to hold stacks in place on the matrices. The Petri dish at the bottom of the stack was denoted as iSMF1.

Similarly, the middle of the stack was iSMF2 and the top of the stack was iSMF3. The height of one Petri dish (12 mm) defined the distance between the layers. Therefore the actual distance from the magnetic surface was z_1=3 mm for layer 1, z_2=15 mm for layer 2, and z_3=27 mm for layer 3. The measured values can be seen in Table **6.2** (in part also presented in Table **3.4**). The SMF-exposure chambers were held in incubators (at 37°C, in 5% CO_2, humidified atmosphere).

Table 6.2. Basic parameters of magnetic exposure conditions.

<table>
<tr><th colspan="4">homogeneous static magnetic field (hSMF) chamber</th></tr>
<tr><td rowspan="2">hSMF</td><td colspan="2">magnetic induction</td><td>comments</td></tr>
<tr><td colspan="2">159.2 ± 13.4 mT</td><td>Average in the 0-50 mm distance from the lower magnetic matrix. Lateral magnetic field scatter was small and regarded ignorable stray field.</td></tr>
<tr><th colspan="4">inhomogeneous static magnetic field (iSMF) chamber</th></tr>
<tr><td>iSMF</td><td>P-P magnetic induction</td><td>lateral gradient of the magnetic induction</td><td>comments</td></tr>
<tr><td>iSMF1</td><td>476.7±0.1 mT</td><td>47.7 T/m</td><td rowspan="3">Measured at the 3, 15, and 27 mm distance from the lower magnetic matrix in the same chamber.</td></tr>
<tr><td>iSMF2</td><td>12.0±0.1 mT</td><td>1.2 T/m</td></tr>
<tr><td>iSMF3</td><td>2.8+0.1 mT</td><td>0.3 T/m</td></tr>
</table>

γ-ray Irradiation

Dose dependency of ionizing radiation has been investigated before [361]. The irradiation doses in our case were: 0.3, 0.5, 1, 2, 3, or 4 Gy. Under our experimental conditions the detectable damage limit for ionizing radiation by the Comet-assay was 0.5 Gy, but significant difference between control and irradiated group was found at doses of 1, 2, 3, and 4 Gy as well. In the present experiment 4 Gy was chosen, because at this level cell damage was strongly expressed and spontaneous repair (and observation period) took another 6 h following irradiation. 4 Gy of γ-ray irradiation (^{60}Co) was performed with a Gammatron 3 with 37.5 cm focus-body middle distance at a dose rate of 0.35 Gy/min at room temperature (*cca.* 11.4 min).

Subjects, Ethics

The effects of homogeneous and inhomogeneous SMF on human whole blood were studied in 4 experiments. The venous blood samples were obtained from 3 healthy, non-smoking volunteers (men aged 26, 26, and 50 y), on 4 different occasions. Participants had not been exposed to chemicals, drugs, or X-rays in the 3 months preceding the blood sampling.

All procedures related to the handling of blood samples were approved by the Local Ethical Committee. Volunteers gave their informed consent *prior* to the experiments.

Blood Sampling

Approximately 30 ml blood was collected from each donor into heparinized vacutainer vials. The samples were then stored in dark at 5°C until use. Blood samples were diluted with RPMI 1640 Medium to 3 times of their original volume before the experiments. The samples were held in Petri dishes (1.5 ml/dish) in an incubator (at 37°C, in 5% CO_2, humidified atmosphere) during the experiments.

Instead of separating blood cells, whole blood was used, because leukocytes remained in their original surroundings, less cell manipulation took place. Our focus in the examination was on the spontaneous repair mechanism of leukocytes in their intact micro-environment in the blood.

Experimental Protocol

The effects of homogeneous and inhomogeneous SMF-exposure on human whole blood were studied in 4 experiments: 2 times for hSMF and 2 times for iSMF. The treatment and sampling time for the different sample groups are shown in Fig. (**6.1**). "Irradiation" stands for the ionizing ^{60}Co γ-radiation and "Exposure" denotes the SMF-exposure of either kind. In the control group (No. 1) samples were neither exposed nor irradiated. Samples of group No. 2 and 3 were exposed to hSMF or iSMF1, 2, or 3 for 24 h, respectively. Samples were taken for Comet-assay at 0.5, 1, 2, 4, 6, 18, 20, or 24 h. Samples of group No. 4 were irradiated with 4 Gy after 24 h of incubation.

Following this, the combined effect of 4 Gy irradiation and 24 h exposure to hSMF (No. 5) or iSMF1, 2, or 3 (No. 6) performed before irradiation was examined. The samples of these groups were measured with Comet-assay only once after the irradiation.

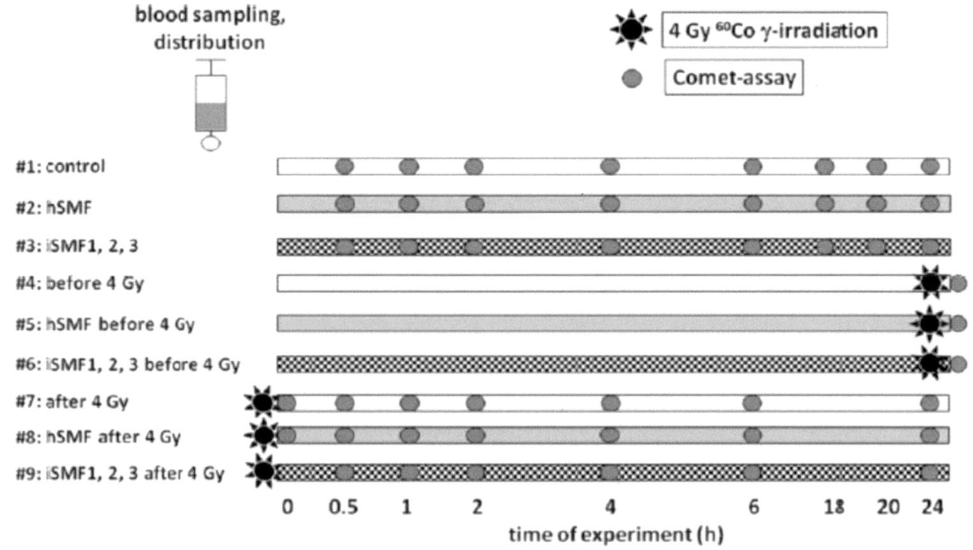

Fig. (6.1). Schematic protocol of different treatments and sampling times. SMF: Static magnetic field-exposure. hSMF: Homogeneous SMF-exposure. iSMF1, 2, 3: Different inhomogeneous SMF-exposure conditions. 4 Gy: 4 Gy ^{60}Co γ-ray irradiation. The time axis is out of scale.

Finally, we studied the situation when irradiation preceded the SMF treatment. The samples of group No. 7 were placed into the incubator immediately after the ionizing irradiation and were incubated for 24 h. Samples in groups No. 8 and 9 were irradiated and then exposed to hSMF or iSMF1, 2, or 3, respectively. Samples were evaluated by Comet-assay at 0.5, 1, 2, 4, 6, or 24 h.

<u>*Chemicals*</u>

Slides and cover slips were purchased from Spektrum-3D, normal melting point agarose from Sigma-Aldrich (A6013), and low melting point agarose from ICN Biomedicals (800259). Lysis buffer contained 2.5 M NaCl (6405), 100 mM Na_2EDTA (Reanal 09171-1-01-38), 10 mM tris(hydroxyl-methyl)aminomethane (Tris, Sigma-Aldrich, T666), 1% Triton X (Sigma-Aldrich, T8532), 10% DMSO

(Sigma-Aldrich, 41640), and was titrated to pH 10. Electrophoresis buffer contained 1 mM Na_2EDTA, 300 mM NaOH (Reanal, 24578-1-01-38), pH 13. Neutralization buffer was 0.4 M Tris, pH 7.5. Ethidium bromide was provided by Sigma-Aldrich (E8751). Blood samples were diluted with RPMI 1640 Medium (GIBCO 12633-012).

DNA Damage Analysis

Alkaline single-cell gel electrophoresis (Comet-assay) was used to investigate the DNA damage (both single and double strand breaks) on human blood cells as basically suggested by Singh *et al.* [362] with minor modifications. Five μl of exposed or control blood was mixed with 75 μl low melting point agarose (0.5%, at 37°C) and pipetted onto slides pre-coated with 1% normal-melting point agarose in 2 parallels. This suspension was immediately covered with a cover glass, and maintained at 4°C until solidification of the agarose. After about 10 min the cover glasses were gently removed, the slides were immersed in freshly prepared cold lysis solution (2.5 M NaCl, 100 mM Na_2EDTA, 10 mM Tris, pH 10, and 1% Triton X-100, 10% DMSO added fresh), and lysed for a minimum of 24 h at 4°C. Afterward, the slides were rinsed in cold electrophoresis buffer and placed in a horizontal gel electrophoresis tank side by side. The tank was filled with cold, fresh electrophoresis buffer (1 mM Na_2EDTA, 300 mM NaOH, pH 13) to a level approximately 0.3 cm above the slides. Slides were left in this solution for 30 min for the unwinding of DNA before the electrophoresis. Electrophoresis lasted 20 min (25 V, 300 mA). Up to this point, the method was conducted in the dark or under dimmed light to prevent additional DNA damage. After electrophoresis the slides were rinsed once in Tris buffer (0.4 M Tris, pH 7.5), placed horizontally and were flooded 3 times with Tris buffer (0.4 M Tris, pH 7.5) for 5 min, and 5 min with ethanol, then allowed to dry at room temperature. Slides were stored at room temperature until analysis.

Slide Scoring

The slides were stained by adding 50 μl ethidium bromide (20 μg/ml) covered with cover glass and examined at 400× magnification using a fluorescence microscope (Carl Zeiss, Oberkochen, Germany). Hundred comets from each sample were analyzed with the Komet 4.0 (Kinetic Imaging) image analysis system with respect to their Tail DNA (tail factor in %).

Statistical Analysis

The results are expressed as means of tail DNA±SEM in %. Statistical analysis of the data was obtained with one-way ANOVA.

Results

For each treated group a control group was prepared. The tail DNA% results of control groups (No. 1) were similar; therefore, their pooled average could be used: 5.32±0.22.

The mean tail DNA% values in group No. 2 were not significantly different from those in group No. 1. There was no significant difference between control and any inhomogeneously exposed groups (No. 3) either.

Effect of 24 h Exposure to hSMF or iSMF on the DNA of Human Blood Cells Before γ-irradiation (No. 4, 5, and 6)

The results of these groups are collected in Table **6.3**. The samples of groups No. 4, 5, and 6 resulted in significantly higher tail DNA% than the control (No. 1). We found significantly fewer DNA strand breaks in the samples of group No. 6 (iSMF2) than in No. 4 (positive control). We also found significantly more DNA strand breaks in samples of the group iSMF3 (in No. 6) than in iSMF2. The number of damaged cells was significantly higher in the samples of group No. 5 than in No. 6.

Table 6.3. Measured values of tail DNA% of control samples (No. 1), positive control samples (No. 4) and samples exposed to homogeneous (No. 5) or inhomogeneous (No. 6) SMF for 24 h before irradiation with 4 Gy ^{60}Co γ-ray. * denotes significant difference (one-way ANOVA).

sample group	tail DNA% ± SEM	*p* values				
		No. 1	No. 4	No. 6		
				iSMF1	iSMF2	iSMF3
No. 1 (negative control)	5.32±0.22					

(Table 6.3) contd.....

sample group		tail DNA% ± SEM	p values				
			No. 1	No. 4	No. 6		
					iSMF1	iSMF2	iSMF3
No. 4 (positive control)		16.73±0.36	<0.001*				
No. 5 (hSMF)		16.61±0.28	<0.001*	>0.05	>0.05	<0.05*	>0.05
No. 6	iSMF1	15.71±0.81	<0.001*	>0.05			
	iSMF2	15.13±0.82	<0.001*	<0.05*	>0.05		
	iSMF3	17.42±0.68	<0.001*	>0.05	>0.05	<0.05*	

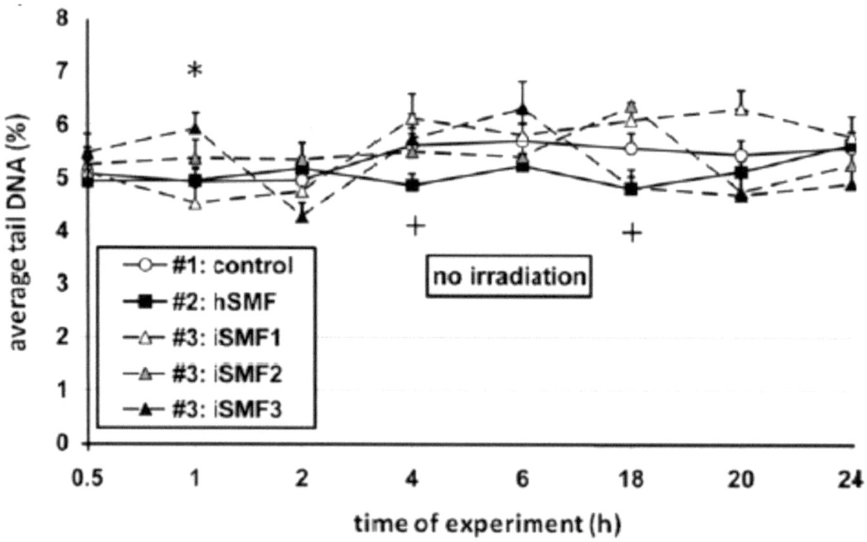

Fig. (6.2). Average tail DNA%±SEM of the control sample and samples exposed to homogeneous (hSMF) or different inhomogeneous SMF (iSMF1, 2, 3) *vs* time of experiment. * denotes significant difference ($p<0.05$) between control sample (No. 1) and hSMF-exposed sample (No. 2). + denotes significant difference ($p<0.05$) between control sample (No. 1) and iSMF3-exposed sample (No. 3) (one-way ANOVA). The time axis is out of scale. Straight lines between markers guide the eye only.

Effect of 24 h Exposure to hSMF on the Repair of DNA Damage of Human Blood Cells Following γ-irradiation (No. 4, 7, and 8)

Fig. (**6.2**) shows the tail DNA%±SEM *vs* exposure time for the control sample (No. 1), the positive control sample (No. 4) and samples exposed to hSMF without or after irradiation (No. 7 and 8). There was no significant effect of the exposure to hSMF on the number of DNA strand breaks in the irradiated and exposed samples, except at the 4th h of exposure. Here the tail DNA% was significantly lower in the 4 Gy irradiated and hSMF-exposed sample than in the positive control group. The tail DNA% in the samples exposed only to hSMF was significantly lower than in the control at the 4th h of the experiment.

Effect of 24 h Exposure to Gradient iSMF on the Repair of DNA Damage of Human Blood Cells Induced by γ-irradiation (No. 4, 7, and 9)

Fig. (**6.3**) presents the tail DNA% *vs* exposure time for the control sample (No. 1) and samples exposed to different gradients (iSMF1,2, or 3 in group No. 9) of iSMF and/or γ-irradiated. The tail DNA% was significantly higher in the iSMF exposed and in the 4 Gy irradiated samples than in the control in the first 2 h of the experiment. In the iSMF exposed samples the repair had gone similar to the positive control (No. 4). The gradient field in iSMF2 significantly delayed the DNA repair at the 1st h of the exposure.

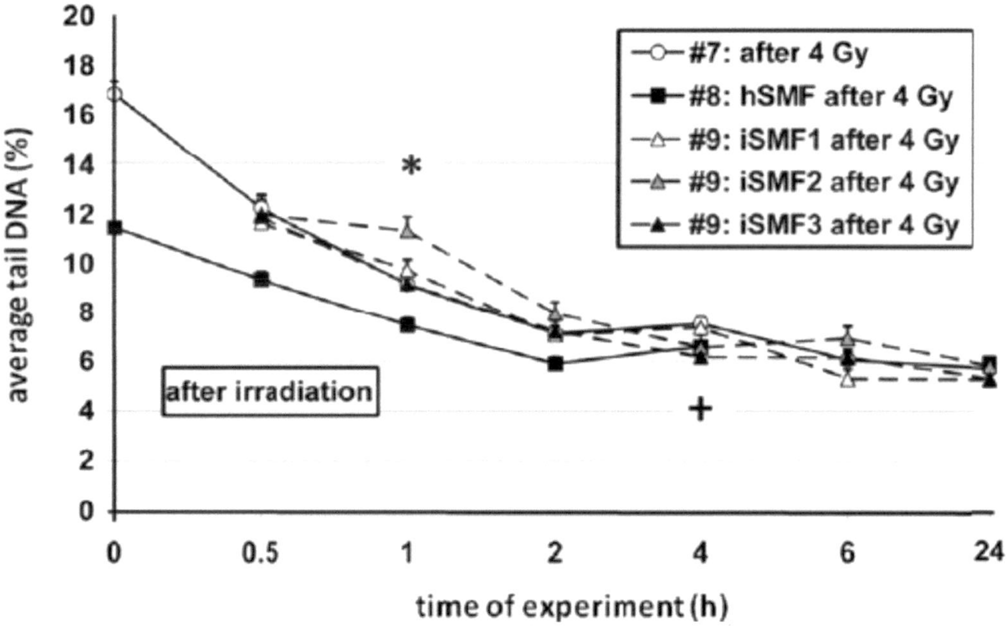

Fig. (6.3). Average tail DNA%±SEM of samples irradiated by 4 Gy ^{60}Co-γ and then incubated without SMF-exposure (No. 7), exposed to homogeneous (No. 8) or different inhomogeneous SMF (No. 9) vs time of experiment. * and +denote significant difference ($p<0.05$) between irradiated sample (No. 7) and hSMF-exposed sample (No. 8) and iSMF2-exposed sample (No. 9), respectively (one-way ANOVA).

Discussion, Conclusions

Effect of Exposure to hSMF or Gradient iSMF on DNA Damage of Human Blood Cells

At the 24 h SMF-exposure, we found no significant differences between either hSMF or any type of iSMF as compared to control in healthy human blood cells. This result is in harmony with those published by Norimura *et al.* [363] and Onodera *et al.* [313] for the instance, when no other stimulation occurred to the blood cells than an exposure to SMF. Norimura *et al.* [363] tested SMF-exposure with inductions below 2 T and found no effect. Hardly could either group identify any effect applying even strong SMF from 4 to 10 T. On the other hand, Gorczyńska [364] found that the percentage of lymphocytes was increased in the peripheral blood of guinea pigs, if exposed to 0.05 T or 0.3 T SMF in 1 h/day for 7 weeks *in vivo* examination. On the contrary, Hashish *et al.* [297] observed a significant decrease in the counts of peripheral lymphocytes. Their exposure system generated an inhomogeneous SMF with ±2.9 μT and was applied for 30 days. No data was published about the gradient. According to recent exposure assessment, the lateral gradient of SMF in the vicinity of MRI devices can reach up to 3.5 T/m [365]. In our studies, the gradient field was more than 10 fold higher in iSMF1 than in iSMF2, and 1 order of magnitude smaller in iSMF3, respectively providing a sufficient dose rate in this context.

Effect of in Advance 24 h Exposure to hSMF or iSMF on the Repair of DNA Damage of Human Blood Cells Induced by γ-irradiation

It is demonstrated in Table **6.3** that 4 Gy irradiation of human blood cells with ^{60}Co-γ causes a serious damage in the DNA including both single and double strand breaks. Irradiation causes a 3 fold increase in the tail DNA% mean values when compared to non-irradiated control. It may be of surprise that in iSMF2 of the inhomogeneous SMF (with magnetic induction 2.8±0.1 mT and magnetic induction gradient 0.3 T/m) as well as the homogeneous SMF (with magnetic induction 159.2±13.4 mT) treatment reduces the damage as compared to positive control (4 Gy irradiated samples), if the treatment is applied for 24 h preceding the irradiation.

A 24 h exposure of human blood cells to hSMF has a slight effect on the DNA tail% of the repaired human blood cells after 4 Gy ^{60}Co-γ irradiation. The only special feature of the curves in Fig. (**6.2**) is the local maximum of both the control and positive controls at 4 h. This behavior remains unexplained even though it occurred several times during earlier Comet-assay experiments. At 4 h exposure hSMF treatment seems to have a slight, but significant beneficial effect on the DNA repair as compared to the positive control. The only reference in the literature we could compare our results to are those of Takatsuji *et al.* [366], who applied 4.9 MeV H^+ or 23 MeV He^+ irradiation to their *in vitro* human peripheral blood cells and looked for the effect of a subsequent SMF-exposure of 1 T. They also found that the intercellular distribution of chromosome aberrations was not significantly influenced by SMF.

In terms of evaluating the results shown in Fig. (**6.3**), we may conclude again that there is no significant effect in any iSMF on the repair of DNA of human blood cells damaged by γ-irradiation other than the feature at the 4th h of exposure. The only result in the literature is that of Hashish *et al.* [297], who used a gradient SMF, but their induction and gradient data were either too low or not specified.

In summary:

i. There is no harmful effect of either hSMF- or any gradient iSMF-exposure on healthy human blood cells in the tested magnetic induction and gradient ranges,
ii. both hSMF- and any iSMF-exposure failed to assist the spontaneous repair process of DNA bond breaks.

Now we can turn our attention to another *in vitro* study of human peripheral blood samples, in which the focus is on the secretion of pro- and anti-inflammatory cytokines from LPS-activated lymphocytes and macrophages.

Anti-inflammatory Effect

In Vitro Analysis of the Anti-inflammatory Effect of Inhomogeneous Static Magnetic Field-exposure on Human Macrophages and Lymphocytes

Preliminaries

Today, due to the preceding research and its dissemination, it is widely accepted that SMF-exposure can achieve well defined and observable responses from cells and living subjects under a broad range of experimental and clinical physiological and pathological conditions [357, 367 - 370]. In contrast to the number of phenomenological observations and descriptions, little knowledge has accumulated about the background mechanisms of action [371], although the elective site of action of SMF seems to be the plasma membrane [372 - 374]. The probable reason for this is the lack of systematic research. Valuable experiments and clinical trials could not contribute to the overall research as much as they would have deserved due to incomplete description of different magnetic inductions and their spatial gradients representing a 6D space, magnet arrangements, *etc*. Missing published data often hinder the replication of otherwise extremely important and promising research projects.

The most frequent use of SMF-exposure occurs in MRI devices nowadays. Although the MRI diagnosis requires 3 different types of magnetic fields, the B_0 component is static. Research concerning the biological effects of SMF-exposure in humans diverges into 2 paths: The compilation of

i. epidemiological evidence that SMF-exposure does not bring health hazards and conversely,
ii. evidence of SMF-exposure's beneficial effects may elevate its status to the level of evidence-based medical therapy options.

Reviews on the topic are available from WHO [12] and more recently from SCENIHR [13]. Russian scientists were specifically devoted to clarify the mechanisms behind magneto-therapy (*i.e.* electromagnetic field irradiation); for a recent review see [375].

In particular, the production of pro-inflammatory cytokines interleukin (IL)-6 and tumor necrosis factor (TNF)-α, and that of the anti-inflammatory cytokine IL-10 was studied in the work of Salerno *et al.* [376] *in vitro* on human peripheral blood mononuclear cells (PBMC) under 0.5 T SMF continuous exposure for 24 h. The authors did not find any significant changes in the release of any cytokines.

Aldinucci *et al.* [377] published similar conclusions based on a similar study to that of Salerno *et al.*'s [376], concerning pro-inflammatory cytokines IL-6 and TNF-α on identical subject cells; the only difference being that the magnetic induction was continuous 4.75 T for 1 h. IL-8 was monitored by Sontag [378] in his *in vitro* study on human promyelocite cells (HL-60) exposed to 0-1.2 mT for a time period of 15 min. He found no significant differences to unexposed control either. Lin *et al.* [304] executed an *in vivo* experimental series on mice. A group of mice was exposed to SMF of 0.25 T for 2 h preceding a 50 mg/kg lipopolysaccharide (LPS) challenge. The authors did not find any significant change in the IL-6 and TNF-α secretion levels compared to positive control (LPS challenge only). On the other hand, Wang *et al.* [379] exposed human embryoid body derived cells to 0.23-0.28 T for 1-4 days continuously and found a significant increase in the release of IL-6.

Goals

If *in vitro* evidence was found on the SMF-exposure induced inhibition or assistance of the release of pro- and anti-inflammatory cytokines, a possible background mechanism of *in vivo* experienced *AE* in invertebrates (**Experiments on invertebrates *in vivo***) and in mice (**Experiments on mammals *in vivo***) would be supported. Therefore, the present set of *in vitro* experiments was designed to prove the null-hypotheses that exposure of PBMC to an inhomogeneous SMF for up to 24 h leads to a significant change in the:

- Production of IL-6, IL-8, TNF-α, and IL-10 compared to negative (unexposed) control,
- LPS-activated production of IL-6, IL-8, TNF-α, and IL-10 compared to positive (LPS-activated, unexposed) control.

Materials and Methods

Ethics Statements

Human blood samples were obtained from buffy coats supplied by the Hospital S. Giuseppe da Copertino (Lecce, Italy). Donors were anonymous to us. Donor consent was waived by the Ethics Committee. The use of buffy coat was acknowledged by the Comitato Etico dell'ASL LE (Ethics Committee of the Health Service of Lecce, Italy). This Ethics Committee is an independent organization that is working under the Declaration of Helsinki and following the rules of Good Clinical Practices according to international and national laws and to the guidelines of the Italian National Committee of Bioethics.

Cells, Chemicals

PBMC (monocytes and lymphocytes) were isolated from human buffy coats of non-smoker healthy male donors between 24 and 45 y of age by Ficoll gradient separation. Over 95% pure peripheral blood lymphocytes were separated from monocytes by overnight adherence to plastic. Cells were cultured in 25 cm^2 flasks at a cell density of 10^5 cells/ml in RPMI-1640 medium supplemented with 10% (v/v) heat-inactivated fetal calf serum, 2 mM L-glutamine, 100 IU/ml penicillin and streptomycin in a humidified atmosphere of 5% CO_2 at 37°C. Some cultures of monocytes and lymphocytes were activated with 1 μg/ml LPS for 3 h first and then were exposed to SMF for 6, 18, or 24 h. Controls cells were cultured under the same culture conditions, but remained unexposed to SMF. All chemicals were of analytical grade and were provided by Sigma-Aldrich unless indicated otherwise. Optical density (OD) values were read by spectrophotometer (Ultrospec 4000 UV/Visible Spectrophotometer) at 450 nm (OD_{450}).

Light Microscope Observations

A Nikon Eclipse TS100 inverted microscope was used to investigate morphological cellular shape changes also at time points 0, 6, 18, and 24 h.

Cytokine Assays

Production of different cytokines: IL-6 (monocytes and lymphocytes), IL-8 (monocytes), IL-10 (monocytes and lymphocytes), and TNF-α (monocytes) were determined by ELISA (R&D Systems, Minneapolis, MN, USA) from the supernatants at time points 0, 6, 18, and 24 h.

Timeline

The timeline of the experiment can be seen in Fig. (**6.4**). Generator 11 (see in **Generators 1-16**) was used in this test series exclusively.

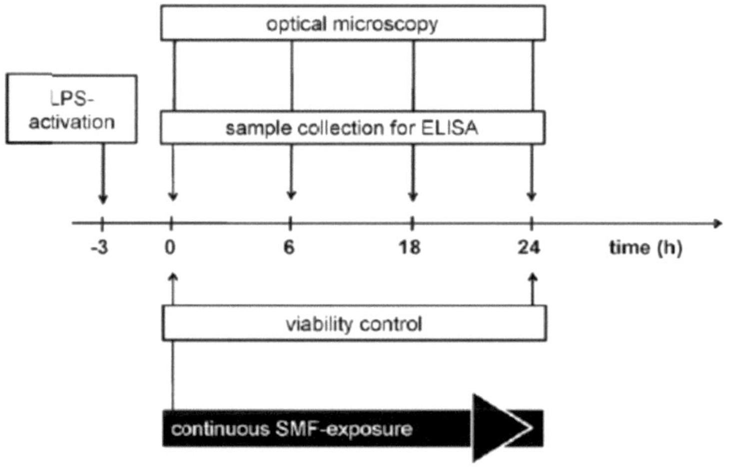

Fig. (6.4). Timeline of the experiment. LPS stands for lipopolysaccharide, and SMF for static magnetic field.

Statistical Analysis

The primary outcome measure was the average OD_{450} value of a specific culture under a certain treatment at a given time point. Concentrations were derived from these values. First the best standard curve (r^2=99%) was set in accordance with the manufacturer's instructions by plotting known concentrations of a certain cytokine expressed in pg/ml *vs* the relative OD_{450} read. Then we interpolated between known average OD_{450} values to get the desired concentration of the given cytokine.

Statistical measures were analyzed in a 2-sided way in accordance with the null-hypotheses. Balanced, self-controlled group analysis of variances (2-way rANO-VA) was applied to get the estimate of the OD_{450} differences due to treatment. The treatment options and the time points were the factors. Treatment options were: None (negative control), LPS (positive control), SMF, or SMF+LPS. Time points were: 0, 6, 18, and 24 h. One-way ANOVA was applied in case of the concentrations. Games-Howell test was used for *post hoc* analysis of binary comparisons within time points (n=9) and also in case of concentrations (n=4 for negative and positive controls, n=3 for SMF and SMF+LPS). A difference between group averages upon different treatments was accepted significant, if p<0.05 at the 95% confidence level. Probabilities below 0.001 are not shown numerically in the text.

Effect between treatment options i and j at a given k time point was defined as $100\left(1-\langle OD_{ik}\rangle/\langle OD_{jk}\rangle\right)$ in percentage, where $\langle OD_{ik}\rangle$ and $\langle OD_{jk}\rangle$ are averages of OD_{450} values at a given k time point, n=9/treatment. i could only be SMF or SMF+LPS, the corresponding j could only be negative or positive (LPS) control, respectively. By definition the effect can be positive (inhibition) or negative (assistance) by definition. Concentrations (pg/ml), viabilities as well as effects (%) are presented in column graphs. Error bars in the figures denote positive standard deviation (SD). Identically scaled y axes were used for the presentation of effects allowing for immediate visual comparison.

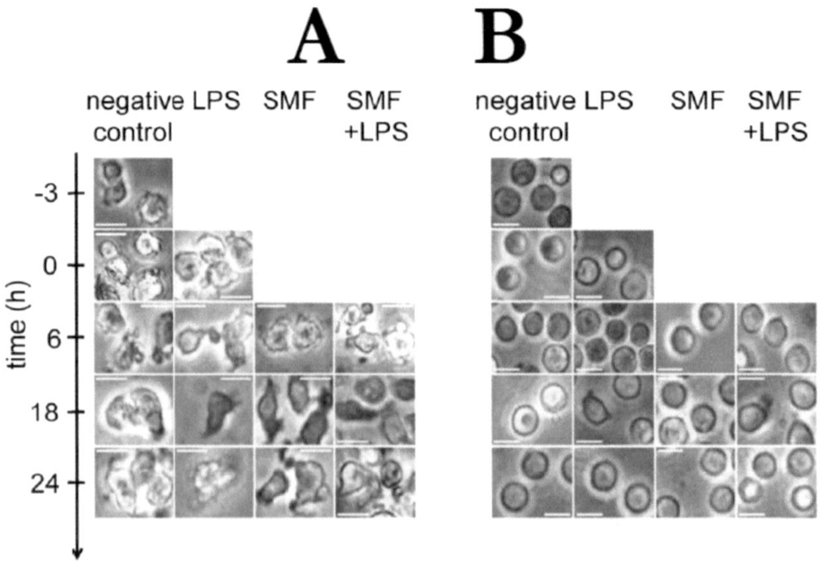

Fig. (6.5). Light microscope images of the morphological changes of **A)** macrophages and **B)** lymphocytes. Negative control: No treatment; LPS: Lipopolysaccharide-activation; SMF: Static magnetic field-exposure; SMF+LPS: SMF-exposure combined with LPS-activation. Bar length=10 µm. The time axis is out of scale.

Results

Time-dependent cell shape modifications have been observed on SMF-exposed cells (on macrophages to a higher extent than on lymphocytes) all through the experiment. Fig. (**6.5A**) and Fig. (**6.5B**) show the morphological changes of macrophages and lymphocytes under different treatment negative control, positive control (LPS), SMF, and SMF+LPS. In particular, at time point 24 h macrophages showed an elongated shape whereas lymphocytes exhibited cell surface ruffling and indentations.

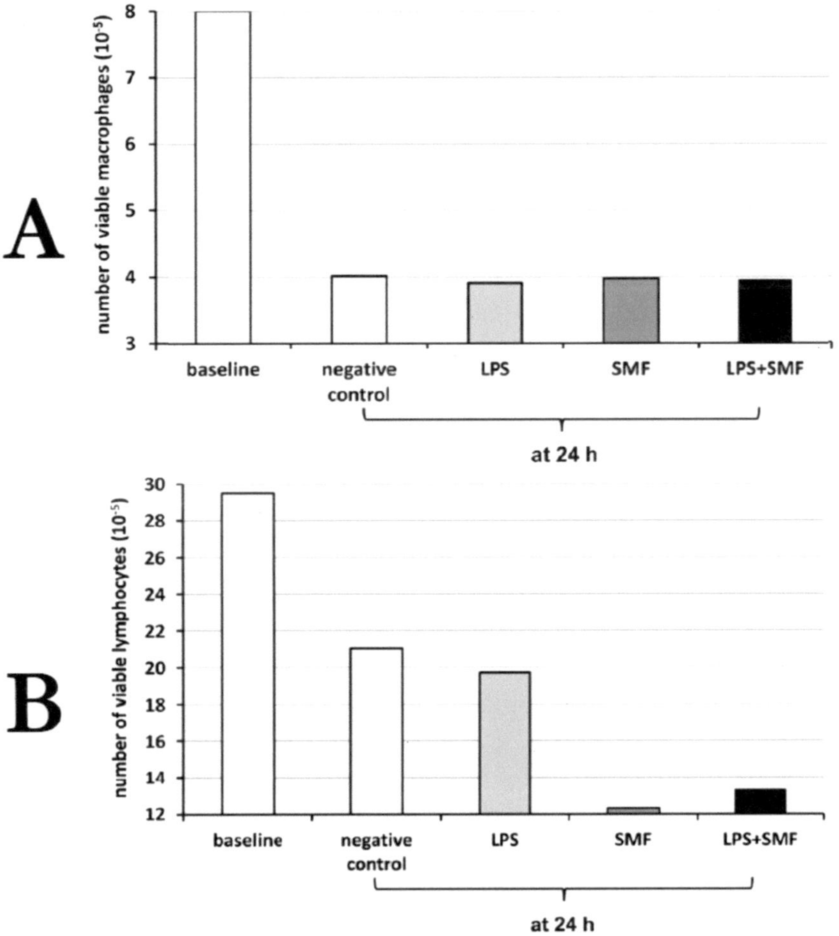

Fig. (6.6). Number of viable **A)** macrophages and **B)** lymphocytes at baseline and at 24 h. Cultures were exposed to different treatments: Negative control: No treatment; LPS: Lipopolysaccharide-activated; SMF: SMF-exposed; LPS+SMF: LPS-activated and SMF-exposed.

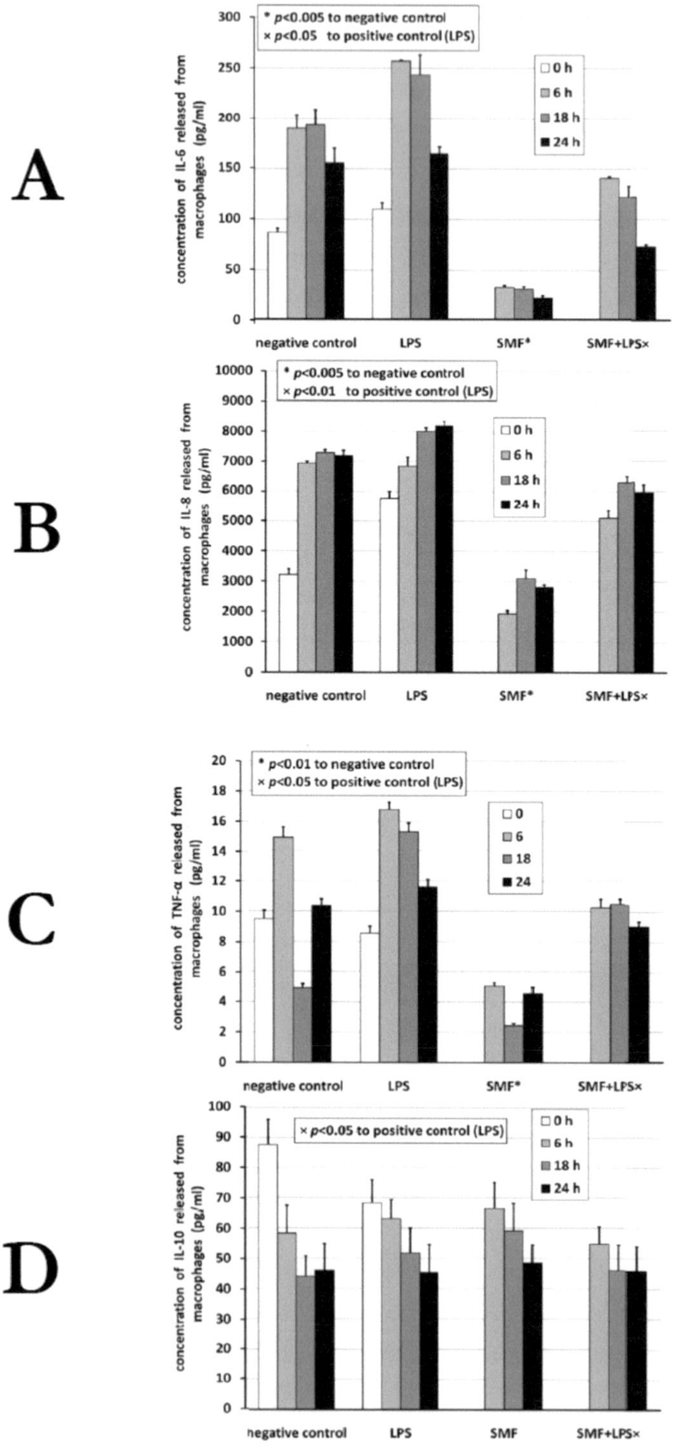
A
* p<0.005 to negative control
× p<0.05 to positive control (LPS)
0 h
6 h
18 h
24 h
concentration of IL-6 released from macrophages (pg/ml)
300
250
200
150
100
50
0
negative control
LPS
SMF*
SMF+LPS×
B
* p<0.005 to negative control
× p<0.01 to positive control (LPS)
0 h
6 h
18 h
24 h
concentration of IL-8 released from macrophages (pg/ml)
10000
9000
8000
7000
6000
5000
4000
3000
2000
1000
0
negative control
LPS
SMF*
SMF+LPS×
C
* p<0.01 to negative control
× p<0.05 to positive control (LPS)
0
6
18
24
concentration of TNF-α released from macrophages (pg/ml)
20
18
16
14
12
10
8
6
4
2
0
negative control
LPS
SMF*
SMF+LPS×
D
× p<0.05 to positive control (LPS)
0 h
6 h
18 h
24 h
concentration of IL-10 released from macrophages (pg/ml)
100
90
80
70
60
50
40
30
20
10
0
negative control
LPS
SMF
SMF+LPS×

Fig. (6.7). Concentration of **A)** IL-6 and **B)** IL-8, **C)** TNF-α, and **D)** IL-10 released by a single macrophage in 24 h under different treatments. Positive error bars show standard deviation (SD) values. * and × denote significant differences ($p<0.05$) to corresponding negative or positive control (LPS), respectively as estimated with Games-Howell post hoc analysis.

Viability of cells was closely controlled. Fig. (**6.6A**) and Fig. (**6.6B**) show the number of viable macrophages and lymphocytes at the baseline and at 24 h, respectively. Even if the spontaneous death of macrophages was about 49.81% during this period, none of the treatment methods seemed to have affected the procedure (they remained between 50.31% and 51.09%). The maximum effect at 24 h between differently treated cultures to each other was 2.54% (LPS to negative control at 24 h). Lymphocytes showed higher sensitivity to the treatment: Apoptosis decreased the number of viable cells to 67.80% of the baseline value at 24 h; LPS caused a reduction of 92.50% only, SMF alone caused 50.83%, and in combination with LPS 56.68% as compared to negative control at 24 h.

Fig. (**6.7A-D**) show time-resolved concentration data for macrophages producing IL-6, IL-8, and TNF-α pro-inflammatory cytokines, and IL-10 anti-inflammatory cytokine, respectively. Different shades of the columns denote different time periods (0, 6, 18, and 24 h); treatment options are the independent variables. * and × mean significant differences $p<0.05$ compared to negative control and to positive control (LPS), respectively. For the 6-24 h time interval ANOVA provided $F_{crit}=4.07$ for all cases analyzed and $F=27.92$ ($p<0.001$), $F=3.13$ ($p=0.087$), $F=4.15$ ($p=0.048$), and $F=0.47$ ($p=0.709$) for IL-6, IL-8, TNF-α, and IL-10, respectively.

Similarly to Fig. (**6.7**), Fig. (**6.8A**) and Fig. (**6.8B**) show the time-resolved concentrations for lymphocytes producing IL-6 and IL-10, respectively. Different shades and marks (* and ×) have the same meaning as in Fig. (**6.7**). ANOVA resulted in $F=4.88$ ($p=0.033$) and $F=3.01$ ($p=0.095$) for IL-6 and IL-10, respectively.

SMF-exposure was more efficient on macrophages than on lymphocytes; macrophages secreted more cytokines than lymphocytes. Without taking the time-dependence into account at baseline, when no SMF treatment was yet used, but LPS had been given for 3 h already, the secretion of IL-6 and IL-8 from macrophages and IL-6 from lymphocytes has started. LPS-activation barely induced TNF-α production in the first 3 h. LPS, as an activator, seemed to work well in the model for macrophages as well as in the model for lymphocytes mimicking the inflammatory situation *in vitro* It enhanced the secretion of IL-6 significantly from lymphocytes (-50.61%, $p<0.001$ estimated by rANOVA), and the secretion of IL-6 (-23.33%, $p<0.001$), IL-8 (-17.04%, $p<0.001$), and TNF-α as well (-23.09%, $p<0.001$) from macrophages. LPS also induced a tendency to increase IL-10 release beyond the first 6 h. LPS-activated cells in the absence of SMF secreted the highest amounts of IL-8 at all times compared to negative control.

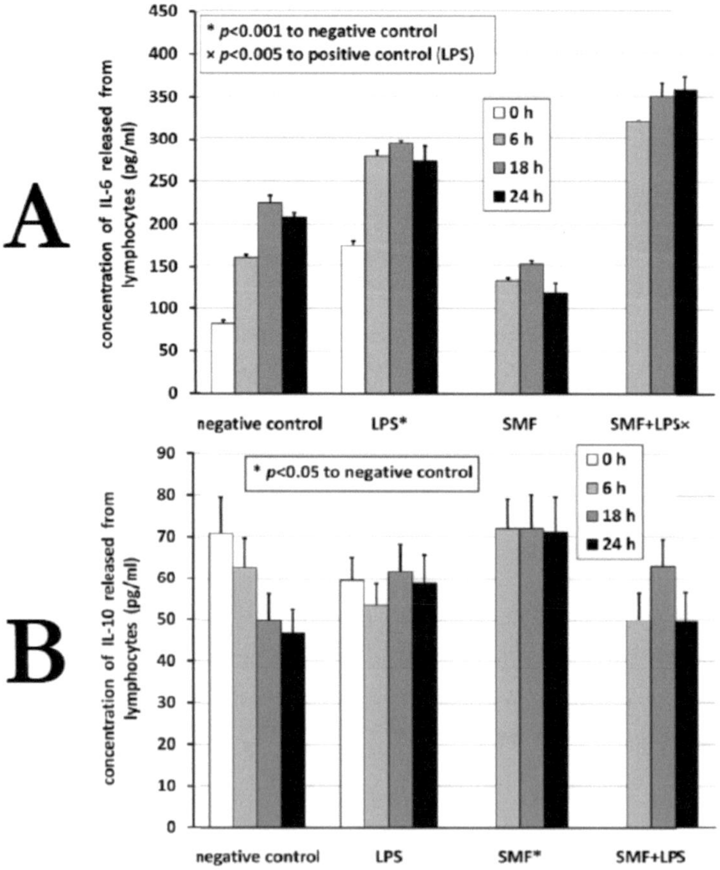

Fig. (6.8). Concentration of **A)** IL-6 and **B)** IL-10 released by a single lymphocyte under different treatment methods. * and × denote significant differences ($p<0.05$) to corresponding negative or positive control (LPS), respectively as estimated with Games-Howell post hoc analysis.

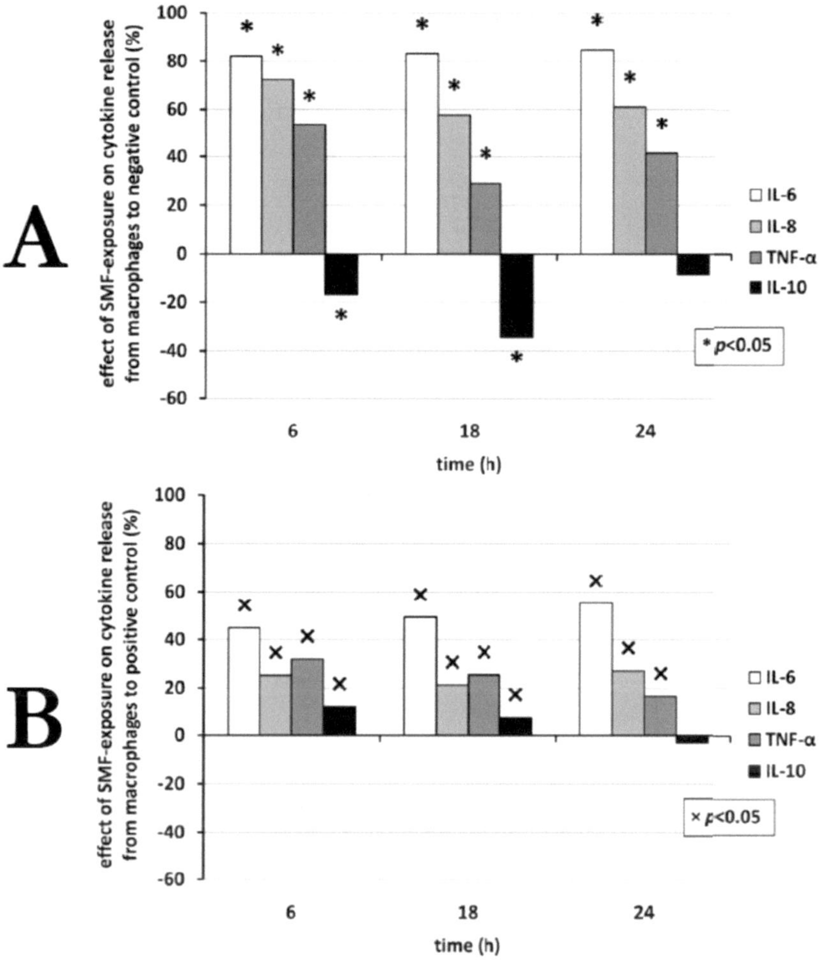

Fig. (6.9). Effect of cytokine release from macrophages under SMF-exposure compared to **A)** negative and **B)** positive (LPS) control, respectively as estimated from OD450 data. * and × denote significant differences ($p<0.05$) compared to negative and positive control, respectively. Positive effect means inhibition, negative effect means assistance. Probabilities of significance can be found in Table **6.4**.

The effect of cytokine release due to SMF-exposure was based on raw OD_{450} data, the time-dependent viability of cells was not considered. Positive or negative effect means if a treatment decreases or increases the OD_{450} values compared to respective control. We would like to remind the Reader of the fact that all figures show a *y* axis with identical scale for easy visual comparison. The effect of SMF-exposure acting on cytokine secretion from macrophages compared to negative and positive control can be seen in Fig. (**6.9A**) and Fig. (**6.9B**). The numerical results of probabilities of significance based on OD_{450} values are collected in Table **6.4**. Similarly to Fig. (**6.9A**) and Fig. (**6.9B**), the effect of SMF on cytokine release from lymphocytes compared to negative and positive control can be seen in Fig. (**6.10A**) and Fig. (**6.10B**).

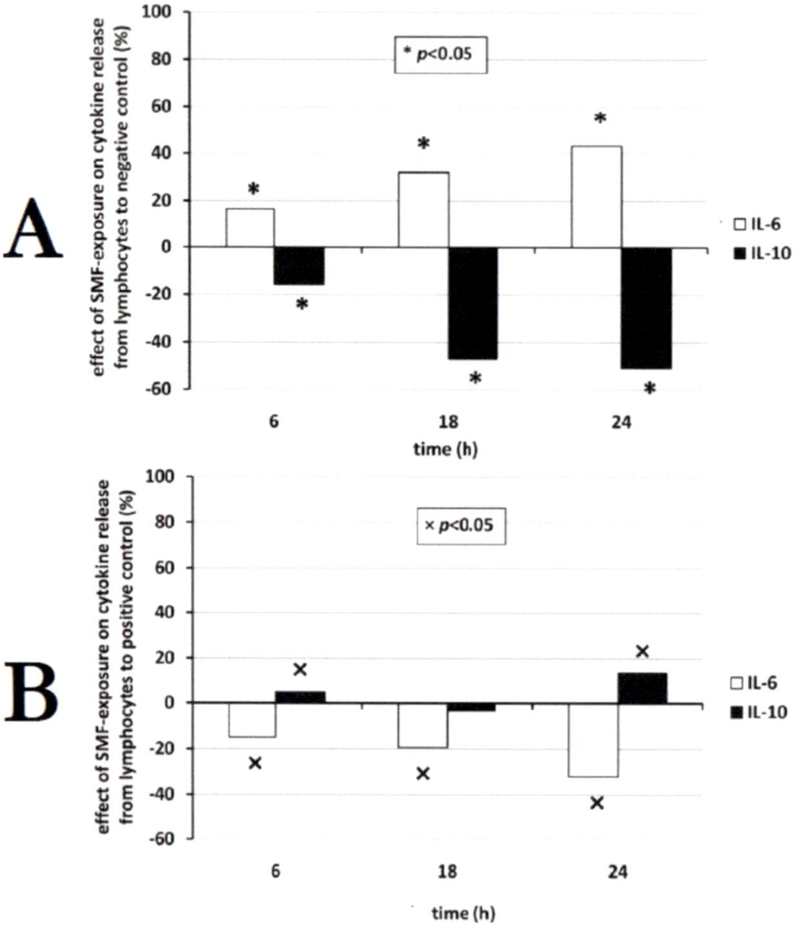

Fig. (6.10). Effect of cytokine release from lymphocytes under SMF-exposure compared to **A)** negative and **B)** positive (LPS) control, respectively as estimated from OD450 data. * and × denote significant differences ($p<0.05$) to negative and positive control, respectively. Positive effect means inhibition, negative means assistance. Probabilities of significance can be found in Table **6.4** and Table **6.5**.

Table 6.4. Effect sizes and corresponding significances for OD_{450} values of pro-inflammatory (IL-6, IL-8, TNF-α) and anti-inflammatory (IL-10) cytokines produced by macrophages or lymphocytes under lipopolysaccharide (LPS) activation and/or SMF-exposure in the 6-24 h time period. * and × denote significant differences ($p<0.05$) compared to negative and positive control, respectively as estimated with Games-Howell post hoc test.

	source	**cytokine**	**treatment to control**	**exposure time (h)**					
				significance *p* range					
				6		**18**		**24**	
effect of SMF-exposure on OD_{450}	**macrophages**	**IL-6**	SMF to negative control	82.06	<0.001 *	83.16 *	<0.001*	84.65 *	<0.001 *
			SMF+LPS to positive control	44.84	<0.001 ×	49.38 ×	<0.001 ×	55.16 ×	<0.001 ×
		IL-8	SMF to negative control	72.33	<0.001 *	57.77 *	<0.001 *	61.07 *	<0.001 *
			SMF+LPS to positive control	25.2	<0.001 ×	21.3 ×	<0.001 ×	27.16 ×	<0.001 ×
		TNF-α	SMF to negative control	53.25	<0.001 *	28.96 *	<0.001 *	41.51 *	<0.001 *
			SMF+LPS to positive control	31.91	<0.001 ×	25.43 ×	<0.001 ×	16.62 ×	<0.001 ×
		IL-10	SMF to negative control	16.92	<0.002 *	34.46 *	<0.001 *	8.58	
			SMF+LPS to positive control	12.27	<0.001 ×	7.89 ×	<0.012 ×	-3.02	
	lymphocytes	**IL-6**	SMF to negative control	16.57	<0.001 *	32.08 *	<0.001 *	43.16 *	<0.001 *
			SMF+LPS to positive control	14.82	<0.001 ×	-19.24 ×	<0.001 ×	-31.91 ×	<0.001 ×
		IL-10	**SMF to negative control**	-15.77	<0.001 *	-46.84 *	<0.001 *	-50.88 *	<0.001 *
			SMF+LPS to positive control	5.47	<0.021 ×	-3.05		13.72 ×	<0.001 ×

SMF-exposure alone induced an anti-inflammatory response from macrophages and lymphocytes by strongly and significantly inhibiting the secretion of pro-inflammatory cytokines IL-6, IL-8, and TNF-α as compared to negative control. The effect of SMF-exposure on IL-10 anti-inflammatory cytokine demonstrated an opposite trend; a moderate, but significant assistance could be seen.

LPS-activated cells in the presence of SMF strongly and significantly inhibited the secretion of pro-inflammatory cytokine IL-6, IL-8, and TNF-α from macrophages. Surprisingly enough, a negative and with time monotonously decreasing effect occurred in the case of IL-6 release from lymphocytes. The production of anti-inflammatory cytokine IL-10 from either macrophages or lymphocytes underwent a slight, hardly significant inhibition as compared to positive control. The production of anti-inflammatory cytokine IL-10 underwent a slight, hardly significant inhibition as compared to positive control from either macrophages or lymphocytes. The time dependence of the effect of cytokine secretion manifested itself in a monotonous rise in the inhibition in the case of IL-6 for both sources compared to either control, but for lymphocytes compared to positive control. IL-8 production barely varied with time following 6 h. TNF-α inhibition basically decreased with time, whereas IL-10 was the only examined cytokine the production of which correlated with the source, the absolute value of the assisting effect decreased in time for macrophages and increased for lymphocytes compared to negative control. LPS-activation in the presence of SMF-exposure had a mild effect (below 20%) on the release of IL-10 for either source. Meanwhile, SMF-exposure of macrophages showed a trend of diminishing action of the release of cytokines with the time of exposure, the action from lymphocytes seemed to be gradually enforced.

Statistical analysis (see Table **6.5** for a comprehensive view) of the concentrations showed that null-hypothesis 1 (*i.e.* effect of SMF-exposure on negative control) held for IL-6, IL-8, and TNF-α for 6-24 h with a significant inhibition between 56.78% and 87.52% for the release of cytokines from macrophages hindering the production of pro-inflammatory cytokines. SMF-exposure basically remained ineffective on the IL-6 release from lymphocytes (< | 12.20% |). SMF-exposure assisted the release of anti-inflammatory cytokine IL-10 from macrophages as well as from lymphocytes (between (183.62% and (6.45%) significantly for

Table 6.5. Similarly to Table 6.4, effect sizes and corresponding significances for concentration values of pro-inflammatory (IL-6, IL-8, TNF-α) and anti-inflammatory (IL-10) cytokines produced by macrophages or lymphocytes under lipopolysaccharide (LPS) activation and/or SMF-exposure in the 6-24 h time period. * and × denote significant differences (p<0.05) compared to negative and positive control, respectively, as estimated with Games-Howell post hoc test.

	source	cytokine	treatment to control	exposure time (h)			significance *p* range
				6	18	24	
effect of SMF-exposure on concentrations	macrophages	IL-6	SMF to negative control	4.91	-3.83	-12.20	<0.005 *
			SMF+LPS to positive control	-26.84	-63.17	-115.15	<0.05 ×
		IL-8	SMF to negative control	72.17	57.35	60.52	<0.005 *
			SMF+LPS to positive control	25.61	21.95	28.17	<0.01 ×
		TNF-α	SMF to negative control	87.52	69.75	56.78	<0.01 *
			SMF+LPS to positive control	49.82	35.47	23.91	<0.05 ×
		IL-10	SMF to negative control	-13.88	-33.42	-6.45	
			SMF+LPS to positive control	12.82	11.55	0.15	<0.05 ×
	lymphocytes	IL-6	SMF to negative control	4.91	-3.83	-12.20	<0.001 *
			SMF+LPS to positive control	-26.84	-63.17	-115.15	<0.005 ×
		IL-10	SMF to negative control	-28.75	-111.18	-183.62	<0.05 *
			SMF+LPS to positive control	-2.69	-37.03	-35.99	

lymphocytes, insignificantly for macrophages. Null-hypothesis 2 (*i.e.* the effect of SMF-exposure on positive control) also held for all pro-inflammatory cytokines. Pro-inflammatory cytokine release was inhibited from macrophages (effect of 0.15-56.03%) by SMF-exposure (significantly for IL-6), while exposure, surprisingly enough, significantly assisted the release of IL-6 from lymphocytes (between (115.15% and (26.84%). Anti-inflammatory cytokine IL-10 release was mildly and insignificantly inhibited from macrophages and assisted from lymphocytes.

Discussion, Conclusions

Normally unstimulated human primary PBMC undergo spontaneous cell death in culture. This is the reason why the decrease in the viability of macrophages as well as lymphocytes in the cultures together with the withdrawal of the release of pro-inflammatory cytokines IL-6, IL-8, TNF-α, and the increase of anti-inflammatory cytokine IL-10 was happening simultaneously in the experiment. In previous studies it was already demonstrated that 6 mT SMF-exposure applied up to 24 h to human U937 promonocytic cells [370] or to freshly isolated human lymphocytes [369] did not significantly exert any toxic or apoptogenic effect. However, in agreement with the data reported here (Fig. **6.5**), 6 mT SMF-exposure affected cell shape [372] as a result of cytoskeleton rearrangements [370] or by influencing the structural components of plasma membrane directly [374].

In our study, the effects observed on macrophages can be directly compared without weighting with the degree of lost viability, since the number of macrophages hardly depended on the treatment options (including no treatment) in the first 24 h period.

It is interesting in itself what strong adverse effect SMF-exposure exerted on the viability of lymphocytes. Although previous *in vitro* studies suggested otherwise for extremely weak SMF (6 mT) on human lymphocytes [369], the authors attribute the effect to the magnetic induction at the target site in the present experimental series which exceeded 6 mT by almost 2 orders of magnitude at average *P-P* value. On the other hand, the elevated level of cell death is in harmony with the results presented by Lee *et al.* [380], who found severe DNA breaks due to exposure with a combined magnetic field of a 3 T clinical MRI running different scanning protocols for durations between 22 and 89 min *in vitro* on human lymphocytes.

There is an opposition in the dependence of the SMF-exposure induced cytokine releasing action on macrophages and lymphocytes as a function of exposure duration. Lymphocytes are fully differentiated cells, whereas macrophages, in the absence of specific inducers, are not fully differentiated. Thus, lymphocytes and (monocytes derived) macrophages have different genetic expression. This is in accordance with the different roles of the cells: Macrophages may produce cytokines immediately upon stress; the production of cytokines by lymphocytes however, is of secondary importance for the lymphocytes. Against macrophages, lymphocytes use receptors to bind antigens and the role of SMF-exposure on some receptors has already been shown [381], **Pharmacological analysis** in this book). Therefore, we might hypothesize that the response evoked by strong SMF-exposure is different for lymphocytes and macrophages as already demonstrated by Tenuzzo *et al.* [357] for 6 mT SMF-exposure.

Needless to remind the Reader that we presented a classical pharmacological analysis of the action of SMF-exposure in **Pharmacological analysis** in a mouse model of acute visceral pain after having employed the same SMF generators as in the present study. We have discovered previously the significant role of opioid receptors, especially that of μ-opioid receptors, and also succeeded in excluding the contribution of κ-opioid receptors. We speculated that the strong *AE* of SMF-exposure may have been due to the release of either/both β-endorphin or/and endomorphin-2 in the spinal cord. We also verified in *Helix pomatia*, in a land snail model in **Experiments on invertebrates *in vivo***, that the thermal nociceptive threshold depended on the preceding 20-40 min long SMF-exposure to either homogeneous SMF of 147 mT or to an inhomogeneous SMF-exposure where, again, SMF was identical to the one used in the present experiment. With the application of naloxone pretreatment we could reveal the mediatory role of opioid receptors in the SMFinduced antinociception. There is also evidence for low-dose naloxone combined with morphine having a similar effect as pro- and anti-inflammatory cytokines presented here [382]. This hints at the fact that the action of SMF-exposure may be similar to that of serum morphine in the sense that naloxone can moderate both, and the secretion of pro- and anti-inflammatory cytokines was also observed.

We also used the same SMF generator in **Peripheral action** as well to prove that the capsaicin-sensitive fibers also mediated the anti-hyperalgesia action of SMF-exposure in a mouse acute peripheral pain model. Carrageenan, TNF-α, IL-6, and IL-8 were reported to induce hyperalgesia [383]. The down regulation of the pro-inflammatory cytokines by SMF-exposure may explain why we observed a significant decrease of hyperalgesia induced by carrageenan in our peripheral pain model. These observations can now be linked to the altered cytokine release characteristics of macrophages and lymphocytes from PBMC.

The up regulation of IL-6 and TNF-α expression in case of chronic constriction injury has been shown recently [384]. If SMF-exposure acts against chronic constriction injury, the extraordinary beneficial effect reported in **Neuropathic pain** in our *in vivo* experiment of a chronic neuropathy mouse model can, at least partially, be understood. Namely, we used nerve ligature to achieve neuropathic pain. The same SMF generator was also shown to significantly prolong the time of LPS induced premature birth occurrence (**Visceral action**). A possible background mechanism for this beneficial effect could be the moderation of the inflammatory response as SMF-exposure acts on the pro-inflammatory cytokine release.

The present results are in fair accord with those of Wang *et al.* [379] who applied 0.23-0.28 T exposure on human embryoid body derived cells continuously for 1-4 days. They experienced a short-term (<24 h) activation of IL-6 involved the coordinate up-regulation of toll-like receptor-4 (TLR4) with complementary changes to NEU3 and ST3GAL5 that reduced ganglioside GM3 in a manner that augmented the activation of TLR4 and IL-6. The authors suggested a plausible mechanism explaining the attenuation of cellular responses to SMF by the loss of GM3. They also observed SMF-mediated morphological changes and biochemical markers indicative of pre-oligodendrocyte differentiation at the cellular level.

In conclusion, the present *in vitro* experiments represent convincing evidence for exposure to a strong, inhomogeneous SMF for up to 24 h having a significant inhibitory effect on the release of pro-inflammatory cytokines IL-6, IL-8, and TNF-α from macrophages as compared to negative, untreated control. The assistance SMF-exposure exerts on the production of anti-inflammatory cytokine IL-10 from lymphocytes was also found to be significant. LPS-activation reduces the differences between treated and untreated cultures; however, IL-6 release from macrophages remains significantly inhibited upon SMF-exposure. The SMF-exposure assisted release of IL-6 from lymphocytes remains a challenging effect to be dealt with in the future. The present experiments may be regarded as proof that SMF-exposure, in fact, has a beneficial effect on human macrophages and lymphocytes *in vitro* and as such, SMF-exposure should be a worthy candidate of further investigation in clinical trials, including diseases with inflammatory background. Now, we have come to the point when it is time to leave phase 1 (*in vitro*) and phase 2 (animal experiment *in vivo*) and proceed to Phase 3; namely, let us have an insight into what SMF-exposure is able to achieve in human trials.

In vivo Trials

On Healthy Volunteers

Exposure to Inhomogeneous Static Magnetic Field Increases Thermal Pain Threshold in Healthy Human Volunteers

Preliminaries

Numerous clinical studies were aimed at assessing the potential *AE* of SMF-exposure. These studies were inspired basically by 2 sources. First, SMF therapies are relatively popular for self-care and treatment of various painful medical conditions. For example, a high variety of magnetic items include arm wraps, necklaces, bracelets, and magnetic mattress pads that are marketed with the purpose of effectively treating the patients' pain problems. Second and more importantly, studies dedicated to the effects of magnets on biological systems have suggested certain biological mechanisms that might induce pain relief. Both the cardiovascular system and the nervous system were found to be affected by SMF. Many animal studies demonstrated that moderate induction SMF have an effect on microvascular functions by triggering vasodilatation and antipressor activity in the skin, and the subcutaneous or muscular tissue [307, 309, 385]. This SMF induced vasodilatation is often argued as a potential mechanism underlying *AE*. In contrast, other investigations either failed to show a benefit from commercially available necklaces with permanent magnets for neck and shoulder pain other than a strong placebo effect [386, 387], or the effects of the magnet or placebo could not be disentangled [42, 351]. However, in a review paper based on the results of 11 out of 15 well-controlled studies, the conclusion clearly stated that SMF-exposure was able to induce *AE* [40]. A different line of research as Saunders [148] reported in a recent review, focused on changes in neurophysiologic responses following exposure to SMF. In general, the results were as follows. On one hand, the authors reported no effects of moderate induction (1 mT-1 T) or high induction (1-5 T) SMF-exposure on action potential conduction velocity, ion channel currents [388, 389], and electroretinogram responses 218. These negative findings seem to support the conclusion of Wikswo and Barach [390], according to which ultrastrong (24 T and above) magnetic inductions are required to produce neurophysiologic changes, especially in axonal conductivity. On the other hand, a series of systematic studies showed positive effects of moderate intensity SMF which resulted in a contrasting conclusion [68, 96, 391 - 393]. For example, during the exposure to SMF, the authors observed reduced visually evoked potentials [391] and lower spontaneous discharge in the lateral geniculate nucleus of cats [392]. In a different study, Wieraszko [159] reported that moderate intensity homogeneous SMF-exposure (2-3 mT) could modify the evoked population spike amplitude in mouse hippocampal slices. Rosen [97] performed a direct measurement of membrane calcium and sodium ion currents in cultured GH3 pituitary cells to reveal whether these effects occur at the level of the cellular membrane. SMF-exposure managed to increase the activation of the time constant of these channels. SMF-exposure managed to increase the activation of the time constant of these channels. These results indicate that moderate SMF induce a rotation of the membrane's phospholipid molecules which influence embedded ion channels [70]. A more general conclusion of these studies is that SMF-exposure effects may be chemically mediated and may have an influence on neurotransmitter release as well [70]. Similar to previous cardiovascular research, neurophysiologic studies also provided well established rationales for testing the beneficial effects of SMF-exposure on both animal and human subjects.

The Reader has already experienced in the sections of Chapter 5 (*In Vivo* Animal Experiments) that mice and rats in pathological condition response to various types of SMF-exposure with *AE*. In contrast to animal studies though, human studies mainly failed to find evidence for *AE* of SMF-exposure. As mentioned in the previous sections a meta-analysis of 29 clinical studies demonstrated that present evidence did not support the use of SMF for pain relief beyond the placebo effect [42]. This conclusion was criticized by Colbert *et al.* [43] in a review of 56 clinical studies. The authors argued that to evaluate the effectiveness of any SMF therapy and to permit protocol replications by other researchers, one must precisely define the SMF dosage and treatment parameters. Their main finding was that most of the SMF therapy studies lack these criteria. More particularly, 34 of the reviewed studies (61%) provided a poor methodological description, especially regarding 3 parameters: The identification of the target tissue, the distance of the magnet's surface from the target tissue, and the physical characteristics of the magnet. In a different paper, Colbert *et al.* [29] extensively discussed why certain parameters are important and they recommended 10 essential dosing parameters for special consideration in future studies (*e.g.* target tissue, distance of magnet surface from target tissue, magnetic field strength or induction, *etc.*).

The above mentioned reviews highlight the essentiality of testing the possible pain relief action of SMF in replicable, non-clinical studies involving human subjects. This claim is all the more relevant since while many aspects of the clinical application of SMF-exposure have been studied, no systematic research with precisely controlled dosimetry has been dedicated to the influence of SMF-exposure on the physiology and psychophysics of pain perception in normal (non-clinical) human participants. The non-clinical human research has to be a crucial part of a comprehensive approach in phase 3, which would allow us to understand the basic biological mechanism behind SMF-exposure and to optimize SMF dosing parameters *prior* to conducting a clinical study. Kuipers *et al.* [394] drew attention to the need of precise dosimetry in a recent study. The authors addressed the question of how a precisely defined 0.06 T SMF-exposure for 1 h alters pain perception using a variety of physiological parameters (sympathetic nerve activity, mean arterial pressure, heart rate, and forearm blood velocity) in healthy human subjects. Their results indicated no effect of SMF-exposure on any of the measured parameters. This finding was in line with their hypothesis that moderate intensity SMF would not alter physiological responses.

Goals

In the current clinically oriented, psychophysical study, our objective was to achieve precise comparability with other human studies and to use an SMF device that was similar to the one previously found to be effective anti-hyperalgesics in animal studies (**Pain and analgesia**). The purpose of the present experiment was to investigate the possible attenuating effects of SMF-exposure on the thermal pain threshold (TPT) measured non-invasively in healthy young adults in a double blind, placebo-controlled manner.

Materials and Methods

Participants

Fifteen undergraduate or postgraduate students (10 females and 5 males between 18 and 30 years of age with a mean age of 21 y) from the University of Pécs participated in the study. They were naïve with regard to the purpose of the experiment. All participants were right-handed and reported normal, medication-free health conditions. They signed a written consent after the nature of the experiment was fully explained to them. The work was conducted in accordance with the declaration of Helsinki and the experimental protocol was approved by the Ethical Committee of the University of Pécs (No.: 3427).

Thermal Stimulus Delivery

Thermal stimuli were randomly delivered through 4 computer controlled miniature piezoelectric heating pads (heating surface 5×5 mm^2) equipped with a 3D motion detector (accelerometer), and a precise digital temperature sensor (Metron Avionics, Pécs, Hungary). One sensor of the heat stimulator device was attached to the inner surface of each fingertip excluding the thumb on the dominant hand of the subjects.

Thermal stimuli were delivered to one finger at a time in a randomized order with approximately 20 s inter-stimulus intervals. The participant's task was to indicate their TPT to a ramp of increasing temperature on the surface of the heating pad (35-55°C temperature range, 1°C/s increase rate). When the participant moved his/her finger, the heating phase was immediately interrupted and the device actively cooled down to the initial temperature level within 2 s. The pad temperature at the moment of the trial termination was logged in a microcomputer (100 Hz sampling rate) and was treated as TPT data for that trial.

Magnetic Exposure Conditions

The SMF-exposure system (**Generator 18**) was used in the experiments. The magnetic matrices formed a treatment chamber of 140×100×50 mm (Fig. **3.7B**), big enough for a human palm and 4 fingers. The thumb remained outside the device.

Table 6.6. Ten essential dosing parameters for the present study following the suggestions of Colbert *et al.* [29].

Target tissue	skin tissue on the ventral surface of the fingertip of 2-5 digits
Site of magnet application	dominant hand
Distance of magnet surface from target tissue(s)	1-3 mm
Magnetic field strength	B_r=1.47 T, 330±0.1 mT at 3 mm from a cylindrical magnet in the isocenter of the matrix along its axis
Material composition of permanent magnet	N50 grade neodymium-iron-boron (NdFeB)
Magnet dimensions	A square lattice (forming a chamber of volume 140×100×50 mm^3) of individual cylindrical magnet blocks of axially magnetized cylindrical permanent magnets of 8×3 mm were fixed on a metal plate. The matrices thus formed a treatment chamber big enough for the human hand.
Magnet polar configuration	Magnetic poles pointed in identical direction within a block. Square lattices facing each other (in the matrices) were of opposite polarity.
Magnet support device	ferrous framing allowing for magnetic coupling
Frequency of magnet application	single experimental session
Duration of magnet application	continuous for 30 min

The induction measurement followed the steps described in **Tools, sampling** for automation. Table **6.6** summarizes the essential magnetic parameters in accordance with the suggestions of by Colbert *et al.* [29] including the following parameters: Target tissue, site of magnet application, magnet dimensions, distance of magnet surface from target tissue(s), magnetic induction or field strength, material composition of permanent magnet, magnet dimensions, polar configuration and support device, frequency and duration of magnet application.

Experimental Procedures

Fig. (**6.11A**) depicts the diagram of the experimental arrangement and Fig. (**6.11B**) shows the schedule of measurement blocks and sets. All participants took part in 4 consecutive recording blocks per session, in 2 sessions 1 week apart. When the participant signed the consent statement, he/she was seated and the stimulation device was attached to the fingertips of the dominant hand. After a block of practicing trials, the participant's dominant hand was exposed to either genuine SMF- or sham-exposure for 30 min in 3 consecutive blocks (blocks A, B, and C) in a double-blind design. In each session, the 4th block (block D) was a control measurement at 30 min post-exposure time (*i.e.* neither SMF nor sham device was used). The order of the genuine SMF- and sham-exposure sessions was counterbalanced across participants. In each block, we stimulated the 4 fingers randomly in 3 sets (Fig. **6.11B**). Thus, each participant performed a total of 48 trials in each session: (4 fingers×3 sets=12 TPT trials)×4 blocks.

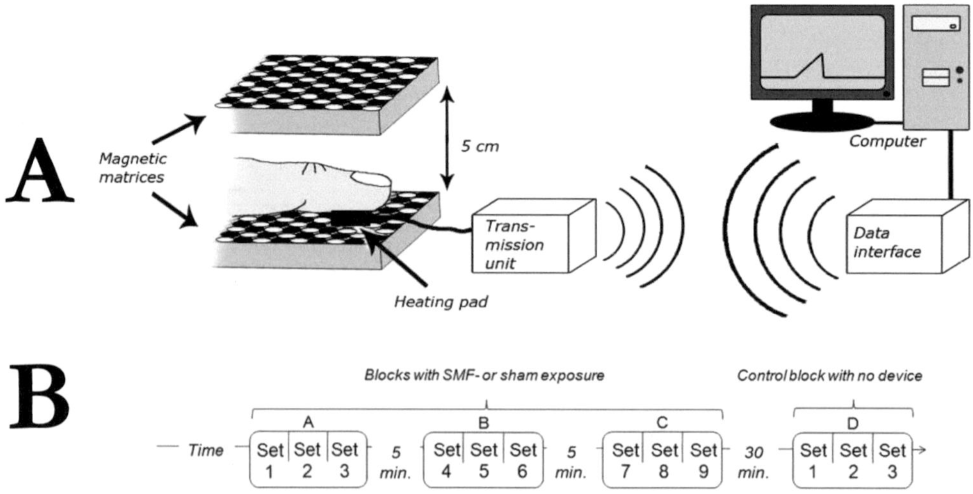

Fig. (6.11). Schematic representation of the **A)** arrangement and **B)** protocol of the experiment. The schedule of a session (at the bottom of the figure) consisted of 4 stimulation blocks (A, B, C, and D) and 12 sets (3 sets of stimuli on each finger per block).

During the first 3 blocks (henceforth device blocks), the participants' fingers were exposed to either SMF or sham (in 2 sessions), in contrast to the control block where no exposure device was used. After each block, subjects marked how painful the stimulus was in a visual analog rating scale (VAS; a 10 cm long line, "no pain" was printed on the left side, "worst possible pain" on the right). Participants' responses were later measured from left to right and subjective pain ratings were expressed in millimeters.

Statistical Analysis

In order to investigate the effect of SMF-exposure, the means of individual TPT measurements were computed first for each set. These data were subjected to repeated measures ANOVA (rANOVA) separately for device and control blocks. In addition, Wilcoxon rank sum tests were performed to test the difference between sets of the 2 sessions (SMF and sham), where appropriate. The threshold for significance was set at $p<0.05$. Results of significant individual comparisons are indicated in the figures below.

Results

TPT data (in °C) were recorded individually for each trial for each participant and were pooled within each set for each subject. Fig. (**6.12**) shows the average threshold data as a function of sets.

To analyze the TPT data, we first performed separate rANOVA for the device blocks and the control block. For device blocks, data were analyzed with a 3 factorial design where session (2 levels: SMF or sham), block (3 levels: A, B, or C), and set (3 levels) were used as independent variables. For the control block, a 2 factorial design was conducted: session (2 levels) and set (3 levels). The results of these calculations are summarized next. For the device blocks, rANOVA revealed a significant main effect of session ($F(1,14)=6.14$, $p=0.02$) and set ($F(2,13)=9.59$, $p=0.003$). There was also a marginal session-set interaction ($F(2,13)=3.56$, $p=0.059$). The main effect of block ($F(2,13)=1.76$, $p=0.21$) and the session-block interaction ($F(2,13)=0.61$, $p=0.56$),however, did not turn out to be significant. For the control block, the only significant result was found in the main effect of set ($F(2,12)=21.03$, $p<0.001$). Neither the main effect of session

($F(1,14)=0.72$, $p=0.41$), nor the interaction between the 2 factors ($F(2,71)=2.23$, $p=0.1$) was found to be significant.

In Fig. (**6.12**), the result patterns are dominated by a cyclic tendency: TPT data show a linear increase within each of the blocks, but drops between consecutive blocks. Whereas this cyclic tendency is highly salient for the sham session, it is much more modest for the SMF session.

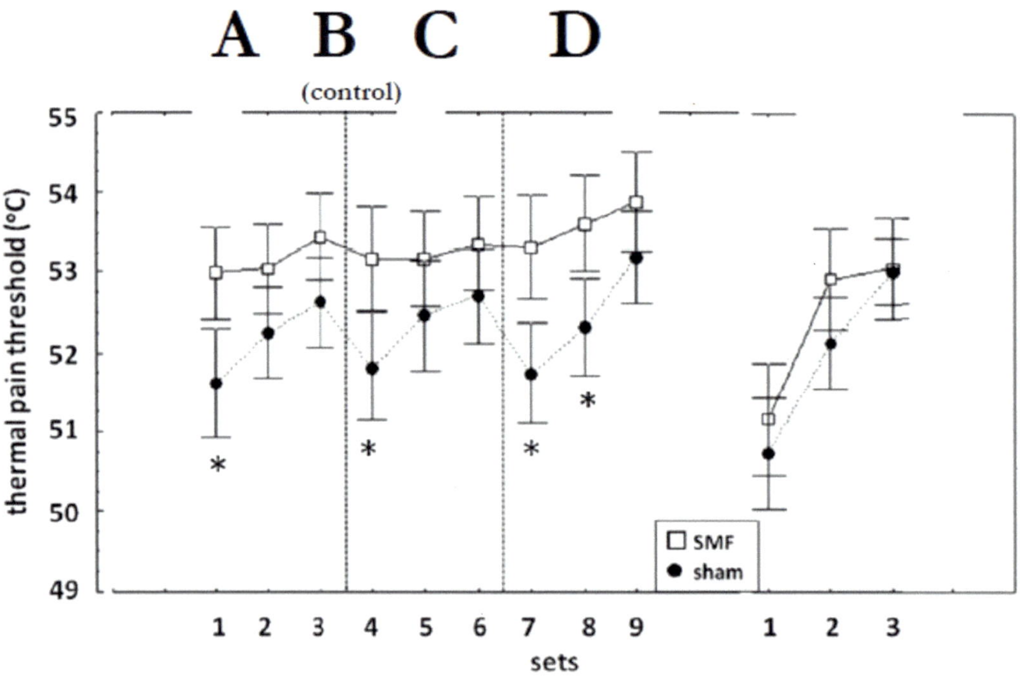

Fig. (6.12). Mean TPT measured in 15 individuals (in °C as a function of sets in each exposure condition (SMF or sham). The borders of the 4 main experimental blocks (A, B, C, and D) are indicated by the vertical dashed lines. Error bars represent SEM. Pairwise comparisons between sets of 2 sessions were performed by the Wilcoxon rank sum test, * designates significant difference $p<0.05$.

For the calculation of the percentage change and the demonstration of significance of the tendency in the data, we further used first set data as the reference point for each block and computed the relative increase (in %) of the TPT data between the 1st and 3rd set within each block. The average relative increase as a function of blocks is indicated in Fig. (**6.13**). Again, rANOVA calculations were performed with factors of session and block separately for the device-blocks and the control-block. For the device-blocks, there was a significant main effect of session ($F(1,14)=7.82$, $p=0.014$), a non-significant main effect of block ($F(2,13)=1.23$, $p=0.32$), and a non-significant 2-way interaction between the factors ($F(2,13) = 0.15$, $p=0.86$). For the control-block, the analysis yielded a non-significant main effect of session ($F(1,14)=0.96$, $p=0.34$).

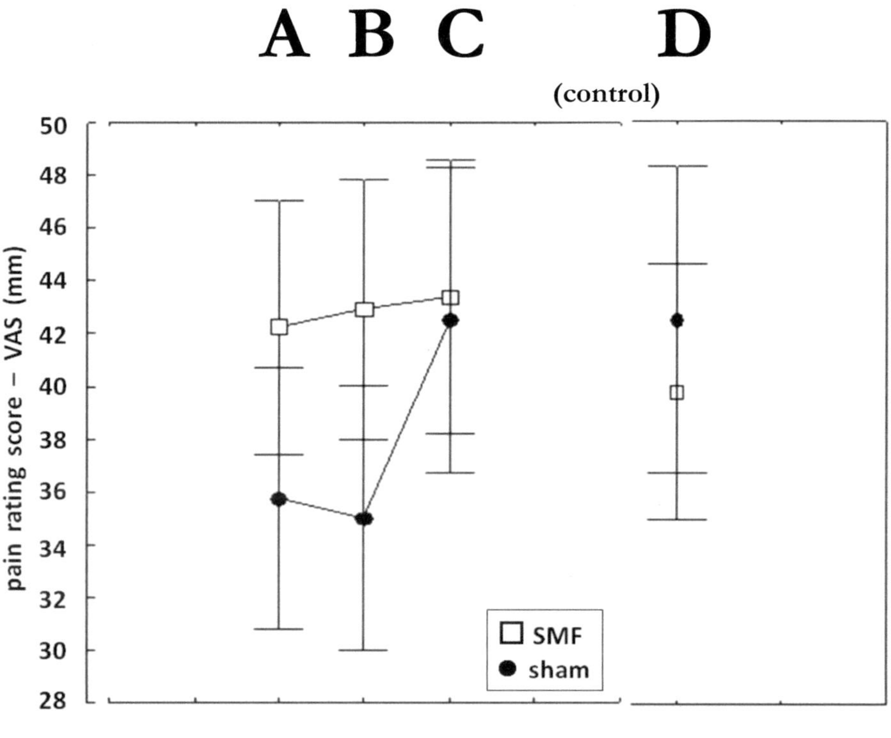

Fig. (6.13). Mean relative increase (in %) in TPT as a function of blocks in each exposure condition (SMF and sham) measured in 15 individuals. Pairwise comparisons between the sets of the 2 sessions were performed by Wilcoxon rank sum test, * designates significant difference $p<0.05$.

The results for the VAS are shown in Fig. (**6.14**). For the device blocks, rANOVA yielded non-significant main effects (session: $F(1,14)=1.37$, $p=0.26$; block: $F(2,13)=2.389$, $p=0.13$), but a significant 2-way interaction between session and block ($F(1,14)=4.28$, $p=0.037$). To analyze this significant interaction in more detail, two more rANOVA calculations were performed separately for 2 sessions. For the SMF session, rANOVA revealed no main effect of block ($F(2,13)=0.07$,

p=0.93). In contrast to this, an identical analysis for the sham session yielded a significant main effect of block ($F(2,13)=6.11$, $p=0.013$). In addition, both the linear ($F(1,14)=8.03$, $p=0.01$) and the quadratic ($F(1,14)=9.11$, $p=0.009$) trends were significant. Finally, for the control block there was no significant main effect of session.

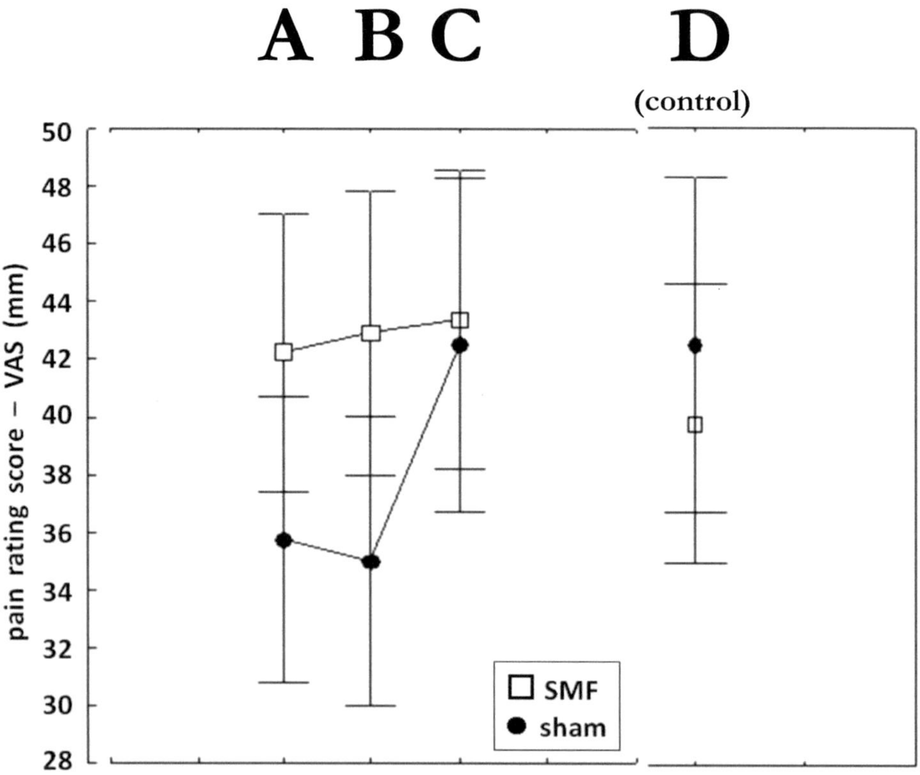

Fig. (6.14). Mean pain rating scores measured in 15 individuals for the VAS (mm) as a function of blocks in each exposure condition (SMF or sham).

Discussion, Conclusions

In the present study, we investigated the possible attenuating effects of a precisely controlled, inhomogeneous SMF-exposure on TPT in healthy young adults. First, we demonstrated that exposure to inhomogeneous SMF increases pain threshold (measured in °C). An ongoing adaptation was observed within each experimental block for pain threshold in the sham condition, which was completely absent under SMF condition. Second, VAS profiles indicated an ongoing increase in pain ratings between measurement blocks in the sham condition, while remaining at a constant level under the SMF condition.

Moreover, a salient (although non-significant) pattern of results was observed for a simultaneous increase in pain threshold (*i.e.* adaptation) and VAS pain rating scores (*i.e.* sensitization). The interpretation of this finding is a little difficult since the adaptation for TPT and the sensitization for VAS pain rating cannot be directly compared. TPT adaptation took place within each block from set to set, whereas VAS rating increased between complete blocks under sham condition. To resolve the issue of increased TPT with increased VAS pain rating, one might consider the increased TPT as a peripheral, receptor or pain fiber level process, and the tendency for the global sensitization represented by the VAS ratings as an indication of the involvement of higher order, overall pain evaluation mechanisms.

As there was no significant decrease in VAS pain rating in the genuine exposure condition, the present data might also imply that peripheral rather than central neuronal mechanisms are involved in the increase in the pain perception level due to SMF-exposure. In the present experimental arrangement, the exposure to SMF was peripheral compared to previous animal studies where whole-body exposure was performed on mice using a similar SMF generator (***In Vivo* Animal Experiments**). In this specific study, although SMF-exposure could not prevent the development of experimentally induced mechanical allodynia, it could inhibit long-lasting processes that normally maintained the increased sensitivity to mechanical stimuli in neuropathic pain. This study could not rule out the effect of possible chronic peripheral neuronal adaptation. Direct evidence for such peripheral pain fiber adaptation mechanism was also reported in a study using the same SMF device on mice, where biochemical transmission was targeted in skin nociceptors (**Peripheral action**). In that particular animal study, *AE* of SMF was completely diminished in either formalin induced pain or carrageenan induced mechanical hyperalgesia unless mice had been previously pretreated with the capsaicin receptor TRPV1 agonist, resiniferatoxin. These results strongly support the notion that such capsaicin receptors are involved in the action of SMF on the perception of mechanically induced pain. It is also known that TRPV1 receptors are involved in heat perception and heat-generated pain processes [395]. This action of SMF-exposure on nociception and the TRPV1 receptor mechanism has been thought to be the consequence of reduced sodium and calcium current influx into the neurons and the resulting reduced potential for spike firing generation which can also be observed under physiological conditions where normal adaptation occurs [396, 397].

It is not clear however, how tactile receptors may be involved in the observed *AE*, because it is known that heat stimuli capable of inducing pain can significantly diminish taction, and *vice versa*; taction can alleviate chronic pain as suggested by Apkarian *et al.* [398, 399].

Another mechanism for physiological adaptation was studied in anesthetized rats, where moderate intensity SMF (below 400 mT, most effective range 10 or 70 mT) acted on L-type Ca channels decreasing the microcirculation and thereby reducing an inflammatory agent induced edema in the skin [166].

In summary, results of the present experiment are not able to support any of the above-discussed conclusions from current animal experimental literature because of the lack of somatic intervention. Non the less, these studies together open up further research possibilities that could shed light on the basic physiological action of SMF-exposure in healthy human subjects.

It is known that the literature widely supports the potential therapeutic benefit of pulsed electromagnetic field application in various areas of medical care (for a list of relevant studies and areas see Morris and Skalak [166]). However, much less direct evidence is available for supporting therapeutic uses of SMF-exposure despite the fact that SMF are much more frequently used than over-the-counter magnetic "healing" products currently on the market [400].

Our study serves as a pioneering work for demonstrating that a positive pain threshold shift may occur in healthy human subjects exposed to SMF under physiological receptor conditions (*i.e.* without inflammation). More specifically, data obtained by using randomized, placebo-controlled trials in a double-blind manner with a precisely tested and controlled dosimetry for inhomogeneous SMF-exposure indicate a positive evidence for an increased pain threshold and a reduced "sensitization" effect between consecutive blocks of trials in a TPT examination. These results may also provide a basis for further testing and possible optimization of SMF parameters relevant for therapeutic applications in pain related to clinical conditions. Would this reduced sensitization manifest itself in anesthesia induced by local exposure to SMF in healthy visitors to a dental office? Would boring and drilling be possible without the injection of potentially allergenic anesthetics? We will explore these questions in the next section.

On Visitors of a Dental Clinic

Effect of Inhomogeneous Sstatic Magnetic Field on Dental Pain in Humans

Preliminaries

Nowadays, due to local anesthesia having become the backbone of pain control techniques in dentistry (*e.g.* [401]), most dental treatments are painless. However, local anesthesia for controlling pain has only temporary effect. Drugs used may be accompanied by adverse side effects (allergy, gastric ulcer, cardiovascular overload, *etc.*). The search for reliable, safe, yet still effective management of pain remains a challenge. As mentioned before, among a number of other treatment strategies, magnetic therapy is increasingly applied to alleviate pain.

Several preclinical studies performed on rodent models testing the effect of analgesic/antinociceptive SMF have been mentioned already in Chapter 5 (***In Vivo* Animal Experiments**). *AE* induced by 10 min SMF-exposure in the writhing test in mice was shown to have a slow fall-off (retard) characteristic after cessation of the exposure. It drops by only *cca.* 10% in the time period 21-30 min following the exposure (**Optimization of SMF parameters**).

I am reminding the Reader of the human trials detailed in the previous section where it was shown that SMF therapy as a self-care intervention has led to the conduct of more than 50 randomized controlled clinical trials [43]. Results obtained from studies that tested *AE* of SMF therapy in pain are inconsistent, though. It has also been mentioned that some authors demonstrated a positive effect of SMF-exposure in achieving anesthesia in neuropathic, inflammatory, musculoskeletal, fibromyalgia, rheumatic, or postsurgical pain [40, 261 - 267]. Others claimed that SMF-exposure had no advantage over sham-exposure in reducing pain intensity in patients with diabetic polyneuropathy, chronic lower back pain, or carpal tunnel syndrome [268 - 273]. Pittler *et al.* [42] published a systematic review and meta-analysis of 29 human studies and concluded that the *AE* of SMF is not supported by experimental data; placebo effect cannot be filtered out adequately. Placebo effect was also shown to liberalize endogenous μ-opioid receptors [35].

A strong motivation of dental studies is the proliferation of MRI in medical diagnosis. The published results concentrated on ferromagnetic materials, such as dental amalgam and prostheses under high gradient magnetic field conditions [402, 403]. Also, orthodontic magnets and implants can be of concern when placed in strong SMF [404]. Bondemark *et al.* [405, 406], for example, examined the effects of orthodontic magnets on the oral mucosa, the dental pulp, and the gingiva. The endpoints of these examinations were morphological and histological alterations of the surrounding tissue. The magnet and the demagnetized control material were bonded on molars on either side of the mouth. The SMF from the implants varied between 10 and 140 mT. Some inflammation was detected in the tissue close to both the magnet and demagnetized magnet but not in other sites. Those were attributed to contact irritation rather than to the SMF-exposure. More recently, a Chinese research group published a series of papers on the effect of SMF on osteoblastic morphology and surface ultrastructure [407], on cytoskeletons of human periodontal ligament cells [408], and on the activity of superoxide dismutase of human gingival fibroblasts [409]. They have also published a paper on the dosimetric considerations of the SMF they had applied [410].

Literature is limited on the dental pain aspects of SMF. Information for dental practitioners is available on phantom tooth pain as a form of neuropathic pain of the oral cavity [411]. The possibility of pain management in neuropathic pain with SMF would be all the more important as today's medicine lacks the general solution for neuropathic pain as such as discussed in **Neuropathic pain**.

Ghione *et al.* [412] conducted a study on the human dental pain threshold modified by 50 Hz, 40 μT electromagnetic fields and they found a significant decrease of the threshold in the treated cases compared to sham control. However,

Ropohl *et al.* [413] reported that dental pain may be induced *via* using repetitive transcranial magnetic stimulation.

The clinical importance of the present study is twofold. To prove or to dismiss one or both of the following assumptions: SMF-exposure may

- replace systemic local anesthesia due to its retard pain inhibitory effect,
- increase pain tolerance threshold in the tooth.

Materials and Methods

Magnetic Exposure Conditions

The exposure system used was **Generator 19**. An identical looking matrix filled with material of equal weight and applied to the same holder was used as a sham arrangement for the placebo-control examinations.

As mentioned in **Generator 19**, the matrix was covered with a thin, soft tissue and was applied

1. on the side of the face closest to the location of the consecutive dental treatment between the maxilla and the mandible in the numerical rating visual analog scale (NRS) test and/or
2. in front of the incisors in the tolerance threshold measurement (TTM) test.

Both SMF and sham device were used for 30 min.

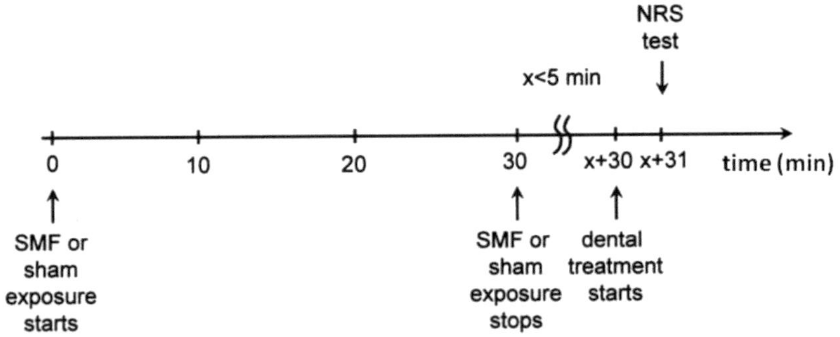

Fig. (6.15). Flow diagram of the NRS test. The dental treatment was either drilling in preparation for caries filling as a pathological situation, or burring in preparation for prosthetic procedure as a physiological situation.

<u>*Assessment of dental pain sensation*</u>

1. NRS group: The primary outcome measure in this examination was the subjective measurement of pain sensation following a 30 min SMF-exposure, 1 min after having a specific dental treatment (either drilling in preparation for caries filling as a pathological situation, or burring in preparation for prosthetic procedure as a physiological situation) started. Before the dental treatment started, the SMF-exposure system was removed from the patient's head (at time point 30 min). A few minutes (not more than 5 min) may have passed between the removal of the device and the commencement of the actual dental procedure. NRS was used for testing. It consisted of a sheet of paper with a single black line of 100 mm length on it with integer Arabic numbers from 0 to 10 in circles above. On the left side of the number scale "no pain" and on the right side "the most intense pain sensation imaginable" were written. Patients were asked to estimate their pain perception after the 1st min of the dental treatment by crossing one of the numbers. One or 2 tests were executed on each patient. One test was conducted in the first session, another (if any) in a follow-up session. Follow-up sessions happened 2-4 weeks after the first session. The dental treatment could be interrupted upon the patient's request even within the 1st min. If the patient asked to do so, systemic anesthesia was applied immediately. Fig. (**6.15**) shows the flow diagram of the examination. Our expectation (null-hypothesis) in this test was an NRS score 0-5 following the 30 min SMF treatment. A baseline would have been a score between 5 and 10.
2. TTM group: The primary outcome measure in this type of examination was the subjective TTM difference between before (pre-) and after (post-) 30 min SMF- or sham-exposure. TTM was tested with a non-invasive tooth pulp tester (Denjoy Dental, model DY310). The instrument gave automatic intermittent bursts of electrical stimuli at increasing voltage through a probe placed on the tooth. The subject had to indicate, by lifting his hand, when the stimulation became painful enough to require interruption, and the corresponding value (ranging from 0 to 80, arbitrary units) on the instrument's display was taken as the tolerance threshold. We used a step width of 10 units. Two healthy, unfilled teeth (two incisors, the right lateral inferior and the left lateral superior) were tested and the average score was used for the subsequent analysis. This

measurement was executed in 2 sessions, twice on each healthy patient in each session; 1 min before and 1 min after 30 min SMF- or sham-exposure; see the flow diagram in Fig. (**6.16**). If the treatment was sham in session 1, then it was SMF in session 2, or the other way round. 2-4 weeks passed between sessions. Our expectation in this test was a TTM score 0-40 before, and 40-80 following the 30 min SMF treatment. We also expected (null-hypothesis) that SMF-exposure will result in higher scores than sham-exposure.

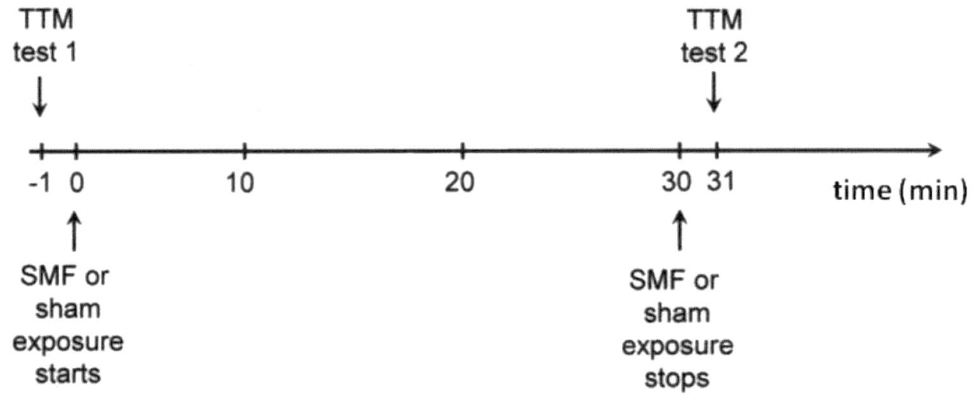

Fig. (6.16). Flow diagram of the TTM test carried out in healthy volunteers.

Subjects and Methodology

The test series lasted for 9 months including recruitment. Tests and treatment were carried out at a dental institute (Dentsana-TA, Sopron, Hungary). We set 10 as the lower limit of the number of participants in each group and left the upper limit open. We planned to recruit as many patients as was needed to achieve 10% relative accuracy of the population mean of the NRS and the TTM primary outcome with 0.95 probability. In the end, we tested 59 participants (26 males + 33 females) altogether, representing 62 cases which was more than necessary due to the little standard deviation of the data. These patients, whose mean age was 43.6 y (73% between 20 to 50 y), were assigned to either the NRS (36 of 62 cases) or the TTM group (23 of 62 cases). The eligibility criteria in both experiments were as follows: Age between 18-72 y, medication free healthiness. The exclusion criteria were as follows:

- Regular use of medication or consumption of alcohol,
- expecting or lactating,
- regular smoking,
- any type of psychological disorder.

Subjects were recruited individually by the dental institute, where later their dental and SMF (or sham) treatment was carried out. Volunteers were allocated to one of the following 4 groups:

NRS: i) Dental problem: Caries, expected treatment: Filling, starting procedure: Drilling, exposure: 30 min SMF, measurement: 1 min after dental treatment started following SMF-exposure, number of participants: 9 females + 6 males
NRS: ii) Dental problem: None, expected treatment: Prosthetic, starting procedure: Burring, exposure: 30 min SMF, measurement: 1 min after dental treatment started following SMF-exposure, number of participants: 13 females + 8 males
TTM: iii) Dental problem: None, measurements: Before and after 30 min SMF treatment, number of participants: 12 females + 11 males
TTM: iv) Dental problem: None, measurements: Before and after 30 min sham treatment, number of participants: 12 females + 11 males (the same 23 people as in iii)

In the case of 3 patients both NRS and TTM were applied. No adverse effects were recorded in either group.

1. NRS group i and ii: After a series of pilot tests, we decided to carry out the testing without placebo-control as all but one subject interrupted the dental treatment asking for systemic anesthesia. Members of group i were volunteers with dental problems. Members of group ii were healthy volunteers with no dental problems. In 3 cases, both caries filling and burring occurred. Dropout rate was 6 out of 42. In 1 case out of 36, we decided to make an exception due to…, and we excluded the corresponding data from the statistical analysis (see Results for details).
2. TTM group iii and iv: Members of this group were healthy volunteers without dental problems. Testing was carried out in a double-blind, placebo-controlled,

randomized manner. When preparing for the randomized trial, we followed the checklist published by the CONSORT (Consolidated Standards of Reporting Trials) group in 2001 [414]. The head of the clinic was in charge of the randomization and control of the double-blind manner. The treatment was either 30 min SMF-exposure (with magnets) or 30 min sham-exposure (without magnets) in each of the 2 sessions. The reason for testing the same person in 2 sessions was to evaluate the reproducibility of the test. A series of random binary numbers (0 or 1, *i.e.* sham or SMF) was generated and assigned to the patient number list. The number determined the order of treatment between sessions. If the number was 0, the treatment was sham-exposure in the first session and SMF in the second. The patient list was concealed from both patients and assistants. Dropout rate in this group was 0 out of 23.

It is rather challenging to ensure blindness in studies including devices with permanent magnets. We advised patients in advance that their sensation would not directly be correlated with the magnetic induction of the device, and the sham device would also be able to increase their tolerance threshold. They were also asked to remove any magnetically anisotropic objects from their reach during the 30 min long exposure period.

Ethical Considerations

Volunteers were informed about the goal of the project, the SMF or sham treatment, and their possible effects. Volunteers in the NRS group understood that if following the 30 min SMF treatment their pain sensation had not been reduced to a tolerable limit during the consecutive dental treatment (drilling or burring), the dental treatment would be interrupted and they would immediately receive an anesthetic drug (2% Ultracain). They all signed a form that they understood the plan and their participation was voluntary (*i.e.* they have given their informed consent). The study was conducted in accordance with the Declaration of Helsinki. In terms of data protection: all personal data were handwritten on paper by one of the heads of the clinic, and the papers were locked in a file cabinet at the dental institute. Only this person was authorized to see and handle these data. They were not opened to or by any third person. Statistical analysis was performed on the basis of patients' numbers and measured scores. In terms of exposure system:

there is no regulation for the use of permanent magnetic devices in the EU whatsoever below 8 T magnetic induction. For potential risks of SMF-exposure we refer the Reader to the SCENIHR report [13].

Statistical Analysis

Data obtained in all 4 groups were evaluated using one-way ANOVA. Two-sample heteroscedastic Dunnett's test was used to compare any binary set of data. If 2 data series of unequal numbers were compared, Bonferroni's correction was applied. The difference between data sets was considered significant at the 95% confidence level, if $p<0.05$.

Results

NRS (Group i and ii)

Fig. (**6.17**) shows NRS raw data for both groups i and ii as obtained patient by patient.

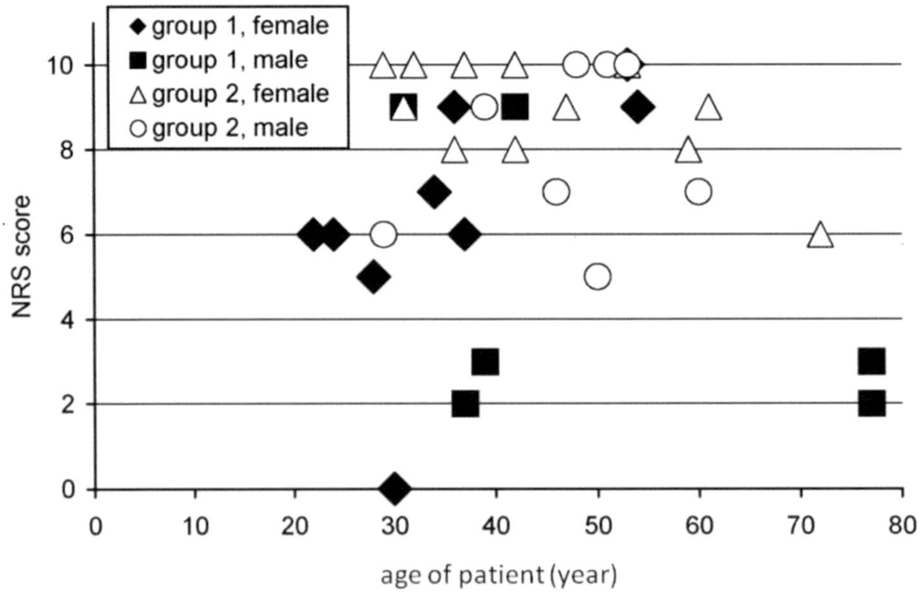

Fig. (6.17). Raw data of the NRS test *vs* age of patient for group i (pathological situation) and group ii (physiological situation) for 36 volunteers (22 females, 14 males).

After the first some experiments, we decided to give up on sham-exposure. We kept executing the test on a group whose members already consented to participation in the study; however, no further members were recruited. 100% failure of pain inhibition in the preliminary tests suggested to us that we might as well do without the placebo-control management. Still, we were interested in comparing the average pain sensation between A) healthy patients and patients with caries, B) sexes, and C) ages even without relying on the pain inhibitory effect of either SMF- or sham-exposure. For the whole group of 36, one single person tolerated the dental treatment without systemic anesthetic. We excluded the data of this patient from the otherwise homogeneous data basis. A histogram of the NRS ratings is presented in Fig. (**6.18**). Both dental treatment procedures (group i and ii) are designated.

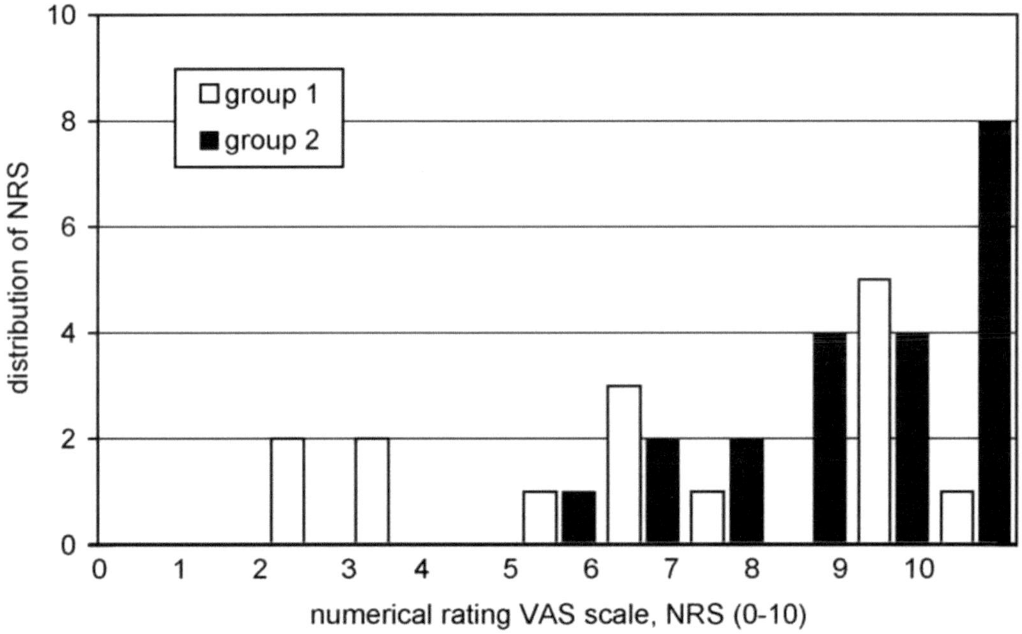

Fig. (6.18). Histogram of the NRS data. NRS was taken after 30 min SMF-exposure in case of group i (pathological situation) and group ii (physiological situation) for 36 volunteers (22 females, 14 males).

Correlation analysis between age and NRS score for group i female and male and for group ii female and male participants showed 82.59%, (51.30%, (55.51%, 22.01%, respectively. Characteristic data including all sexes, ages, and types of dental treatment were: Mean 7.52, median 8.00, mode 9.50, range 8.00, SEM 0.37. Drilling and burring caused an average NRS of 6.39±0.61 (mean±SEM) and 8.52±0.34, respectively. Females tolerated drilling better and burring worse than did males. For drilling, the ratio was 8.52 to 5.29, meanwhile for burring: 8.85 to 8.00. The NRS scores obtained in double (first plus follow-up) sessions were identical; no dynamic variation of the pain sensation could be identified in a time range of 2-4 weeks.

The effect of SMF-exposure including group i and ii, females and males is represented in Table **6.7**. The only potential candidate for pain inhibition due to 30 min SMF-exposure was the group of males with caries. Even in this group patients interrupted the dental treatment within the 1st min asking for systemic anesthesia. In this group, the percentage of NRS scores below 5 was 66.67% of all scores which could refer to a beneficial SMFinduced effect if the participant number were higher. Score for males was 4.67±1.38 *vs* 6.44±0.99 for females in this group still yielding an insignificant difference (p>0.3).

Table 6.7. NRS scores below 5 (in % to all in section) on a scale of 0-10 as tested in the 1st min after having dental treatment started following a 30 min SMF-exposure in the NRS groups i (drilling) and ii (burring).

section			number of cases	NRS scores below 5 (in % to all in section)
overall			36	17.14
	group i		15	35.71
		females	9	12.50
		males	6	66.67
	group ii		21	4.76
		females	13	0.00
		males	8	12.50

The exceptional case mentioned above was that of a 30 y old female patient who visited her dentist complaining of dental pain. The dentist diagnosed caries and a developed pulpitis. Following a 30 min SMF-exposure, a complete anesthesia was achieved; her NRS score in the 1st min of the tooth drilling was 0. No drug was used throughout the dental treatment.

TTM (Group iii and iv)

TTM values below the age 50 y (90.91% of all data for females, 81.82% of all data for males) were 50% for both sexes (40 in the arbitrary unit scale), pre- and post-SMF or -sham treatment. The average TTM value was identically 41.5±1.5 for both SMF- and the sham-exposure (pre- and post-exposure) for females, whereas 42.9±2.0 for SMF-exposure (pre- and post-exposure) and 42.2±1.6 for the sham-exposure (pre- and post-exposure) for males. Characteristic data for all sexes and ages are collected in Table **6.8**. ANOVA resulted in p=0.74 (F_{crit}=3.95) for the difference between SMF and sham treatment including both pre- and post-treatment values. The p values were united when pre- and post-treatment TTM values (including SMF and sham treatment) were compared. The correlation between age and tolerance threshold was 54.82% and 72.67% for females and males, respectively. The only case when difference was found between SMF and sham-exposure was that of a 53 years old male. In his case, SMF-exposure seemed to have a more beneficial effect with regard to the tolerance threshold value than placebo (by 14.29%).

Table 6.8. Characteristic statistical data of the TTM experiment for all sexes and ages in the TTM groups iii (SMF) and iv (sham). Pre- and post-exposure values proved to be identical.

	pre-(and post-) exposure	
	SMF	**sham**
mean	42.4	41.6
median	40	40
mode	40	40
range	16	16
SEM	0.8	0.8

The lady who was mentioned before as a special case for the NRS group also participated in the TTM measurement 1 month after having the caries filled. She was exposed to SMF treatment for 30 min. There was no difference in her tolerance threshold value pre- and post-exposure.

Discussion, Conclusions

The *AE* of an inhomogeneous SMF produced by a one-sided arrangement of magnets was shown to achieve 24.39% in the writhing test in mice as opposed to 81.81% in the case of the arrangement of the highest effect (**Optimization of SMF parameters**). However, in the setup of animal experiments with mice, the place of action was estimated at 20 mm from the surface of the magnets. In the present arrangement, the distance between the tooth and the magnets' surface was always smaller than an estimated 10 mm. At this distance the *P-P* value of the magnetic induction is 4.7 times bigger than in the animal experiments; also the gradient field is more intense. Consequently, we expected a significant pain inhibitory effect.

The finding that exposure to an inhomogeneous SMF did not significantly alter either pain sensation or pain tolerance threshold in subjects is in contradiction with the results presented by Ghione *et al.* [412] as well as the observation made on sensitization in the previous section **On healthy volunteers**. It is noteworthy though that direct comparison is not possible since Ghione *et al.* [412] applied a 50 Hz, 40 μT electromagnetic field, whereas the previous section **On healthy volunteers** included the testing of response to thermal stimulus. The lack of comparability also holds for the transcranial magnetic stimulation study of Ropohl *et al.* [413] where dental pain was reported to be induced by the electromagnetic field.

Common dental disorders often involve an inflammatory state in the oral environment. Although the relatively low participant number and the uncontrolled manner in the case of the NRS examination did not allow us to draw unambiguous conclusions, it seemed that SMF-exposure failed to have an effect on healthy patients (group ii, iii and iv); thus, we should drop the corresponding null-hypothesis. The only potential candidate for an effect was when an inflammatory situation occurred at (or under) the place where the SMF-exposure was targeted. In our case, the male participants with caries (group i) responded most positively to the SMF treatment. This finding is in harmony with previous observations in *in vivo* animal experiments detailed in Chapter 5 (***In Vivo* Animal Experiments**) where SMF-exposure did not induce any effects in healthy animals. The retard effect was also observed in animals with pathologic conditions (**Optimization of SMF parameters**). However, recent studies applying strong SMF (*e.g.* MR devices with B_0 component above 1.5 T) show that this statement should not be taken for granted either. Exposure to strong SMF may have an effect on healthy organisms as well [415, 416].

Although the average age in group iii and iv (TTM) was 39.71 y only, 3 people in the group were over 68 y. There was still hope that the electrically measurable tooth sensitivity remains normal even in elderly patients. Petrikas *et al.* [417] have reported that normal sensitivity is maintained even in severe periodontitis when measured with electroexcitability.

The case of the lady with caries and pulpitis with complete anesthesia achieved following the 30 min SMF-exposure (0 NRS score) was extraordinary; however, this case is to be regarded as an exception. It was her case that encouraged us to carry out a complete double-blind study on dental patients with diseases of inflammatory background (to be presented in **Stomatological pain**).

In conclusion; when a 192 mT (maximum *P-P* amplitude by 19 T/m gradient) inhomogeneous SMF was applied 30 min *prior* to a dental procedure, it failed to significantly reduce pain associated with drilling or burring of the teeth. Would local exposure to a similar SMF apparatus have beneficial effects under inflammatory conditions in patients?

On Patients

Inflammation

We shall now focus on non-lethal diseases with a high impact on the quality of life such as acute or chronic inflammatory diseases (*e.g.* alveolitis, aphta, temporomandibular joint disorders, and erosive gastritis). We expected that our research would develop improved pathology and intervention strategies with the expected impact of an effective therapy and improving quality of life.

Chronic inflammation is a pathological, persistent, and acute inflammation condition due to non-degradable pathogens, persistent foreign bodies, or autoimmune reactions characterized by concurrent active inflammation, tissue destruction, and attempts at repair. Chronicallyinflamed tissue can be described as the infiltration of mononuclear immune cells (monocytes, macrophages, lymphocytes, and plasma cells), tissue destruction, and attempts at healing that include angiogenesis and fibrosis. Its primary mediators are INF-γ and other cytokines, growth factors, reactive oxygen species (ROS), and hydrolytic enzymes. Its duration may be months or even years. Its outcomes are tissue destruction and fibrosis. The chronic diseases that involve the highest number of patients are: chronic pain, pulmonary diseases (*e.g.* asthma and chronic obstructive pulmonary disease, or COPD), autoimmune conditions (among others rheumatic diseases as rheumatoid arthritis), chronic intestinal inflammation (*e.g.* erosive and hemorrhagic gastroduodenitis, peptic ulcer, and Crohn's disease), and post infarction health challenges.

Chronic inflammatory diseases afflict millions of people across the world leading to untold suffering, economic loss and premature death. Arthritis alone is a problem of about 1/6 of the world's population. Despite the importance of these diseases and the intensive global research, there have been relatively few innovative breakthroughs into their cause, treatment or cure.

Therefore, the need to understand and develop treatment options for inflammatory diseases is of primary importance. On the one hand, in the treatment of the syndromes of *e.g.* rheumatological diseases, steroid and no-steroid anti-inflammatory drugs (*e.g.* SAIDs, such as betametazon, prednisolon, and hydrocortisone, or NSAIDs, such as diclofenac, piroxicam, or naproxen) are preferred and used worldwide. Even though their efficiency and mechanism of action are different, they all inhibit inflammation. Their usage and dosage constitute real concern, though. Other than adverse side effects, the involved system of interactions should also be taken into account (see *e.g.* gastric and duodenal ulcer). Bacteria and viruses are implicated in the development of some inflammatory diseases. The exacerbation of these diseases is frequently caused by infections. It is currently estimated that within the next 10 years many antibiotics, currently employed for treating bacterial infections, will no longer be effective due to microbial resistance. Also, very few treatments for viral infections exist to this date.

Stomatological Pain

Effect of Local Exposure to Inhomogeneous Static Magnetic Field on Stomatological Pain Sensation – a Double-Blind, Randomized, Placebo-Controlled Study

Preliminaries

In the following 3 areas of therapeutic applications of SMF the published results are contradictory: the healing of damaged joints, inflammation, and wound healing. Segal *et al.* [265] compared the effect of a 4block arrangement of permanent magnets with that of a single magnet (no placebo control) fixed to the knee of 64 patients with rheumatoid arthritis. Exposure continued for 1 week. Different rheumatologic indices and subjective pain assessment showed a significant improvement in both groups wearing magnets compared to baseline data and also to untreated control. SMF was tested on pathologic joint healing by Hsieh *et al.* [418] who reported that 3 T magnetic induction of a clinical MRI combined with RF electromagnetic field for 1 h suppressed cell growth and induced apoptosis *in vitro* in human chondrocytes. They also presented the results of an *in vivo* experiment with the same exposure system for 1 h applied on the surgically damaged knees of 6 Lee-Sung pigs on a single occasion. SMF plus RF hindered cartilage repair. On the contrary, Chen *et al.* [419] presented the effect of magnetic knee wraps on joint position sense in 50 individuals with knee osteoarthritis. The applied continuous exposure was 35 mT for 12 weeks. The wearing of magnetic wraps did not show a significant effect in the joint position sense compared to placebo control. Jaberi *et al.* [420], however, examined the effect caused by permanent cylindrical magnets of 40 mT induction implanted in the right medial femoral condyle of 30 rabbits. The condyles had been defected by drilling. After 12 weeks the group with implanted magnets showed a Mankin's score about 1/5 of that of the sham or the control group. We also presented in **Peripheral action** that SMF-exposure significantly diminished the duration of formalin-evoked behavioral responses in both phase I (acute somatic nociception) and phase II (acute inflammatory nociception) in mice. Selective inactivation of capsaicin-sensitive sensory fibers by high dose resiniferatoxin pre-treatment decreased nocifensive behaviors in phase II of the formalin test which indicates that pro-inflammatory neuropeptides, such as substance P and CGRP released from these fibers are involved in this inflammatory reaction. An acute *AE* of SMF-exposure was observed by Morris and Skalak [166]. They induced inflammation with the help of injecting inflammatory agents, λ-carrageenan or histamine, into rat hind paws alone or in conjunction with pharmacological agents. Application of a 10 or 70 mT, but not 400 mT, SMF for 15 or 30 min immediately following histamine induced edema resulted in a significant reduction in the edema formation. In addition, a 2 h, 70 mT SMF-exposure to λ-carrageen-aninduced edema also resulted in significant edema reduction. The authors found if exposure was applied immediately after histamine injection, edema was reduced by 40-65%. This background was reinforced by the research of Lin *et al.* [304] who studied the effect of 0.25 T homogeneous SMF on the production of IL-1ra (interleukin-1 receptor antagonist) in *in vivo* in BALB/cByJ male mice that were exposed to SMF for 2 h before the intraperitoneal injection of 50 mg/kg lipopolysaccharide. They found that both the survival rate and the plasma IL-1ra level in the SMFexposed group were by almost 100% higher than in the sham-exposed group. The authors claimed that the possible mechanism by which SMF-exposure prevents the development of disseminated intravascular coagulation is *via* the up regulation of IL-1ra rather than *via* the down regulation of pro-inflammatory cytokines. In **Anti-inflammatory effect**, we also said that SMF-exposure has a direct inhibitory effect on the release of pro-inflammatory cytokines and an assisting effect on IL-10 anti-inflammatory cytokine from human lymphocytes and macrophages.

Klepetko *et al.* [421] reviewed results of SMF-exposure (foils) on heart surgery scars. Although patients treated with these foils showed faster improvement than control, the effect was not significant. However, Eccles and Hollinworth [422] performed a study on 26 patients with chronic leg ulcers. What they did was apply a magnetic or mock wrap of unknown magnetic induction for 12 weeks continuously and regularly recorded ulcer size, level of pain, and function. They found a significant positive effect of the magnetic wrap over the mock one in wound healing. Nursal *et al.* [423] exposed 50 rats to continuous 39-42 mT magnetic induction. They used sham and control groups as well. Authors performed assessment of 4 quantities of healing on postoperative day 3 and 7 and could not establish any significant differences between the healing parameters of the groups. However, Henry *et al.* [424] published an experimental study on 33 rats with standardized cutaneous wounds on their back. They applied magnets (2.3 mT) or "mock" magnets for continuous exposure beyond negative control. Magnets significantly reduced the gross healing period to 15.3 days in contrary to sham-exposed and negative control groups where this period exceeded 20 days. Shen *et al.* [425] confirmed that in 48 rats exposed to either 160 or 320 mT continuous SMF for 12 days promoted deep wound healing. On the other hand, there was no significant difference between either group to control in the vascular endothelial growth factor. Also, Jing *et al.* [426] reported that the healing rate significantly increased and the gross healing time reduced in 48 rats with wounds or diabetic wounds upon the application of continuous 180 mT SMF compared to sham control in the examination period of 19 days.

In the previous section **On visitors of a dental clinic**, both volunteers and patients were included. For the SMF-exposure the same SMF generator was applied then as in the present study. Healthy volunteers were tested for their dental pain tolerance threshold resulting in no significant difference between sham- and SMF-exposure. Patients, on the other hand, expected a dental treatment either because of a pathologic situation (drilling in preparation for caries filling) or a physiologic situation (burring in preparation for prosthetic procedure). No significant effect of SMF- over sham-exposure was observed here either with the exception of a single case (out of 62) where there was an inflammatory reason behind the (female) patient's pain sensation. Local anesthesia with SMF-exposure was complete in her case; no further pain killer was needed during the dental treatment.

The present authors decided to check the above results in stomatological patients in an evidence based (randomized, double-blind, placebo-controlled) manner that allows replication. For this very reason, patients with temporomandibular disorders, alveolitis, or aphta in the oral mucosa were recruited and treated with a local SMF-exposure that had been optimized and validated in earlier experiments (Chapter 5 ***In Vivo* Animal Experiments**). One of the inclusion criteria was a diagnosed inflammatory reason for the pain sensation. Our null-hypothesis in this trial was: SMF-exposure decreases pain more effectively than placebo.

Materials and Methods

Trial Design, Participants, Recruitment and Ethics

Our trial was a placebo controlled, double-blind, randomized, 1:1 parallel-group, single center clinical trial complying with the recommendations of the CONSORT Group for RCT-NPT (Randomized, Controlled Trial extended to Nonpharmacological Treatments) [427]. Fig. (**6.19**) shows the CONSORT flow diagram of the trial.

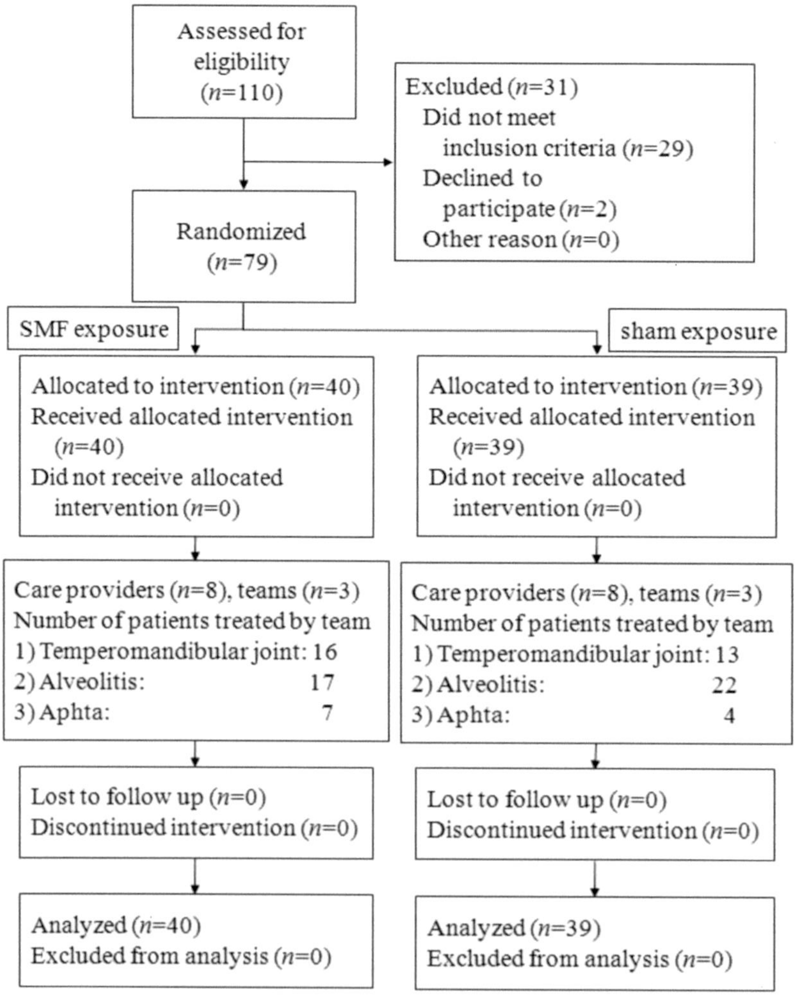

Fig. (6.19). CONSORT flow diagram of the trial.

Recruitment, tests, and treatment were carried out at the Central Institute of Stomatology (Center henceforth). Subjects were recruited individually by the Center where later their stomatological treatment was carried out. Based on the 3 different health condition backgrounds, 3 groups of patients were defined:

1. Patients with temporomandibular disorders (29 participants, 37% of all cases including 21 females and 8 males),
2. Patients with alveolitis (39 participants, 49% of all cases including 29 females and 10 males),
3. Patients with aphta in the oral mucosa (altogether 11 participants, 14% of all cases including 7 females and 4 males).

No patient belonged to more than one group. The eligibility criterion in the experiments was: Age between 15-79 y. The exclusion criteria were:

- Regular use of medication,
- regular consumption of alcohol,
- pregnancy or lactation,
- regular smoking,
- any type of psychological disorder,
- cardiovascular disease (pacemaker),
- oncological disease,
- any kind of skin irritation or irritability at the place of the local treatment,
- fever, or
- magnetically anisotropic object in the temporomandibular joint or in the teeth.

The test series lasted for 14 months including recruitment. There was no follow-up in any of the groups. All participants confirmed that they understood the plan and participated on a voluntary basis (*i.e.* an informed consent was signed). Volunteers were informed about the goal of the project, the SMF or sham treatment, and their possible effects. Patients understood that if during the 5 min SMF or sham treatment their pain sensation would not lessen, the treatment would be discontinued. Both SMF and sham treatment could immediately be interrupted upon the patient's request. These cases would be counted as dropouts.

The study was conducted in accordance with the Declaration of Helsinki. The

Center had permission from the Regional Institute of Central Hungary of the National Public Health and Medical Officer Service (No.: 9432-4/2009), and from the Scientific and Ethical Committee of the Medical Research Council (No.: 8-159/2009-1018EKU) to perform the study.

Magnetic Exposure Conditions

Generator 19, used in previous dental trial, was applied here again. Colbert *et al.*'s [29] description of the standardization of clinical study reports, including SMF was employed here again. Table **6.9** contains the relevant data.

Table 6.9. Ten essential dosing parameters for the present study following the suggestions of Colbert *et al.* [29].

Target tissue	facial
Site of magnet application	mainly between maxilla and mandible
Distance of magnet surface from target tissue(s)	1-3 mm
Magnetic field induction	B_r=1.2 T (remanent induction), 192, 10, and 3 mT (*P-P* magnetic induction, averaged for all neighbors) and 19, 1, and 0 T/m (lateral magnetic induction gradient of the main induction component, averaged for all neighbors) at 3, 10, and 15 mm from a cylindrical magnet in the isocenter of the matrix along its axis, respectively
Material composition of permanent magnet	N35 grade neodymium-iron-boron (NdFeB)
Magnet dimensions	rectangular matrix (39×39 mm) containing 3×3 pieces of 10×10 mm cylindrical magnets fixed on the headband of a headphone
Magnet polar configuration	neighboring magnets are placed with alternating poles (checkerboard configuration)
Magnet support device	ferrous plate beneath the magnets, plastic framing around and soft coverage on the contact site
Frequency of magnet application	single session
Duration of magnet application	5 min continuous

Outcomes: Pain Sensation on a Visual Analogue Scale

The primary outcome measure in this examination was the difference between subjective pain sensation before and after a 5 min SMF or sham-exposure. A standard VAS was used for testing. It consisted of a sheet of paper with a black line of 100 mm length on it. On the left side of the number scale "no pain" and on the right side "the most intense pain sensation imaginable" were written. Patients were asked to estimate their pain perception by making a cross on the line. TheVAS score was defined by the distance between the crossing mark and the zero point measured in mm and rounded to the next integer. All patients were tested in 4 turns (see Fig. (**6.20**) for the timeline of the examination). Turn 1 was the baseline VAS testing (before placing the device on the head), turn 2 occurred right after placing the device on the head, turn 3 occurred 5 min later before the device was removed from the head, and turn 4 right after that the removal. The pre-treatment VAS value was defined by the average VAS of turn 1 and turn 2. Similarly, the post-treatment VAS was defined by the average VAS of turn 3 and turn 4. Differences between VAS values of turns 1-2 and turns 3-4 were supposed to provide information whether the wearing of the device caused any discomfort in itself. Before we began the stomatological treatment, the SMF- or sham-exposure system was removed from the patient's head (at time point 5 min).

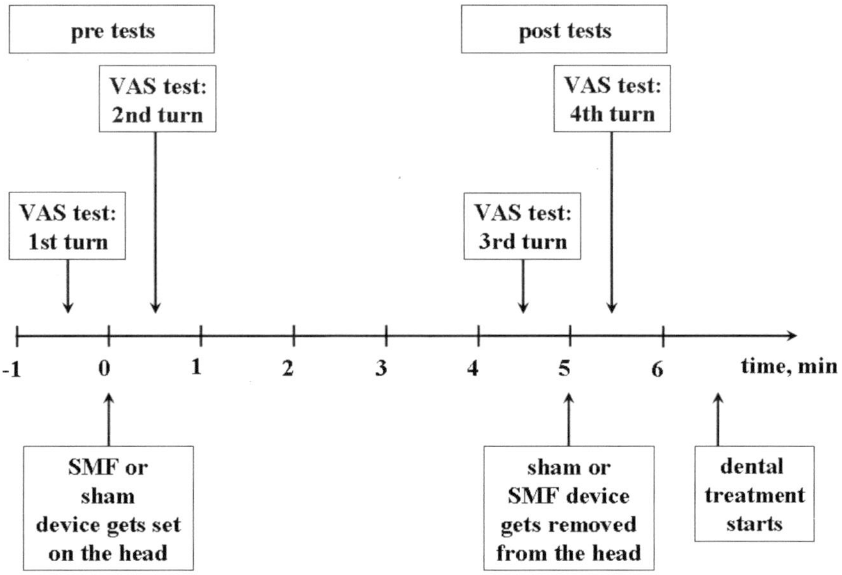

Fig. (6.20). Schematic protocol for VAS testing. Between 2 pairs of VAS testing either sham- or SMF-exposure for 5 min was executed.

Randomization Sequence Generation

The head of the Center was in charge of the randomization and control of the double-blind manner. Within the groups, a series of random binary numbers was generated and assigned to the patient number list in the given group. If number 0 was allocated to a patient, he/she received sham-exposure, if number 1, then SMF-exposure.

Allocation Concealment

The numbered patient list together with the assigned binary numbers remained concealed from both patients and care providers. A table with patient numbers, age, gender, medication taken, diagnosis (identifying group), number of exposure device (identifying sham or SMF), and 4 VAS scores per patient was provided to the statistician who was in charge of the assessment of the results. He was the only person to whom these data were revealed; however, he did not receive the corresponding name list of patients.

Implementation

All personal data were handwritten on paper by the care takers, and the papers were locked in a file cabinet at the Center. Only the head of the Center was authorized to see and handle these data later. They were not opened to or by any third person.

Two lead care takers were in charge of the 3 teams providing care; the 3 teams enrolled and assigned patients to different groups according to diagnosis. The head of the Center generated the allocation sequence; he was in charge of determining the appropriate intervention device for the selected patients. Altogether 6 SMF and sham generators were used; only the device provider and the head of the Center knew which of them was SMF and which was sham. The head of the Center did not participate in the treatment of patients himself.

Blinding

We first informed the care providers in all 3 teams in writing as well as orally that the subjective pain perception the patients would describe following the interventions would not be directly correlated with the magnetic induction of the device the patients had on their head. We emphasized that the sham device would also be able to increase the patients' pain tolerance threshold. We also advised patients about this in writing and orally in advance. Care providers as well as patients were asked to remove any magnetically anisotropic objects from their reach during the time period of the 4 turns of the test.

Statistical Methods

Pain reduction for each subject was defined as the difference between the VAS scores before and after treatment. Mean pain reduction in the SMF and sham group was compared by 2-sample Student's t-test allowing for unequal variances (Welch test). Placebo effect was estimated by comparing mean pre- and post-treatment VAS scores for the sham groups by paired Dunnett's test. The 3 groups of patients with different diseases were analyzed separately. For the statistical computation the program R (version 2.11.1) was used.

Results

Participant Flow

Table **6.10** summarizes the age characteristics of patients.

Table 6.10. Age characteristics of patients.

group	mean±SEM (y)
1	41.79±3.00
2	35.15±2.43
3	33.55±4.37

Baseline Data

Baseline data from turn 1 did not significantly differ from those of turn 2; neither did turn 3 data differ from turn 4 data in any the groups. For gender differences see point Effect of gender.

Outcomes and Estimation

Raw data can be seen in Fig. (**6.21**). For temporomandibular disorders the trend line for the sham- is above the SMF-exposure trend line for $x \geq 2$. For alveolitis the 2 trend lines are parallel, the sham line is above the SMF line. For aphta the sham trend line is above the SMF trend line only $x \geq 5.5$. The regression coefficients show bigger standard deviation for SMF- than for sham-exposure. Baseline VAS scores (mean±SEM) data in all 3 groups were similar to each other for both sham and SMF treatment. These data were the following. Group 1: 3.8±0.6 for sham (n=13) and 4.4±0.5 for SMF (n=13, p=0.427), for group 2: 6.2±0.3 for sham (n=22) and 6.8±0.3 for SMF (n=17, p=0.256), for group 3: 6.0±0.8 for sham (n=4) and 6.4±0.5 for SMF (n=7, p=0.655).

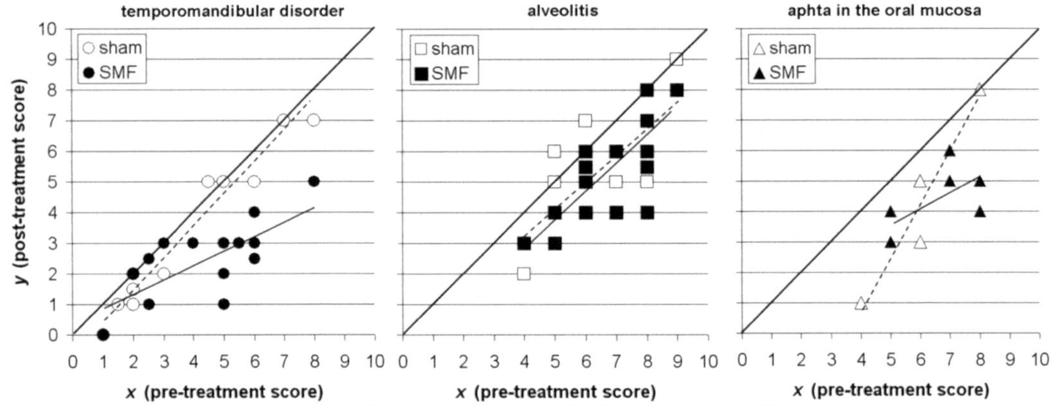

mark	group	exposure	trend line style	slope	offset (y_0)	regression parameter (r^2 in %)
○	temporomandibular disorder	sham	dashed	1.0	-0.6	95.5
●		SMF	solid	0.5	0.4	51.1
□	alveolitis	sham	dashed	0.9	-0.3	57.2
■		SMF	solid	0.9	-0.8	57.3
△	aphta in the oral mucosa	sham	dashed	1.8	-6.3	91.6
▲		SMF	solid	0.5	0.9	43.4

Fig. (6.21). VAS data for the 3 groups of patients. Pre-exposure values (turns 1-2 averaged) are shown on the x axis, post-exposure values (turns 3-4 averaged) on the y axis. Open and dark markers denote sham- and SMF-exposure, respectively. 45° thick solid lines are the "no effect" lines; values below this line mean that the SMF treatment was effective. Thin solid and dashed lines represent trend lines for SMF- and sham-exposure, respectively.

Placebo effect, measured by comparing the mean pre- and post-treatment VAS scores for the sham treatment, was significant in group 1 and 2, but not in group 3.

In group 1 the mean pre- and post-treatment VAS scores were 3.8±0.6 and 3.3±0.7 (n=13, p=0.008), in group 2 they were 6.2±0.3 and 5.2±0.4 (n=22, p<0.001), and in group 3 they were 6.0±0.8 and 4.3±1.5 (n=4, p=0.102).

The decrease of the VAS score between the SMF-exposed group (mean=2.0±0.3, n=16) and the sham-exposed group (0.5±0.1, n=13) in group 1 showed a significant difference (p<0.001), see in Fig. (**6.21**). In group 2 the corresponding values were not significantly different, 1.4±0.3, n=17 *vs* 1.1±0.2, n=22, p=0.319. Similar values in group 3 showed no significant difference either: 2.1±0.4, n=7 *vs* 1.8±0.8, n=4, p=0.623.

Effect of Gender

There was no significant baseline difference between the VAS scores for females and males in any of the groups. Namely, in group 1 VAS for females were 4.5±0.4 *vs* 3.3±0.7 for males, in group 2 these data were 6.4±0.3 *vs* 6.7±0.3, and in group 3 5.9±0.5 *vs* 7.0±0.7.

Female patients from all 3 health condition groups together were responsible for the statistically significant difference between SMF and sham treatment. The number of females was by 2.6 larger than the number of males. For females SMF-exposure appeared in a VAS score mea$n$=1.9±0.2 (n=25) *vs* the sham-exposure 0.9±0.2 (n=32). The Welch-test resulted in p<0.002. For males these numbers were 1.6±0.3 (n=15) *vs* 1.1±0.4 (n=7), respectively with a corresponding non-significant inhibitory effect.

Harms

No adverse effects were recorded in any of the groups that could be attributed to the applied sham or SMF interventions. The 5 min long trial was never interrupted or discontinued for any reason. No dropouts were registered.

Discussion, Conclusions

Limitations

Limitations in the design of the study did not allow us to distinguish between the fundamental reasons behind the exposure effect, if any. Local SMF-exposure may influence pain sensation either because it causes pain inhibition directly, or because it increases the pain tolerance threshold. Our own experience presented in **Pain and inflammation** supports the former theory. The measurements carried out in our previous experiment on the effect of local SMF-exposure with the same SMF generator as in the present study on the dental tolerance threshold in healthy volunteers (**On healthy volunteers**) made us believe that the tolerance threshold did not change upon exposure to SMF.

The literature is expanding in terms of the gender dependence in pain perception (for a review, see Fillingim *et al.* [428]). In general, we might accept a higher prevalence in women than in men in the area of oral pain (see references in [428]). Our baseline data did not show significant difference between female and male VAS scores in any groups. It is worth noting though that a higher number of females than males visited the Center with an oral problem.

The observed gender effect of SMF-exposure did not allow us to draw conclusions on the SMF- and sham-exposure effect difference between genders because none of the groups were balanced in gender. It is likely that the number of patients, rather than the gender, caused the significant difference knowing that an overall increase of the number of male patients by a factor of 7 would already result in a significant effect.

Further studies with more subjects are required to estimate how the pain inhibitory effect depends on the time- and spatial distribution of SMF, its magnetic induction, its lateral gradient, *etc.* For future applications we also need to establish the dynamics of the effect in order to propose an evidence-based complementary or alternative method for local anesthesia.

Strengths

While the size of the study was small, results allow for the conclusion on the primary outcomes of our study; and thus provide evidence that local exposure to inhomogeneous SMF-exposure failed to cause any adverse effects. The results also support that SMF-exposure affects the sensation of pain in the temporomandibular joint under pathological conditions in a beneficial way.

Comparison with Other Studies

The previously published results concerning stomatology concentrated on ferromagnetic materials, such as dental amalgam and prostheses under high gradient magnetic field conditions (see *e.g.* the paper of Tenforde and Budinger [402]), or the report of the American Society for Testing and Materials [403]. Also orthodontic magnets and implants can be of concern, when placed in strong SMF [404]. Bondemark *et al.* [405, 406] examined the effects of orthodontic magnets on the oral mucosa, the dental pulp, and the gingiva. The endpoints of these examinations were morphological and histological alterations of the surrounding tissue. The magnets and the demagnetized controls were bonded on molars on either side of the mouth. The SMF from the implants varied between 10 and 140 mT. Some inflammations were detected in the tissue close to both the magnet and the demagnetized magnet, but not in other sites. Those were attributed to contact irritation rather than to the SMF.

Possible Background Mechanisms

A potential background mechanism for analgesia at the receptor level was proposed in **Pharmacological analysis**. We tested several receptor antagonists in mice before exposing them to SMF and concluded that the most likely effect of SMF-exposure in mice is the release of either β -endorphin or endomorphin-2. Since inflammation was shown to increase the expression of opioid peptides both *in vivo* and *in vitro* [253, 254], it can be hypothesized that SMF-exposure may be beneficial for a tissue in inflammatory condition. We also presented *in vitro* evidence that SMF-exposure inhibits the release of pro-inflammatory cytokines and assists that of anti-inflammatory cytokine IL-10 in **Anti-inflammatory effect**.

At the electron spin level we believe that the positive action of SMF-exposure on pain may be based on the modified lifetime of free radical pairs [429]. This explanation relies on the fact that an external SMF can enhance the interconversion of such pairs from singlet (S) to triplet (T) states [430 - 433]. Radicals of the pair cannot recombine in the T state *in loco*, they must react elsewhere. If they react with DNA, undesirable free radical damage can occur or to the contrary, beneficial effects can be observed. Radical pair mechanism seems to govern the magnetoreception in birds [434].

When a 192 mT (maximum *P-P* amplitude by 19 T/m lateral gradient at 3 mm from the magnets) inhomogeneous SMF-exposure was applied locally for 5 min *prior* to a stomatological procedure on pain originating from the sickness of the temporomandibular joint, it significantly reduced pain sensation. Sham-exposure was demonstrated to also affect pain perception. The SMF generator itself did not cause any discomfort in its present form. The clinical importance of the present study is relevant to stomatologists, who should consider exposure to SMF as a viable method for drug free local anesthesia in situations where systemic anesthesia is contraindicated. We have now seen that whole-body SMF-exposure may be beneficial in pathological situations in rodents when a visceral organ has inflammation and also in humans when applied locally. Let us now see whether this advantage could be maintained in pain perception and bone turnover in osteoporosis patients.

Pain Perception and Bone Turnover

Exposure to static magnetic field on pain perception and bone turnover of osteoporotic patients

Preliminaries

We have already mentioned in **Inflammation** how chronic pain influences the quality of life of millions around the globe. Especially chronic back pain is a common medical condition in developed countries affecting one third of the world's population, not to mention its management costs. Osteoporotic back pain is mostly related to vertebral fractures especially in women during or following menopause [435]. For many patients, pain produces continued distress and disrupts their quality of life. Current treatments have limited effectiveness and may cause side effects or abuse potential [259]. SMF-exposure is an alternative therapy that has proliferated, although its mechanism of action had not been fully clarified, and its effectiveness had not been convincingly proven in randomized controlled trials (RCT) [38]. Commercially available medical devices, using a combination of SMF and electromagnetic field, are frequently utilized by patients without their effectiveness having been proven in randomized trials. Furthermore, the individual effect of the components is virtually impossible to separate given the nature of the devices. Instruments with permanent magnets are appealing because they promise a safe, drug-free, durable, and non-invasive solution for pain relief. The interpretation of published trials is rather difficult due to the incomplete description of the trial and the SMF-exposure conditions [29]. Animal studies using whole-body exposure as seen in Chapter 5 (***In Vivo* Animal Experiments**) suggest that SMF improves pain perception threshold and produces *AE* in short-term experiments of acute pain and in long-term experiments of chronic pain.

Human studies are equivocal regarding the pain relief of SMF-exposure. Some studies were unable to prove any effect over placebo [264, 272, 436]. Some other researchers reported improvements on particular measures of pain but no change in other markers [266, 437]. Yet others reported no improvement in short-term but some improvement in longer follow-up [438].

Fortunately, there is accumulating literature on the effect of SMF-exposure on bone metabolism. *In vitro* studies mostly talk about increased differentiation and calcification in osteoblast and dental pulp cell cultures [334, 439 - 441], while some authors found negative or no effects in cell cultures [442, 443]. Animal studies further support the hypothesis that SMF-exposure could be beneficial in bone metabolism. Fracture healing studies and studies in animals with increased bone resorption showed faster healing or less bone loss, better bone mineral density (BMD), and higher calcium content in bones exposed to SMF either as an implant in the fractured bone [444 - 448], or as an implant over the exposed bone [424, 449], or even where SMF was outside the animals' cage [312, 450, 451]. Human evidence regarding SMF-exposure on bone health is limited and provides no firm conclusions [452, 453]. All the above-mentioned studies investigated the effects of long-term (days or weeks), continuous SMF-exposure on bone health.

The above evidence from *in vitro* and *in vivo* animal studies suggests that SMF-exposure could be of benefit to osteoporotic patients both for bone turnover markers and in reducing pain related to osteoporotic fractures. In the current double-blind RCT study we sought to investigate the effect of repeated, local, inhomogeneous SMF-exposure of 196 mT (at the target distance) compared to sham-exposure to the back on subjective measures of pain in the short-term (hours) and in the long term (weeks) and also to measure changes in markers of bone formation (osteocalcin) and bone resorption (β-crosslaps) over 10 weeks in osteoporotic postmenopausal women with vertebral deformity and back pain.

Materials and Methods

Trial Design, Participants, Recruitment, and Ethics

Participants were recruited, and measurements were taken at the 1st Department of Medicine, Semmelweis University (Budapest, Hungary). Females between 50 and 70 y of age with postmenopausal osteoporosis, vertebral deformity (thoracic 11-12 and/or lumbar 1-4), and chronic back pain taken care of in the Department were eligible to participate in the trial.. We excluded women who fell in any of the following categories:

- regular alcohol consumption (>2 units/day),
- current smoker,
- having psychological disorders,
- any known cardiovascular disease,
- those using a pacemaker device,
- any current or past oncological disease,
- skin irritation/irritability on the place of local treatment,
- fever at the time of recruitment, or
- magnetically anisotropic implant in any joint.

All 11 women assessed were randomized and subjected to treatment in the following groups:

Sham-exposure (sham, n=5): n=1 lumbar deformity only, n=2 thoracic deformity only, n=2 lumbar + thoracic deformity;
SMF-exposure (SMF, n=6): n=2 thoracic deformity only, n=4 lumbar + thoracic deformity.

Each week from visit 1-10 a 30 min treatment session was carried out. During visit 11 (follow-up) no treatment was given, only the outcomes and safety measures were recorded. No changes in concomitant medications were allowed during the study.

Two women were lost to follow-up (18.2%). Fig. (**6.22**) shows the CONSORT 2010 flow diagram for the trial [454]. The Regional and Institutional Committee of Science and Research Ethics of Semmelweis University reviewed and approved the study (No.: 63/2008) and written informed consent was obtained from each participant before study-related procedures began.

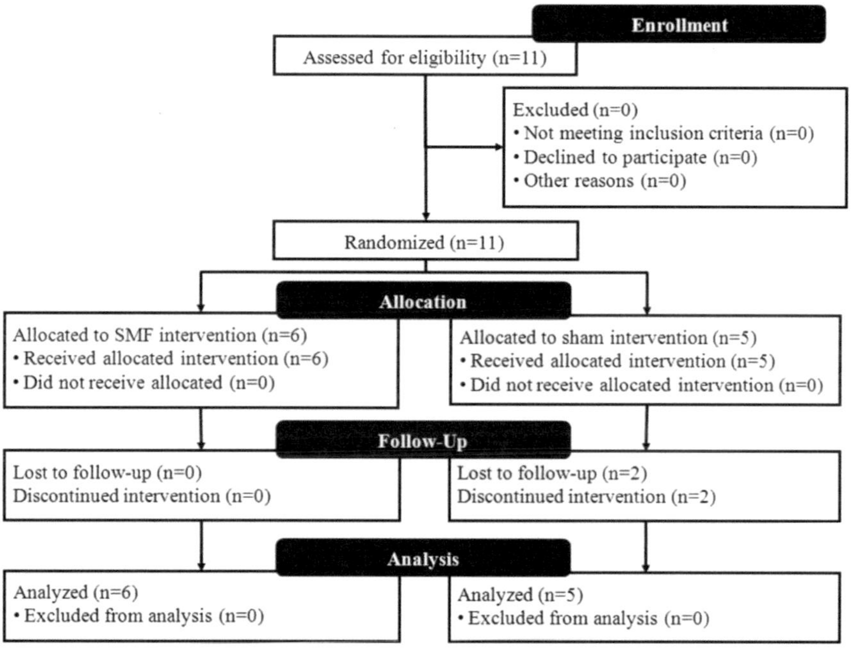

Fig. (6.22). CONSORT flow diagram of the trial.

Magnetic Exposure Conditions

The exposure system used was generator 3 (see **Generators 1-16** and Table **6.11** for reference). The magnetic matrix was covered with a thin, soft tissue, and was applied on the side of the pain sensation in the thoracic or lumbar region. Patients were in a prone position with the matrix on their back during treatment. An identical looking, unmagnetized ("mock") matrix of equal mass was applied to the same holder and was used as placebo control. Both SMF and sham matrices had an on/off switch that made a clicking noise. The matrices were illuminated by a green light during treatment Fig. (**6.23**). The standardized description of SMF-exposure (according to [29]) is provided in Table **6.11**.

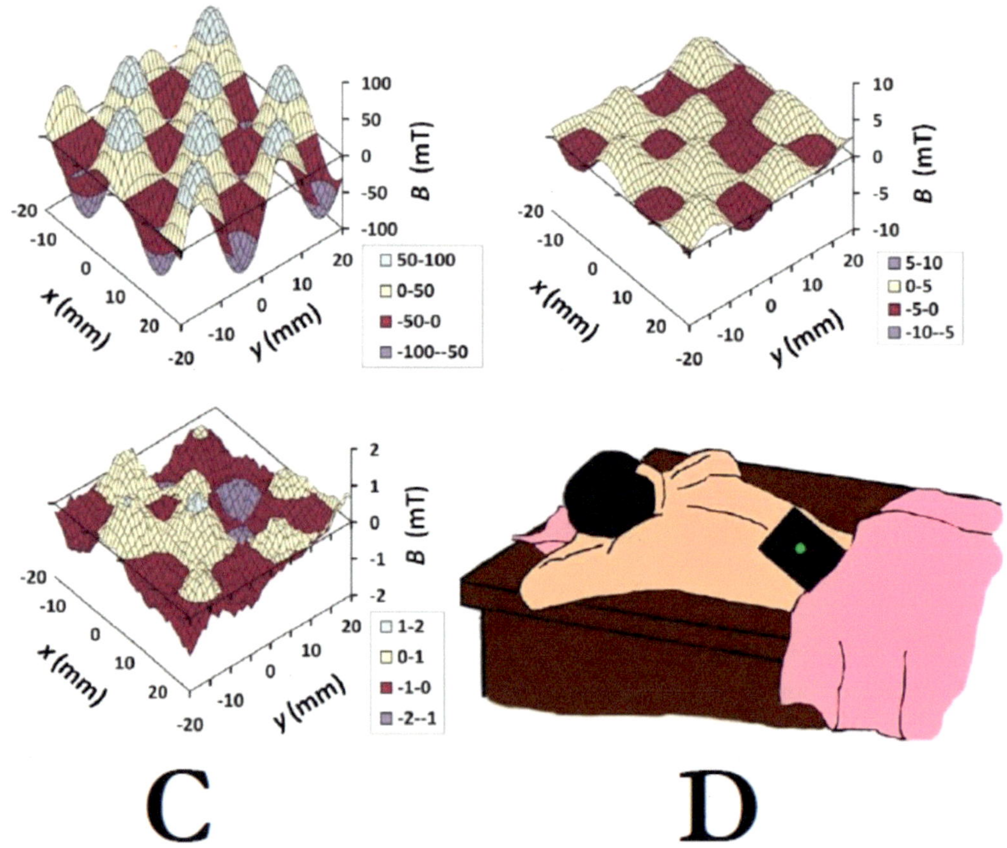

Fig. (6.23). Magnetic induction scans measured in the center of the magnet arrangement (A-C, where the distortion of SMF is minimal) and its placement on the patients (D). The presented magnetic induction is the component perpendicular to the magnets' surface at A) 3, B) 10, and C) 15 mm from it.

Table 6.11. Ten essential dosing parameters for the present study following the suggestions of Colbert *et al.* [29].

Target tissue	skin
Site of magnet application	thoracic and/or lumbar part of the back
Distance of magnet surface from target tissue(s)	3-15 mm

(Table 6.11) contd.....

Magnetic field induction	B_r, remanent magnetic induction 1.2 T; 192, 10, and 3 ;mT *P-P* magnetic induction and 19, 1, and 0 T/m lateral gradient at 3, 10, and 15 mm from a cylindrical magnet in the isocenter of the matrix along its axis, respectively
Material composition of permanent magnet	N35 grade neodymium-iron-boron (NdFeB)
Magnet dimensions	rectangular matrix (140×140 mm) containing 14×14 pieces of 10×10 mm cylindrical magnets
Magnet polar configuration	neighboring magnets placed with alternating poles (checkerboard configuration)
Magnet support device	ferrous plate beneath the magnets, plastic framing around, soft coverage on the contact site
Frequency of magnet application	in 11 visits during 10 weeks, 1 visit/week
Duration of magnet application	continuous for 30 min at each visit

Outcomes: Pain Sensation on a Visual Analogue Scale, Bone Transport Markers

The primary outcome was pain sensation reported by the participant on a VAS from 0-10 centimeter (cm) (higher values corresponding to more severe pain) immediately before and after intervention on each visit [455]. We investigated both acute changes in pain sensation (VAS results before and after each visit: primary outcome), and long-term changes in pretreatment VAS scores from visit 1-10 (secondary outcome). Tertiary outcomes were bone turnover markers at baseline (visit 1) and at the last follow-up visit (visit 11). All blood samples were drawn in the morning in a fasting state. Osteocalcin (bone formation measure) was determined by electrochemiluminescence immunoassay (Elecsys N-MID Osteocalcin, Roche Diagnostics), coefficient of variation, CV=8%. The osteocalcin immunoassay detects a stable 43-amino-acid fragment of the N-terminal end (NMID (N-terminal midfragment)). For bone resorption, β-crosslaps (CTX) was measured by an electrochemiluminescence immunoassay (Elecsys β-CrossLaps), coefficient of variation CV=10%.

Safety Measures

Anthropometrics were measured at visit 1, 5, 10, and 11. Height was measured to the nearest 0.1 cm on a stadiometer. Weight was measured on a Metripond Plus

BW 150 scale. Body mass index (BMI) was calculated as (mass in kg)/(height in m)^2. Blood pressure and heart rate were measured using an automated system (Omron M4). During visit 1, blood samples were collected for thyroid stimulating hormone (TSH), 25-OH vitamin D (25(OH)D3; LIASON 25 OH Vitamin D Total Assay), parathyroid hormone (PTH), alkaline phosphatase (ALP), creatinine, serum calcium, phosphate, and albumin to exclude any secondary causes of metabolic bone disease. All the above-mentioned procedures were carried out in the central laboratory of the Department. Dual-energy X-ray absorptiometry was used (Lunar Prodigy) to determine lumbar (L2-L4) and femoral BMD at baseline (coefficient of variation 1%). T-scores (the number of SD above or below the young adult mean BMD) were calculated with reference to a local normative population BMD database.

Sample Size

The sample size was calculated based on the assumption that a 1.5 point difference on the visual analogue pain scale is clinically relevant. Based on previous studies, we estimated a standard deviation (SD) of 2.5 of the pain scores. For the primary outcome of acute pain relief, we needed 44 pairs of measurements to have 80% power with a 2-sided α of 0.05 that translates into 5 patients in each study group, all with 10 pairs of measurements [455 - 457].

Randomization-Sequence Generation, Implementation, Allocation Concealment

The lead care taker was the one generating the randomization table. The list of the random numbers was accessible to her alone. She enrolled patients and assigned a sequential number to each participant. After enrolment, she assigned an intervention device to the patient using the randomization table. One SMF and one sham generator were used, and only the lead care taker knew which device was which (SMF or sham). All patient data were stored separately from the random number list in the Department.

Blinding

Study participants and care providers were both blinded to the intervention. At each visit the lead care taker selected the appropriate device but was not allowed to communicate with the participants. The difference between sham and SMF devices could not be revealed by looking, hearing, weighing, or touching. To minimize bias on the secondary outcome, we informed patients and care providers in writing and orally that the lack of acute change in pain sensation did not exclude the possibility of having had received active treatment. Care providers and patients were asked to remove any magnetically anisotropic objects from their reach during the tests.

Statistical Analysis

Statistical analyses were undertaken using SPSS 14.0 statistical software (SPSS, Chicago, IL, USA), statistical significance was inferred at a 2-tailed $p<0.05$. Baseline comparisons between groups were done using independent samples t-tests, Mann-Whitney test for continuous variables, and χ^2 tests for categorical parameters as appropriate. For the primary analysis we used an intention-to-treat strategy, with patients analyzed in their assigned groups. To increase statistical power, we used all measurement points in building different linear mixed models. Data were structured so that measurements were nested within subjects and the non-independence of the observations (the same individuals contributed to more than one observation) was taken into account in assessing standard errors.

For the investigation of acute effects we modeled the pre- and post-treatment VAS scores, hypothesizing a uniform difference between these scores irrespective of the visit number. Thus, the models, apart from the intercept, included a treatment effect (pre-/post-treatment), a treatment allocation term (sham/SMF), and their interaction.

For the investigation of chronic effect we hypothesized a linear change in VAS scores from visit 1-10 and modeled pretreatment VAS scores accordingly. The model thus included a treatment effect (visit number 1-10, the change in VAS score from one visit to the next visit), a treatment allocation term, and their interaction. For the changes in bone turnover markers we used similar models to estimate these values for visit 1 and visit 11 using the following terms: Treatment effect (visit 1/visit 11), treatment allocation term, and their interaction.

Two sets of ancillary analyses were performed:

i. On the subset of participants with complete data, and
ii. primary outcomes were further adjusted for vitamin D levels (as main effects) as there was a significant group difference in vitamin D levels at baseline.

Results

Participant Flow

Eleven subjects were assessed, all of whom were randomized and took part in at least one session of their assigned intervention. Two subjects were lost to follow-up, both from the sham group. One of them took part in the first 3 visits, the other one only in the first visit. All available data from all participants were used in the subsequent evaluation.

Recruitment

Participants were recruited between September and December, 2008. The last visit occurred in January 2009.

Baseline Data

Details of the baseline characteristics of the participants by treatment allocation are provided in Table **6.12**. Participants in the groups were similar regarding age, height, weight, BP, bone turnover markers, serum calcium, PTH and albumin levels, and similar proportions received vitamin D supplementation as well (all $p>0.15$). We found higher vitamin D and phosphate levels among SMF treated participants compared to controls (mean difference for vitamin D 10.7, 95% confidence interval (CI) 3.1-18.2 ng/ml, for serum phosphate 0.17, 95% CI 0.03- 0.31 mM/l). The SMF group had significantly lower VAS scores compared to the sham group (mean difference 2.8, 95% CI 0.47-5.2 cm) at baseline.

Table 6.12. Baseline characteristics of patients by treatment allocation: Mean±SD; VAS: Visual analogue scale. Groups were compared using t-tests and χ^2-tests as appropriate.

	sham-exposed	SMF-exposed	*p*
age (y)	64.60±0.51	62.83±2.17	NS
body mass (kg)	66.40±4.82	73.17±1.80	NS

(Table 6.12) contd.....

body height (cm)	161.20±1.50	157.17±2.56	NS
body mass index (kg/m^2)	29.8±1.5	25.61±1.9	NS
systolic BP (Hgmm)	140.00±4.74	139.67±5.51	NS
diastolic BP (Hgmm)	83.00±5.15	77.33±2.47	NS
heart rate (1/min)	82.80±3.06	76.00±2.83	NS
lumbar bone mineral density (g/cm^2)	0.928±0.082	1.114±0.160	NS
femoral bone mineral density (g/cm^2)	0.736±0.040	0.814±0.030	NS
femoral T score	-2.0±0.4	-2.4±0.2	NS
lumbar T score	-1.5±0.5	-2.4±0.7	NS
thyroid stimulating hormone (mIU/l)	0.93±0.39	0.93±0.38	NS
β-crosslaps (pg/ml)	510.00±89.88	337.17±70.40	NS
osteocalcin (ng/ml)	36.01±10.76	24.88±7.00	NS
25 (OH) D-vitamin (ng/ml)	18.14±2.92	28.82±1.84	=0.011
parathyroid hormone (pg/ml)	42.80±3.69	38.50±5.06	NS
alkaline phosphatase (U/l)	194.20±13.04	225.33±28.65	NS
serum creatinine (mM/l)	61.20±5.02	69.50±3.37	NS
serum calcium (mM/l)	2.45±0.03	2.44±0.03	NS
serum phosphate (mM/l)	1.08±0.04	1.25±0.04	0.023
serum albumin (g/l)	47.12±0.60	46.78±0.77	NS
number of vitamin D treatments	3	5	NS
VAS score, cm	5.2±1.5	8.0±2.0	0.024

Numbers Analyzed

For the analyses of the acute changes in VAS scores all participant with complete data provided 10 pre- and 10 post-treatment values. The 2 participants who were lost to follow-up provided 1 and 3 pairs of measurements, respectively. Thus the final sample included 120 (SMF-exposure) and 68 (sham-exposure) measurement points. For the analysis of the chronic changes in VAS scores all participants with complete data provided 10 pretreatment values. The 2 participants who were lost to follow-up provided 1 and 3 measurement points, respectively. The final sample, thus, included 60 (SMF-exposure) and 34 (sham-exposure) measurement points. For the bone turnover analysis all participants with complete data provided 2 data points, the participants lost to follow-up provided 1 data point each. Altogether 20 data points were included (12 in the SMF group, 8 in the sham group).

Outcomes and Estimation

According to the multilevel models of change, VAS scores acutely decreased by 0.47, 95% CI 0.07-1.01 (p=0.092) cm in the SMF-group and by 1.06, 95% CI 0.35-1.17 cm (p=0.004) in the sham group from pre- to post-treatment. The amount of decrease, however, was not different between the groups (0.6, 95% CI 0.3-1.5, p=0.195) yielding a similar effect in the sham and the SMF treatment (Table **6.13**).

Table 6.13. The short-term effect of SMF- and sham-exposure on VAS scores and their long-term effect (visit 1 to visit 10) on osteocalcin and β-crosslaps levels. Differences (between before and after values), exposure effects (interaction between treatment and time), and p values were calculated using multilevel models of change. Mean±SD or mean (95% confidence interval).

	SMF-exposure	sham-exposure	exposure effect	*p*
pre-treatment VAS score (cm)	4.2±1.9	4.6±2.2		
post-treatment VAS score (cm)	3.7±2.4	3.5±2.3		
difference (cm)	0.5 (-0.1-1.0)	1.1 (0.4-1.2)	0.6 (–0.3-1.5)	0.195
osteocalcin levels at baseline (ng/ml)	24.9±17.1	36.0±24.1		
osteocalcin levels at visit 10 (ng/ml)	18.6±9.3	28.6±5.1		
difference (ng/ml)	6.2 (0.7-13.2)	0.9 (–8.8-10.7)	–5.3 (–6.7-17.4)	0.329
β-crosslaps at baseline (pg/ml)	337±172	510±201		
β-crosslaps at visit 10 (pg/ml)	285±196	507±26		
difference (pg/ml)	51(–62-164)	3 (–152-157)	–54 (–138-246)	0.528

The models describing the long-term effect of treatments on VAS scores showed a non-significant decrease in the SMF group from visit to visit (0.04, 95% CI 0.09-0.17 cm/visit) and a significant decrease in the sham group (0.31, 95% CI 0.13-0.50 cm/visit). The amount of change was significantly larger in the sham group compared to the SMF group (0.27, 95% CI 0.04-0.50 cm, p=0.021) meaning that the sham treatment was more effective in reducing pain than the SMF treatment (Fig **6.24**).

Osteocalcin levels were similar at baseline and decreased non-significantly up until visit 10 in both groups without any difference in the amount of change (5.3,

95% CI 6.7-17.4 ng/ml, p=0.329) according to similar multilevel models (Table **6.13**).

β-crosslaps levels were also similar at baseline and changed non-significantly in both groups without any difference between the groups (54, 95% CI 138-243 pg/ml, p=0.53) according to similar models (Table **6.13**).

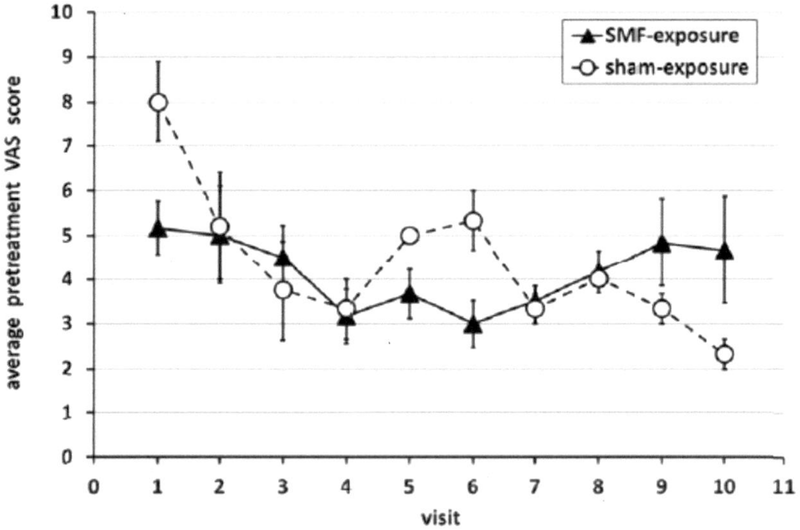

Fig. (6.24). Mean VAS±SEM scores before each treatment. Dark triangles represent VAS scores for SMF-exposure, and open circles represent VAS scores for sham-exposure at each visit. Straight lines between markers guide the eye only.

Ancillary Analyses

The models after exclusion of the participants lost to follow-up gave similar results to the main analysis on the short term effect of treatment yielding no significant difference between the groups (p=0.134). The results on long-term effects on VAS scores were also in line with the findings of the main analysis showing a significant decrease in the sham group and a non-significant change in the SMF group, however the between group difference was non-significant (0.22, 95% CI 0.02-0.46 cm, p=0.066).

We have also run analyses after adjustment of the observed baseline difference in vitamin D levels. Regarding the short-term changes in the VAS scores, we found no significant difference between the groups (0.59, 95% CI 0.30-1.49, p=0.195). As for the long-term effects on the VAS score, a significant between-group difference remained with a more prominent decrease in the sham compared to the SMF group (0.26, 95% CI 0.03-0.49 cm, p=0.03).

Harms

No serious adverse events were reported. None of the investigated safety measures (body mass, height, systolic and diastolic BP, and heart rate) changed significantly from baseline up to visit 10 (all p=0.2).

Discussion, Conclusions

In the present randomized controlled trial in postmenopausal women with vertebral deformity and back pain we found a non-significant reduction of pain sensation with SMF treatment on VAS in the short-term (after 30 min treatment session), whereas pain perception significantly decreased after sham treatment; with no difference between the acute effect of SMF and sham treatments (primary outcome). During a series of 10 visits we found no change in pain perception in the SMF group and a significant decrease in the sham group, with a larger decrease in pain perception in the sham compared to the SMF treatment (secondary outcome). We found no change in bone turnover markers in either group or between groups. However, our study was rather underpowered to allow for any far-reaching conclusion on these tertiary outcomes.

Limitations

Due to the limited number of participants, we had to apply a strong hypothesis to improve statistical power, according to which the acute change in VAS scores after treatment are similar at the first and the last visit, and VAS scores linearly decrease during a 10 session series. Whereas the first hypothesis seems to be plausible, the latter might easily be false; therefore, our findings in terms of the secondary outcome may be less valid.

To improve the interpretation of the secondary outcome, participants were informed that the lack of effect immediately after a treatment session did not exclude the possibility of active SMF treatment. While this may have modified the effect size of the primary outcome, it is an unlikely source of bias as both treatment groups had received the same information.

There was a baseline difference in VAS scores that may have influenced the changes observed throughout the study. Although we did adjust this difference during analysis, it is possible that some members of the sham group had higher scores due to some acute reason (such as inflammatory processes) that regressed during the study spontaneously. This scenario is easily possible taking into account the small number of participants and the fact that this might have led to an unbalanced randomization. The difference in baseline VAS scores is extremely important with regard to long-term changes in VAS scores, since the sham group started with a very high pain sensation (8 out of 10 on the VAS score) that makes regression to the mean more probable during repeat measurements.

As only Caucasian women enrolled in our study, generalizability may be limited. Furthermore, generalizability is also hindered by the low number of participants. An additional limitation is related to the fact that back pain in osteoporotic women with a vertebral fracture of undetermined duration could also be due to factors other than bone deformity, such as myofascial pain or nerve compression.

Strengths

While the size of the study was small, the statistical methods (multilevel modeling) used for analysis gave us confidence to conclude on the primary outcome of our study and, thus, exclude the effect of SMF on short-term pain sensation in the current setting.

A further strength of our study was that our primary and ancillary analyses (on participants with a full set of data and those adjusted for baseline vitamin D level differences) gave corresponding results. It should be noted, however, that the observed significant difference in vitamin D levels may also indicate the possibility of an unbalanced randomization.

Comparison with Other Studies

Our negative findings on the primary outcome are quite surprising especially in light of the results of the *in vivo* animal studies described in Chapter 5 (***In Vivo* Animal Experiments**) that almost consistently reported decreased pain in different models of acute pain. Most of these studies used acute pain models that may be less relevant to the target population of our study. One out of 2 studies of chronic pain (**Neuropathic pain**) showed an extreme improvement of mechanical allodynia in Seltzer-operated mice a fortnight after the operation provided that mice were repeatedly exposed to an inhomogeneous SMF for 30 min/day following the challenge.

Moreover, another study suggests that the effect of SMF-exposure could be related to an improved circulation and decreased inflammatory environment in rats with adjuvant arthritis [312] that might also be less relevant to osteoporotic pain. Important differences between our study setting and the animal models were that animals exposed to SMF treatment

i. had a whole-body exposure and
ii. they were freely moving within the SMFinducing electric currents in their bodies.

Magnetic and electric effects could both have affected the findings.

The results of human reports are more controversial. Most of the studies with proper control groups found no differences between placebo exposure and SMF in healthy volunteers [272]; in people with sensitive teeth (section **On visitors of a dental clinic**), in people with neck pain [436], and in patients with fibromyalgia [264].

The study presented in the section **On healthy volunteers** came to the conclusion that VAS may not be sensitive enough to identify the effect of SMF treatment since thermal perception threshold improved significantly while no change in the VAS scores were observed. Brown *et al.* [266] claims that other methods for measuring pain sensation may be more sensitive to...(pain disability index, clinical global improvement severity).

Other common factors in the positive studies that are different from our setting are the continuous use of SMF treatment as well as the much larger scale of the studies [266, 267, 437]. It does not seem feasible to use the magnet from our study continuously due to its mass. Our trial was powered to show clinically meaningful improvements of 1.5 cm on the VAS scale. This, of course, does not exclude a smaller effect. The finding on the secondary outcome of long-term pain relief is totally contrary to any of the studies reported previously. We attribute the implausibility of these findings to residual confounding related to the low number of participants.

The effect of SMF on bone metabolism seems to be supported by several *in vitro* experiments [334, 439 - 441]. These studies report enhanced osteoblast differentiation and increased production of bone morphogenic protein 2 (BMP-2) and type 1 collagen. *In vivo* animal experiments support these findings too: BMP-2 production was increased in both experimental periodontitis [449] and in ovariectomized animals [444, 451]. Furthermore, in an ischemic bone model, the decrease in BMD values was also prevented [445, 446], in addition to the effect on BMP-2. Prompt healing after fracture or osteotomy also observable in several models [447, 448, 450]. Human studies also corroborate this by showing improved fracture healing and a decreased loss of periodontal tissues [452, 453]. Our negative findings on the tertiary outcomes are not contradictory to these results as our study was not equipped to show changes in these markers. Another possible explanation for our negative findings may lie in the difference in the duration of SMF-exposure. Namely, we used short-term weekly exposure, whereas most of the other studies applied continuous SMF-exposure (for days or weeks). We are of the opinion that larger studies with longer follow-up and repeat BMD measurements are required to prove or disprove any effect of SMF on bone turnover.

Our results suggest that a repeated 30 min local exposure to a special inhomogeneous SMF has no clinically meaningful effect on pain sensation. Therefore, we cannot recommend SMF, as was used in this study, to be employed in the treatment of back pain in postmenopausal women with bone deformity. The finding that sham treatment was more effective in long-term pain relief is very implausible in the mirror of previous studies and, as has been mentioned before, is likely to be related to residual confounding. Merely based on our results, an effect of SMF on bone turnover cannot be excluded.

CHAPTER 7

Summary

The Author as a positive skeptic has certainly learned an awful lot in the course of the experiments and trials described in this book. Beyond personal gain though, let us guide the Reader through the most important findings. *In vitro* experiments are summarized in Table **7.1**.

Table 7.1. *In vitro* experiments described in this book with reference chapter or point within this book, subject, outcome measure, exposure conditions, other treatment if applies, and the observations.

reference link in this book	subject of measurement	observed quantity, model	SMF-exposure conditions	other treatment (if any)
***In Vitro* Experiments on Microorganisms**	microorganisms: *Bacillus circulans, Escherichia coli, Micrococcus luteus, Pseudomonas fluorescens, Saccharomyces cerevisiae, Salmonella enterica serovar Enteritidis, Serratia marcescens, Staphylococcus aureus*	endpoint viability, standard incubation	3 different iSMF (all in generator 11) for 10, 30, 50 min, or 24 h	
Result: No significant difference between SMF-exposed and sham cell numbers was found at the 95% confidence level for any strain, for any exposure time or layer with the exception of *P. fluorescens* 30 min, layer 2 (p<0.001), *B. circulans* 30 min, layer 3 (p<0.05) and layer 4 (p<0.05), and *E. coli* 50 min, layer 1 (p<0.05).				
DNA damage	human leukocytes	DNA analysis, single-cell gel electrophoresis	3 different iSMF (all in generator 11) or hSMF (generator 15) for 0.5, 1, 2, 4, 6, 18, 20, or 24 h	^{60}Co-γ irradiation

(Table 7.1) contd.....

reference link in this book	subject of measurement	observed quantity, model	SMF-exposure conditions	other treatment (if any)
Result: Statistically significant differences were found at 1 h (iSMF), and 4 or 18 h (hSMF) if samples were exposed to only SMF, compared to control. When the SMF-exposure followed the ^{60}Co-γ irradiation, statistically significant differences were found at 1 h (iSMF) and 4 h (hSMF). If exposure to SMF preceded γ irradiation, no statistically significant difference was found compared to γ irradiated group.				
Anti-inflammatory effect	human macrophages and lymphocytes	endpoint analysis of IL-6, IL-8, TNF-α, and IL-10, enzyme-linked immunosorbent assay	iSMF (generator 11) for 6, 18, or 24 h	lipopoly-saccharide
Result: Exposure caused visible morphological changes on macrophages as well as on lymphocytes, and also seemed to be toxic to lymphocytes (37-42%, $0.308<p<0.444$), but not to macrophages (<1.43%, $p>0.987$). Analysis of concentrations showed a significantly reduced production of pro-inflammatory cytokines IL-6, IL-8, and TNF-α from macrophages compared to negative control (57-88%, $p=0.031$) and IL-6 compared to positive control (45-56%, $p=0.035$). The production of anti-inflammatory cytokine IL-10 from macrophages and from lymphocytes was enhanced compared to negative control, significantly from lymphocytes ((-184%)-(-28.75%), $p=0.042$). The secretion of IL-6 from lymphocytes was significantly decreased compared to positive control ((-115%)-(-27%), $p=0.039$).				

Conclusions from the *in vitro* studies: Microorganisms have not been activated by any means of external agent; they have remained in their normal habitat. Under such circumstances, they were not affected by the SMF-exposure in the dose range applied. Neither was the repair of DNA-damaged human leukocytes influenced by the exposure. However, when macrophages and lymphocytes were activated with LPS, SMF-exposure exerted an anti-inflammatory action in the release of different cytokines. This latter study has an extremely important lesson for us. SMF-exposure itself without any kind of induced electric phenomenon has the capability of significantly affect cytokine secretion.

Similarly to Table **7.1**, Table **7.2** contains similar results for the *in vivo* animal experiments.

Table 7.2. *In vivo* animal experiments described in this book with reference chapter or point within this book, subject, outcome measure, exposure conditions, other treatment if applies, and the observations.

reference link in this book	subject of measurement	observed quantity, model	SMF exposure conditions	other treatment (if any)
Experiments on invertebrates *in vivo*	land snail, *Helix pomatia*	response latency to thermal stimulus, hot plate test	hSMF (generator 15), or iSMF (generator 11) for 20, 30, or 40 min	naloxone and/or serotonin, or tryptamine
Result: Both hSMF and iSMF-exposure increased the thermo-nociceptive threshold: 40%, 29%, or 42% after hSMF-exposure for 20, 30, or 40 min by $p<0.001$ for all, and 33% or 46% after iSMF-exposure for 20 or 40 min by $p<0.05$ or $p<0.001$, resp. The response latency depended on the day-night cycle; response latency was higher by 51% ($p<0.001$) during the night. This trend also held for SMF-exposure (29%, $p<0.001$). Serotonin alone increased response latency (56%, $p<0.001$), whereas serotonin antagonist tryptamine decreased it (-98%, $p<0.001$). Using naloxone, response latency decreased (-52.5%, $p<0.001$); however, both SMF-exposure and serotonin in combination with naloxone rose it back to above the control level (117% or 150%, resp. by $p<0.001$ either).				
Locomotor activity and anxiety behavior in healthy mice	CFLP mouse	number of entries, EPM test; time of walking, running, rearing, and immobility in locomotor activity test	iSMF (generator 11) for 30 min	acetic acid
Result: Exposure failed to affect anxiety behavior and hyperlocomotion-inducing effect of morphine.				
Peripheral action	BALB/c mouse	MWT, resiniferatoxin-, formalin-, carrageenan-test, resiniferatoxin desensitization, von Frey and rotarod test	iSMF (generator 11) for 5, 20, 30 min	resiniferatoxin, formalin, carrageenan
Result: SMF-exposure reduced the number of formalin-evoked paw lickings and liftings in both phase I and phase II (30-60%, $p<0.05$). It diminished mechanical hyperalgesia evoked by *i.pl.* injection of carrageenan (26%, $p<0.05$) as well as the TRPV1 capsaicin receptor agonist resiniferatoxin (27%, $p<0.05$). Selective inactivation of capsaicin-sensitive sensory fibers by high dose resiniferatoxin pretreatment decreased nocifensive behaviors in phase II of the formalin test to a similar extent. Significant inhibitory effects of SMF on formalin-induced nociception and carrageenan-evoked hyperalgesia were absent in resiniferatoxin-pretreated mice. No significant difference was found in the rotarod performance.				
Optimization of SMF parameters	CFLP mouse	number of writhings, writhing test	hSMF or iSMF (generators 1-16) for 5, 20, 30, or 40 min	acetic acid, Epsom salt

(Table 7.2) contd.....

reference link in this book	subject of measurement	observed quantity, model	SMF exposure conditions	other treatment (if any)
Result: Inhibition of pain reaction: The number of writhings decreased from 9, 32, and 30 to 2, 15, and 14, respectively, measured in 0-5, 6-20, and 21-30 min following the acetic acid challenge. The pain reaction during the total observation period was reduced by 57% (p<0.005). Exposure significantly diminished the Epsom salt-induced number of writhings (26%, 39%, or 52% in the 3 time intervals, resp.) *AE* could be identified 10-30 min following SMF-exposure (61-91%, p_{max}<0.003).				
Clinical MRI	CFLP mouse	number of writhings, writhing test	hSMF (generator 20) for 5, 20, or 30 min	acetic acid, naloxone
Result: *AE* of 68±2% (p<0.001) was found in a clinical MRI. Subcutaneous injection of naloxone in the mice reversed the SMF-induced *AE*.				
Lateral gradients	CFLP mouse	number of writhings, writhing test	hSMF (generator 2) or iSMF (generator 11) for 5, 20, or 30 min or iSMF (generators 17a-e) for 5, 20, or 30 min; different sized cages protruding out of the SMF	acetic acid
Result: No significant difference was found in the site preference (hSMF, iSMF *vs* sham) indicating that SMF is neither aversive nor favorable. Comparison of writhings observed in the sham *vs* SMF side of the cage revealed that SMF-exposure resulted in significantly fewer writhings than sham (64%, p<0.004 and 81 %, p<0.03 for hSMF and iSMF, resp.). Deeper statistical analysis clarified that the lateral SMF gradient between SMF and sham sides could be responsible for most of the analgesic effect (91%, p<0.02 and 54%, p<0.02, respectively). The best possible partition for *AE* was 3×3. Motion-induced electric current density may make antinociception more effective and/or has a preventive manner as compared to the nerve stimulatory effect leading to pain sensation. Regarding MR equivalent switching rate *AE* may not exclusively be related with the inhomogeneity of SMF. The higher the MR equivalent slew rate, the more expressed *AE*.				
Pharmacological analysis	CFLP mouse	number of writhings, writhing test	iSMF (generator 11) for 5, 20, or 30 min	acetic acid, naloxone, naltrindole, norbinaltor-phimine, β-funaltrexamine, morphine
Result: *AE* induced by SMF was inhibited by *s.c.* administration of naloxone, irreversible μ-opioid receptor antagonist β-funaltrexamine, and δ-opioid receptor antagonist naltrindole, but the *x*-opioid receptor antagonist norbinaltorphimine failed to affect the SMF-induced *AE*. In contrast to *s.c.* administration, *i.c.v.* injected naloxone did not antagonize *AE* of SMF.				

(Table 7.2) contd.....

reference link in this book	subject of measurement	observed quantity, model	SMF exposure conditions	other treatment (if any)
Neuropathic pain	BALB/c mouse	MWT, neuropathic pain model	iSMF (generator 11) for 30 min/day for 14 days starting post operation day 1 or 15	partial nerve ligature
Result: Exposure failed to prevent the decrease of MWT in the first postoperative week. Thirty min/day SMF treatment started just after the nerve ligation elevated MWT values to a modest extent after 14 days. However, the effectiveness of a daily exposure to SMF was prominent when applied between postoperative days 15 and 28. In this case, MWT was already noticeably increased after the first treatment and it practically reached the control values by the end of 14 days.				
Neuropathia diabetica	CD1 mouse	blood glucose level, laboratory; TPT, diabetes model	iSMF (generator 11) for 30 min/day for at least 42 days	streptozotocin
Result: Exposure failed to affect TPT, it statistically significantly (23%, $p<0.001$) reduced blood glucose level in the 200 mg/kg streptozotocin group.				
Neuropathia diabetica	CFLP mouse	body mass, weighting	iSMF (generator 11) for 30 min/day for 40 days	
Result: Exposure failed to affect body mass.				
Visceral action	timed-pregnant C57BL/6 mouse	time of PTB, PTB test	iSMF (generator 11) for 40 min/day for 3 or 17 days	lipopoly-saccharide
Result: The fetal development and the delivery were normal in animals that were exposed to SMF but not treated with LPS. SMF in these cases did not influence the term of delivery. In LPS-challenged animals, exposure prolonged the time of PTB occurrence from 18 to 22 h after the challenge ($p<0.05$). The higher the dose, the longer the prolongation.				

Conclusions from the *in vivo* studies: A long series of experiments had been performed to optimize the SMF-exposure system preceding most of the experiments with SMF. According to the results the obtained generator had the flair of influence different biological response in a well measurable fashion. The locomotor activity and anxiety behavior of healthy mice have not been influenced by pre-exposure to SMF. Hyperlocomotion induced by morphine was also no subject to change upon exposure. However, whole-body exposure had a significant effect on the response if the mouse was in patho(physio)logical condition. The effect was observable if different irritating chemical agents were administered either peripherally or viscerally. Even a disease of the CNS could be beneficially affected by repetitive SMF-exposure. Acute as well as chronic types of illnesses have been modeled and were found to respond beneficially to SMF-exposure. Both mechanical and thermal pain sensitivity were decreased, the latter also in invertebrates. From the pure physical viewpoint, a special result was obtained through investigations with inhomogeneous SMF. Gradients seem to have an almost as high importance to different biological responses than the magnetic induction itself. The tested responses were less dependent on exposure times. Concerning the background mechanism of action beyond those found about the anti-inflammatory effect in the *in vitro* studies, we established that *AE* of SMF-exposure acts primarily *via* μ-opioid receptors. The beneficial behavior of exposure was proven in allergic response as well.

Similarly, Table **7.3** contains similar results for the human trials.

Table 7.3. Human trials described in this book with reference chapter or point within this book, subject, outcome measure, exposure conditions, other treatment if applies, and the observations.

reference link in this book	subject of measurement	observed quantity, model	SMF exposure conditions	other treatment
On healthy volunteers	healthy volunteers	thermal pain threshold (TPT), visual analog scale, heating pads under 4 fingers (4 blocks of 12 TPT trials)	iSMF (generator 18) for 15 and 30 min	
Result: Exposure resulted in a statistically significant increase in TPT during the entire exposure duration and diminished within-block thermal habituation leaving pain perception unchanged.				
On visitors of a dental clinic	dental patients	subjective pain index, numerical rating visual analogue scale (NRS); pain tolerance threshold measurement (TTM), pulp meter	iSMF (generator 19) for 30 min	dental treatment
Result: Exposure failed to significantly reduce pain perception in the NRS group and to enhance tolerance threshold in the TTM group.				

(Table 7.3) contd.....

reference link in this book	subject of measurement	observed quantity, model	SMF exposure conditions	other treatment
Pain perception and bone turnover	postmenopausal osteoporotic women with bone deformity and back pain	pain sensation, visual analogue scale; bone turnover markers, laboratory analysis	iSMF (generator 3) for 30 min/day for 10 days	osteoporosis treatment
Result: Both SMF- and sham-exposure similarly reduced short term pain (sham-SMF: 0.59, 95%CI 0.30-1.49 centimeter, p=0.195). VAS did not change in SMF-, while it decreased in the sham-exposed group (between-group difference 0.27, 95%CI 0.04-0.50 centimeter/visit). Bone turnover markers remained unchanged after 11 visits.				

Conclusions from the human *vivo* studies: In the tested situations the response of humans was systematically less expressed than that of animals. This might have something to do with the kind of exposure: For humans the exposure was always local, while in case of *in vivo* studies, it was whole-body. No positive result was found in healthy volunteers other than the change of peripheral thermal threshold.

CHAPTER 8

Plans

I must admit at this point that although the book is close to its end, there is much more research ahead of us than behind us. As already mentioned, we have learned a lot and through this process of cognition doors opened, where no openings had been assumed. Here are some doors I plan to close behind me in the future. This Chapter may be the most relevant for those, who are thinking of initiating research in this field.

SHORT-TERM ISSUES

At this time, when the Reader is holding this book, 3 journal articles have been published all of which I kindly refer the Reader to kind attention with the abstracts of the papers. An *in vivo* animal model, experimental autoimmune encephalomyelitis (EAE), a model for human multiple sclerosis (MS) was used in rodents [458]. Static magnetic field (SMF)-exposure was shown to be beneficial in specific cases of inflammatory nature, where it could suppress symptoms. The null-hypothesis was that animals with induced EAE exposed to SMF would show different seriousness of symptoms, than those in the sham-exposed control group. Three replicated series of repetitive, 30 min/day whole-body exposure to SMF with 477 mT magnetic induction and 48 T/m lateral induction gradient were conducted on female CSJLF1 mice with a mild, mouse spinal cord homogenate emulsion-induced EAE. Conventional scores of animal response to EAE were compared between sham- and SMF-exposed groups. Following a pilot test, we used 18 animals/group. The primary outcome measure was the daily group average of standard EAE scores. Results show that SMF-exposure has a strong, reproducible, and significantly beneficial effect up to 51.82% (p<0.001) over sham-exposure on symptoms of EAE throughout the 25 days of the experiment. This study aimed at laying the experimental research foundation for a later therapy option for SMF-exposure in the clinical management of MS.

Another experimental series published includes an *in vivo* mouse allergy model

János F. László

and a skin prick human test under SMF-exposure [459]. Previous observations suggest that static magnetic field (SMF)-exposure acts on living organisms partly through reactive oxygen species (ROS) reactions. In this study, our goal was to determine the impact of SMF-exposure on ragweed pollen extract (RWPE)-induced allergic inflammation closely associated with oxidative stress. Inhomogeneous SMF was generated with an apparatus validated previously providing a peak-to-peak magnetic induction of the dominant SMF component 389 mT by 39 T/m lateral gradient in the *in vivo* and *in vitro* experiments, and 192 mT by 19 T/m in the human study at the 3 mm target distance. Effects of SMF-exposure were studied in a murine model of allergic inflammation and also in human provoked skin allergy. We found that even a single 30min exposure of mice to SMF immediately following intranasal RWPE challenge significantly lowered the increase in the total antioxidant capacity of the airways and decreased allergic inflammation. Repeated (3 consecutive days) or prolonged (60 min) exposure to SMF after RWPE challenge decreased the severity of allergic responses more efficiently than a single 30 min treatment. SMF-exposure did not alter ROS production by RWPE under cell-free conditions, while diminished RWPE-induced increase in the ROS levels in A549 epithelial cells. Results of the human skin prick tests indicated that SMF-exposure had no significant direct effect on provoked mast cell degranulation. The beneficial effects of SMF are likely due to the mobilization of cellular ROS-eliminating mechanisms rather than direct modulation of ROS production by pollen NAD(P)H oxidases.

The third paper was devoted to the effect of static magnetic field (SMF)-exposure on erosive gastritis [460]. The randomized, self- and placebo-controlled, double-blind, pilot study included 16 patients of the 2nd Department of Internal Medicine, Semmelweis University diagnosed with erosive gastritis. The instrumental analysis followed a qualitative (pre-intervention) assessment of the symptoms by the individual patients, which included lower heartburn (in the ventricle), upper heartburn (in the oesophagus), epigastric pain, regurgitation, bloating, and dry cough. Medical diagnosis included a double-line upper panendoscopy followed by 30 min local inhomogeneous SMF-exposure intervention at the lower sternal region over the stomach with peak-to-peak magnetic induction of 3 mT and 30 mT/m gradient at the target site. A qualitative (post-intervention) assessment of the same symptoms served as the closing of the examination. Sham- or SMF-exposure was used in a double blind manner. The authors succeeded in justifying the clinically and statistically significant beneficial effect of SMF- over sham-exposure on the symptoms of erosive gastritis the average effect of inhibition being 56% by p=0.001, n=42+96. This pilot study was meant to encourage gastroenterologists to test local, inhomogeneous SMF-exposure on erosive gastritis patients in order for this intervention to become an evidence-based alternative or complementary method in the clinical use, especially in cases when conventional therapy options are contraindicated.

Voltage-gated sodium channels play an important role in the transport of frequency-coded information in generating the action potential. CNS develops primarily Nav1.1, Nav1.2, Nav1.3, and Nav1.6 subtypes; the expression of Nav1.2 neuron is specific. Nav1.2 is essential in the pathogenesis of not only neurodegenerative diseases like epilepsy, but also of inflammatory illnesses implying high fever. Evidence shows that exposure to an external SMF can alter the permeability of ion channels [70], thus may modify Nav1.2 expression [70, 461]. The biophysical characterization of conformation changes in the course of the opening-closing of a channel by an experimental series concerned with human embryonic kidney (HEK) 293 cells may then be informative.

Diffusion and segregation processes as well as solidification are seriously dependent on the magnetic induction and geometry of an external SMF [462 - 465]. We have good reason to hypothesize that SMF-exposure may equally contribute to such changes in living matter. Confocal laser scanning microscopy could provide a solution in looking for induced cell death in slices of rat *cornu ammonis* 3 (CA3) hyppocampal regions either untreated, treated with kainic acid, and/or exposed to SMF. Even the diffused depth profile of propidium iodide (PI) dye can be monitored this way.

Strong assumptions hint at exposure to SMF interacting with the orientation or the result of the differentiation of developing cells [360, 466 - 469]. The effect of SMF-exposure on the rate of sympathetic preganglionic axonal outgrowth could be investigated on a grid where neurons can grow only along parallel channels while they are treated with BDNF and/or SMF.

One task of GIT is to absorb nutrients. GIT has not been included in SMF-exposure research other than in [470] where the authors reported that exposure to 0.317 T for 60 min resulted in decreased chemotaxis of human peripheral phagocytes. The, so far, one and only human trial is presented in this book. In a study of Ohata *et al.* [471], KCl solution and ion transport through regenerated cellulose membrane was measured before and after 0.24 T SMF-exposure. Exposure significantly enhanced the rate of ion transport, especially after the first exposure ($p<0.05$), whereas the increased ion transport rate did not return to the initial basal level after exchange of the aqueous medium. Cell proliferation and mitogenic signal transduction showed a decrease in thymidine incorporation and in second messenger formation after 0.2 T exposure for 60 min as reported by Pacini *et al.* [353]. The Caco-2 (human epithelial colorectal adenocarcinoma) monolayer model for absorption could be useful for predicting whether SMF-exposure can affect the transport rate of taxol, a plant alkaloid, in everyday usage as a chemotherapy drug and PEG-4000 (polyethylene glycol, macrogol with molecular mass 4000) between the apical and the basal chamber. Especially the absorption of ribose and glucose would be interesting under external SMF-exposure in practice [472].

Transdermal drug delivery (TDD) systems (for a review see [473]) have become exclusively important also due to the development of magnetophoresis [474, 475]. Magnetic nanoparticles may guide the active substance through the layers of skin in an interactively controlled fashion.

Since Grace Kimball's examination of yeast in 1938 [476], several research studies have suggested that exposure of plant seeds to strong SMF influences the growth characteristics of plants. Exposure might affect germination rate, seedling length, and other characteristics. Such application of exposure would serve as an extremely important biotechnological development for both industry and commerce since priming the seeds by SMF-exposure may decrease the hydration of seeds, which, by extension, would allow for easy storage. It is crucial to prove in a series of experiments whether a single 10-30 min long homogeneous or inhomogeneous SMF-exposure created with the generators discussed in this book (especially generator 11, 15, and 22, see in sections **Generators 1-16** and **Generator 22**) would affect the subsequent development of the plant. Although it seems reasonable to assume that plants have been developing sensors just as animals have, research is scarce in this field [477]. Possibly, the best approach so far has been put forward by Ahmad *et al.* [478] who suggested that cryptochrome, a special protein in the plant tissue, would be a good candidate for detecting SMF in the presence of blue light. The background mechanism of this action probably lies in radical-pair interactions.

According to the literature and our own experiments, there is an ideal duration of homogeneous SMF-exposure at a certain magnetic induction from the viewpoint of pathophysiological action. To test this assumption, we should use a species evolutionary more developed than microbes. Among invertebrates we find the nematode called *Caenorhabditis elegans* (*C. elegans*). *C. elegans* is a widely used model animal. With the pioneering work of Kimura *et al.* [479], the group of Huang became active studying this model under SMF-exposure [480 - 482]. However, the optimal duration and magnetic induction have not yet been discovered.

Another capable model in looking for the origin of SMF sensors would be the zooplankton. As mentioned before, magnetotactic bacteria perceive the geomagnetic field. Magnetites, to assist their taxation, have been shown to be synthesized by these bacteria [483]. The relevant question here would be if zooplankton possessed SMF sensors. Zooplankton found in quantity in Lake Balaton (*e.g.* nauplius, cyclopoida, calanoida, cladocera, and rota) might easily be the subject of an experiment searching for the answer to the question whether the spontaneous site preference of these animals would reveal any difference between exposure to geomagnetic field and to strong artificial SMF, including subgroups exposed to light or to elevated water temperature.

As the land snail invertebrate model was appropriate to show the responses to thermal stimulus under SMF-exposure conditions, a promising idea would to develop the model toward either mechanical stimulus or TRP ion channels. This latter direction would also reveal differences in the activity of C fibers under SMF-exposure between invertebrate and mammal models.

By now, it is presumably evident to the Reader that most of our experiments have been done in *in vivo* animal models of acute visceral pain. Another interesting point in this area would be to investigate whether the positive effects of local SMF-exposure in the human trial with gastritis patients could also be applicable in case an alcohol induced gastric ulcer model in mice. In 1982, FONAR, the company of Raymond Damadian, introduced its patented iron-core technology which was the basis for the open-field MRI scanners used nowadays. The epidemiological concern with regard to this strong field open-field MRIin which the dominant component of the SMF is ventral-dorsal, thus, perpendicular to the main blood vessels, is whether it would jeopardize the patient's health through magnetohydrodynamic action. In this respect, the most sensitive part of the mammalian body is the heart with its intricate electricity based power system. If we investigated the SMF-proof ECG of an isolated rodent heart [484] under SMF-exposure, we would be able to judge at least in a small, particular part of the concern.

There was much said in this book already about the effect that SMF-exposure may exert on (micro)circulation. Probably Mészáros was the one who started this kind of investigation in 1991 [485] looking for the effects of 40 mT SMF-exposure on BP in rats. I would complement the since then published studies with an experiment on mice anesthetized with a matter that does not influence the cardiac output [486]. In the course of the experiment, constant body core temperature should be taken care of in the sense that anesthesia, through the regulation of core temperature, may contribute to dropping BP. In conscious animals, body cooling excites the homeostatic thermoregulation in the preoptic area of the anterior hypothalamus trying to maintain the temperature and raise the BP accordingly [487]. BP was shown to alter with body temperature as 1.6 mmHg/°C in anesthetized mice [488]. The topic of BP was reviewed in [489]. This test would be a BP test in the brain measured *via* a tracheal cannula and a tapered catheter placed into the femoral artery connected to a BP sensor.

Much debate has been devoted in this book also to the potential effect of Faraday currents in freely moving rodents, the specific issue being whether these interact with the response to SMF-exposure? A method to verify the assumption that motion induced currents do not influence the response is to compare these in conscious and anesthetized animals within the same model. The mustard oil (allyl-isothiocyanate) induced ear edema model seems suitable for this study [490]. Separate animal groups exposed whole-body or locally in the lower back region, on the treated ear, or on the head including both ears would eliminate the controversy surrounding the exact place of action of the SMF-exposure.

SMF- and ELF magnetic field-exposure interferes also with cancer. Tumor growth inhibition and increased apoptosis was observed in human colon adenocarcinoma, breast carcinoma, and non-transformed embryonic lung fibroblast cell lines [491]. SMF-exposure affected murine mammary tumors induced by 7,12-dimethylbenz(a)anthracene in rats [492] and enhanced the action of adriamycin against mammary tumors transplanted into female B6C3F1 mice [493]. The combined effect of SMF-exposure and anti-cancer drugs was investigated as well [494]. SMF-exposure to 25-150 mT affected cellular immunity in C57BI/6 mice [495]. The increased apoptosis of thymic cells (16) and reduced red blood cell velocity in tumor microvessels has been observed as well [496]. Blood vessel formation under continuous exposure to inhomogeneous SMF (0.2-0.4 T by 2.09 T/m) and to homogeneous SMF-exposure was compared in the literature [379]. Effect of low (6 mT) or moderate (705 mT) SMF-exposure on normal or malignant lymphocytes (human leukemic TK6 cells) has been discussed [497]. With all the sources available on these various issues, the effect of SMF-exposure on tumor progression has not been fully clarified yet. Daily, repetitive, whole-body exposure to SMF created by generator 11 would be of great interest on immune-deficient NSG (non-obese diabetic *scid* gamma) mice engrafted with HT199 or on C57BL/6 mice engrafted with B16 melanoma cells.

With regard to human studies, one of the most intriguing problems, at least to the Author, is whether or how direct, local SMF-exposure can influence nerve conduction *in vivo*. In the past 10 years, serious research has been conducted in this area. Compound-evoked potentials did not show any difference in response latency during, before, or after SMF-exposure, but there was a small, statistically significant, decrease in amplitude [498]. A single trial on patients with carpal tunnel syndrome ended in the conclusion that SMF-exposure was beneficial to the symptoms [499]. No significance was demonstrated between-group differences for change in the primary endpoint for Symptom Severity Scale (SSS), Function

Severity Scale (FSS), or median nerve conduction parameters. For the SSS and the FSS, each group showed a reduction at 6 weeks indicating improvement in symptoms. The values of the nerve conduction velocity of C fibers were significantly reduced by B_{max} of 0.7 T SMF during the 4 to 6 h exposure period compared to unexposed control [500]. B_{max}=0.21 T SMF-exposure for 6 h failed to result in significant differences. The changes predicted in [97] in terms of speed of conduction and refractory period are very small [501]. The trial could include patients with critical illness polyneuropathy. Measuring both nervous medianus and ulnaris with electroneurography on both arms with SMF- or sham-exposure randomly might be able to answer our questions.

Shellock *et al.* [502] investigated whether the 1.5 T SMF of an MRI applied for 20 min would alter the surface skin temperature of humans as measured with fluoroptic thermometry during the exposure. They found no significant difference when compared to control. Mayrovitz and Groseclose published the results of a human trial in which they measured skin blood perfusion by laser Doppler in the dorsum skin of healthy volunteers [503]. They applied 90 or 400 mT for 15 min. A significant difference could be detected between exposed and unexposed fingers. The difference was attributed to SMF-exposure. Moreover, case studies appear on the internet showing dramatic improvements in the color of ecchymosis/hematoma already a few hours following the placement of a permanent magnet on the injured surface [504 - 507]. An international study might be warranted to clear up the issue of local SMF-exposure with a permanent magnetic device having a quantitative effect on the surface area of ecchymosis, presupposing that the SMF-exposure affected the regeneration of the damaged tissue. A permanent magnet, a non-magnetic (sham) device, and the combination of SMF-exposure with mechanical pressure exerted on the area of the ecchymosis must all be tested. While the extension of the ecchymosis should be analyzed quantitatively, the shape should be done in a qualitative way. A free internet software application would be useful to process image data and unravel the time development of the bruise.

Our study with PTB calls for a phase III study to provide evidence that PTB can be prevented by the repetitive use of local SMF-exposure on those expecting mothers who are compromised.

Simulation wise, I am still intrigued by the RADAR mouse phantom described in [508]. Some more work is needed for preparing the model to include organs of the mouse with appropriate magnetic susceptibilities. Such measured values are available in the literature. Then we shall pose the following question: A glass sphere of radius R moves with a constant velocity v_0 along the x axis where it suddenly enters an SMF of $\vec{B} = B_z\vec{k}$. Sodium ions (i) are distributed evenly along the surface of the sphere, (ii) fill up the globe uniformly representing the total of Q electric charges in a $-Q$ charged, also uniformly distributed but frozen background medium on the surface (i) or in the bulk (ii). Ions can move without any kind of energy loss over the surface (i) or in the bulk (ii). Now the question is how does the surface and the volume distribution of ions change after a longer period of time within the SMF *($\tau > 2R/v_0$)?* What kind of electromotive forces (*εmf*) develop between the upper and lower, front and back, and left and right hemispheres? If we know the answer to this question, we could apply it to other, more elaborate and realistic shapes and materials (of organs) and use these in RADAR to predict possible motion-induced electric parameters in rodents moving in(to) an SMF.

LONG-TERM COMMITMENTS

The most important commitment of the Author is to the contribution of the standardization of how experiments and trials including SMF-exposure in all research phases are reported. Following the foundation of this subject by the Consolidated Standards of Reporting Trials Group for Randomized, Controlled Trials extended to Nonpharmacological Treatments in 2001 [414], this group developed the idea in 2008 [427]. Later, they reported on the improvements of the standardization in 2010 [454], and further updating is currently in progress. Especially for SMF-exposure, an outstanding effort was that of Colbert *et al.* [29] cited on several occasions in this book. Standardization would not only serve the goal of reproducibility, but would also provide intercomparability between tests including SMF-exposure; and, further on, comparability with tests including other methods of intervention.

A very practical as well as fundamental aspect of SMF-exposure is whether the exposure exerts its effect at the supraspinal level. This issue is in need of much more work involving a lot of animal experiments and also human trials with clinical MRI devices.

One of the most challenging parts of this area of research is certainly the transition from SMF-exposure to ELF radiation. From a physics point of view, motion-induced currents in an SMF environment are identical to that of ELF acting on a static subject. We need to map this transition, the involved frequency range, the amplitudes of magnetic induction, *etc*.

This is about as much as I can say at the moment about the state of the art of our present research. There are still a lot of unanswered questions and a lot of achievable challenges remaining. The more doors we open, the more interesting discoveries we may make. Let us explore what is behind these doors together.

References

[1] Lengyel J. Die Wirkung des magnetischen Kraftfeldes auf die Faserbildung und auf das Gewebewachstum. Archiv für Experimentelle Zellforschung 1933; 14: 255.

[2] Barnóthy J. Rejection of transplanted tumors in mice. In: Barnóthy M, Ed. Biological Effects of Magnetic Fields. New York, NY, USA: Plenum Press 1964; pp. 100-8.

[3] NOAA. (National Oceanic and Atmospheric Administration, National Geophysical Data Center): Simulation model for Earth's magnetic field. 2014. Available at http://www.ngdc. noaa.gov/geomag-web/#igrfwmm.

[4] Jogler C, Lin W, Meyerdierks A, *et al.* Toward cloning of the magnetotactic metagenome: identification of magnetosome island gene clusters in uncultivated magnetotactic bacteria from different aquatic sediments. Appl Environ Microbiol 2009; 75(12): 3972-9. [http://dx.doi.org/10.1128/AEM.02701-08] [PMID: 19395570]

[5] Harada Y. The relation between the migration function of birds and fishes and their lagenal function. Acta Otolaryngol 2008; 128(4): 432-9. [http://dx.doi.org/10.1080/00016480701724920] [PMID: 18368579]

[6] Meyer CG, Holland KN, Papastamatiou YP. Sharks can detect changes in the geomagnetic field. J R Soc Interface 2005; 2(2): 129-30. [http://dx.doi.org/10.1098/rsif.2004.0021] [PMID: 16849172]

[7] Holland RA, Kirschvink JL, Doak TG, Wikelski M. Bats use magnetite to detect the Earth's magnetic field. PLoS One 2008; 3(2): e1676. [http://dx.doi.org/10.1371/journal.pone.0001676] [PMID: 18301753]

[8] Prato FS, Wills JM, Roger J, *et al.* Blood-brain barrier permeability in rats is altered by exposure to magnetic fields associated with magnetic resonance imaging at 1.5 T. Microsc Res Tech 1994; 27(6): 528-34. [http://dx.doi.org/10.1002/jemt.1070270607] [PMID: 8012055]

[9] Gmitrov J, Ohkubo C. Artificial static and geomagnetic field interrelated impact on cardiovascular regulation. Bioelectromagnetics 2002; 23(5): 329-38. [http://dx.doi.org/10.1002/bem.10020] [PMID: 12111753]

[10] Kovats RS, Campbell-Lendrum D, Matthies F. Climate change and human health: estimating avoidable deaths and disease. Risk Anal 2005; 25(6): 1409-18. [http://dx.doi.org/10.1111/j.1539-6924.2005.00688.x] [PMID: 16506971]

[11] Damadian R. Tumor detection by nuclear magnetic resonance. Science 1971; 171(3976): 1151-3. [http://dx.doi.org/10.1126/science.171.3976.1151] [PMID: 5544870]

[12] WHO. World Health Organization: Environmental Health Criteria 232: Static Fields. 2006. Available at http://who.int/peh-emf/publications/EHC_232_Static_Fields_full_document.pdf

[13] SCENIHR. Scientific Committee on Emerging and Newly Identified Health Risks: Health effects of exposure to EMF. 2009. Available at http://ec.europa.eu/health/ph_risk/committees/04_scenihr/docs/scenihr_o_022.pdf

[14] Tilke B. Alliance for MRI gains delay, but new European rules still loom. 2007. Available at https://www.myesr.org/html/img/pool/Auntminnie_26072007.pdf

[15] Dimbylow P. Quandaries in the application of the ICNIRP low frequency basic restriction on current density. Phys Med Biol 2008; 53(1): 133-45.
[http://dx.doi.org/10.1088/0031-9155/53/1/009] [PMID: 18182692]

[16] Tomasi DG, Wang R. Induced magnetic field gradients and forces in the human head in MRI. J Magn Reson Imaging 2007; 26(5): 1340-5.
[http://dx.doi.org/10.1002/jmri.21143] [PMID: 17969175]

[17] Schenck JF. Physical interactions of static magnetic fields with living tissues. Prog Biophys Mol Biol 2005; 87: 185-204.
[http://dx.doi.org/10.1016/j.pbiomolbio.2004.08.009]

[18] Brandt T. Vertigo: its multisensory syndromes. London, UK: Springer 2003.
[http://dx.doi.org/10.1007/978-1-4757-3801-8]

[19] Wang Z, Yang P, Xu H, Qian A, Hu L, Shang P. Inhibitory effects of a gradient static magnetic field on normal angiogenesis. Bioelectromagnetics 2009; 30(6): 446-53.
[http://dx.doi.org/10.1002/bem.20501] [PMID: 19405043]

[20] Galluzzi KE. Management of neuropathic pain. J Am Osteopath Assoc 2005; 105(9) (Suppl. 4): S12-9. [PMID: 16273720]

[21] Weingart SN, Ship AN, Aronson MD. Confidential clinician-reported surveillance of adverse events among medical inpatients. J Gen Intern Med 2000; 15(7): 470-7.
[http://dx.doi.org/10.1046/j.1525-1497.2000.06269.x] [PMID: 10940133]

[22] Xu J, Kochanek KD, Murphy SL, Tejada-Vera BS, Tejada-Vera B. Deaths: final data for 2007. Natl Vital Stat Rep 2010; 58(19): 1-135.
[PMID: 25075874]

[23] Adair RK. Constraints on biological effects of weak extremely-low-frequency electromagnetic fields. Phys Rev A 1991; 43(2): 1039-48.
[http://dx.doi.org/10.1103/PhysRevA.43.1039] [PMID: 9905119]

[24] Adair RK. Static and low-frequency magnetic field effects: health risks and therapies. Rep Prog Phys 2000; 63: 415-54.
[http://dx.doi.org/10.1088/0034-4885/63/3/204]

[25] Hore PJ. Rapporteur's report: sources and interaction mechanisms. Prog Biophys Mol Biol 2005; 87(2-3): 205-12.
[http://dx.doi.org/10.1016/j.pbiomolbio.2004.08.005] [PMID: 15556659]

[26] Hofmann S. Quantitative depth profiling in surface analysis - a review. Surf Interface Anal 1980; 2(4): 148-60.
[http://dx.doi.org/10.1002/sia.740020406]

[27] Prato FS, Robertson JA, Desjardins D, Hensel J, Thomas AW. Daily repeated magnetic field shielding induces analgesia in CD-1 mice. Bioelectromagnetics 2005; 26(2): 109-17.
[http://dx.doi.org/10.1002/bem.20056] [PMID: 15672364]

[28] Okano H. Effects of static magnetic fields in biology: role of free radicals. Front Biosci 2008; 13: 6106-25.
[http://dx.doi.org/10.2741/3141] [PMID: 18508647]

[29] Colbert AP, Markov MS, Souder JS. Static magnetic field therapy: dosimetry considerations. J Altern Complement Med 2008; 14(5): 577-82.
[http://dx.doi.org/10.1089/acm.2007.0827] [PMID: 18532897]

[30] Kangarlu A. High-field magnetic resonance imaging. Neuroimaging Clin N Am 2009; 19(1): 113-28.
[http://dx.doi.org/10.1016/j.nic.2008.09.008] [PMID: 19064204]

[31] Heinrich A, Szostek A, Nees F, Meyer P, Semmler W, Flor H. Effects of static magnetic fields on cognition, vital signs, and sensory perception: a meta-analysis. J Magn Reson Imaging 2011; 34(4): 758-63.
[http://dx.doi.org/10.1002/jmri.22720] [PMID: 21751291]

[32] Yamaguchi-Sekino S, Sekino M, Ueno S. Biological effects of electromagnetic fields and recently updated safety guidelines for strong static magnetic fields. Magn Reson Med Sci 2011; 10(1): 1-10.
[http://dx.doi.org/10.2463/mrms.10.1] [PMID: 21441722]

[33] Ueno S. Studies on magnetism and bioelectromagnetics for 45 years: from magnetic analog memory to human brain stimulation and imaging. Bioelectromagnetics 2012; 33(1): 3-22.
[http://dx.doi.org/10.1002/bem.20714] [PMID: 22012916]

[34] Collins H, Pinch T. The hole in the heart of medicine: The placebo effect Dr Golem. Chicago, IL, USA: University of Chicago Press 2005.

[35] Zubieta JK, Bueller JA, Jackson LR, *et al.* Placebo effects mediated by endogenous opioid activity on mu-opioid receptors. J Neurosci 2005; 25(34): 7754-62.
[http://dx.doi.org/10.1523/JNEUROSCI.0439-05.2005] [PMID: 16120776]

[36] Zubieta JK, Stohler CS. Neurobiological mechanisms of placebo responses. Ann N Y Acad Sci 2009; 1156: 198-210.
[http://dx.doi.org/10.1111/j.1749-6632.2009.04424.x] [PMID: 19338509]

[37] Pollo A, Benedetti F. The placebo response: neurobiological and clinical issues of neurological relevance. Prog Brain Res 2009; 175: 283-94.
[PMID: 19660663]

[38] Salomonowitz G, Friedrich M, Güntert BJ. [Medical relevance of magnetic fields in pain therapy]. Schmerz 2011; 25(2): 157-60.
[http://dx.doi.org/10.1007/s00482-010-1005-0] [PMID: 21258821]

[39] Shapiro AK, Chassan J, Morris LA, Frick R. Placebo-induced side effects. J Oper Psychiatr 1974; 6(1): 43-6.

[40] Eccles NK. A randomized, double-blinded, placebo-controlled pilot study to investigate the effectiveness of a static magnet to relieve dysmenorrhea. J Altern Complement Med 2005; 11(4): 681-7.
[http://dx.doi.org/10.1089/acm.2005.11.681] [PMID: 16131292]

[41] Bjordal JM, Johnson MI, Lopes-Martins RA, Bogen B, Chow R, Ljunggren AE. Short-term efficacy of physical interventions in osteoarthritic knee pain. A systematic review and meta-analysis of

randomised placebo-controlled trials. BMC Musculoskelet Disord 2007; 8: 51. [http://dx.doi.org/10.1186/1471-2474-8-51] [PMID: 17587446]

[42] Pittler MH, Brown EM, Ernst E. Static magnets for reducing pain: systematic review and meta-analysis of randomized trials. CMAJ 2007; 177(7): 736-42. [http://dx.doi.org/10.1503/cmaj.061344] [PMID: 17893349]

[43] Colbert AP, Wahbeh H, Harling N, *et al.* Static magnetic field therapy: a critical review of treatment parameters. Evid Based Complement Alternat Med 2009; 6(2): 133-9. [http://dx.doi.org/10.1093/ecam/nem131] [PMID: 18955243]

[44] Langford DJ, Crager SE, Shehzad Z, *et al.* Social modulation of pain as evidence for empathy in mice. Science 2006; 312(5782): 1967-70. [http://dx.doi.org/10.1126/science.1128322] [PMID: 16809545]

[45] McEntee J. MRI in Europe: it's time to end the uncertainty. Medical Physics Web 2007. Available at http://medicalphysicsweb.org/ cws/article/opinion/31320.

[46] de Vocht F, Stevens T, van Wendel-de-Joode B, Engels H, Kromhout H. Acute neurobehavioral effects of exposure to static magnetic fields: analyses of exposure-response relations. J Magn Reson Imaging 2006; 23(3): 291-7. [http://dx.doi.org/10.1002/jmri.20510] [PMID: 16463303]

[47] Potenza L, Ubaldi L, De Sanctis R, De Bellis R, Cucchiarini L, Dachà M. Effects of a static magnetic field on cell growth and gene expression in *Escherichia coli.* Mutat Res 2004; 561(1-2): 53-62. [http://dx.doi.org/10.1016/j.mrgentox.2004.03.009] [PMID: 15238230]

[48] Stansell MJ, Winters WD, Doe RH, Dart BK. Increased antibiotic resistance of *E. coli* exposed to static magnetic fields. Bioelectromagnetics 2001; 22(2): 129-37. [http://dx.doi.org/10.1002/1521-186X(200102)22:2<129::AID-BEM1016>3.0.CO;2-L] [PMID: 11180259]

[49] Chow K, Tung WL. Magnetic field exposure enhances DNA repair through the induction of DnaK/J synthesis. FEBS Lett 2000; 478(1-2): 133-6. [http://dx.doi.org/10.1016/S0014-5793(00)01822-6] [PMID: 10922484]

[50] Stasiuk GA. [Effect of a steady magnetic field on *Mycobacterium tuberculosis.*]. Probl Tuberk 1974; 7(7): 75-7. [PMID: 4212632]

[51] Khar'kova NA, Kazanin VI, Volkova ZS, Red'ko AF. [Effect of a steady magnetic field on several properties of a pathogenetic *staphylococcus*]. Zh Mikrobiol Epidemiol Immunobiol 1976; 1(1): 145-6. [PMID: 961235]

[52] Grosman Z, Kolár M, Tesaríková E. Effects of static magnetic field on some pathogenic microorganisms. Acta Univ Palacki Olomuc Fac Med 1992; 134: 7-9. [PMID: 1364971]

[53] Benson DE, Grissom CB, Burns GL, Mohammad SF. Magnetic field enhancement of antibiotic activity in biofilm forming *Pseudomonas aeruginosa*. ASAIO J 1994; 40(3): M371-6. [http://dx.doi.org/10.1097/00002480-199407000-00025] [PMID: 8555541]

[54] Kohno M, Yamazaki M, Kimura I, Wada M. Effect of static magnetic fields on bacteria: *Streptococcus*

mutans, Staphylococcus aureus, and *Escherichia coli*. Pathophysiology 2000; 7(2): 143-8. [http://dx.doi.org/10.1016/S0928-4680(00)00042-0] [PMID: 10927195]

[55] Binhi VN, Alipov YD, Belyaev IY. Effect of static magnetic field on *E. coli* cells and individual rotations of ion-protein complexes. Bioelectromagnetics 2001; 22(2): 79-86. [http://dx.doi.org/10.1002/1521-186X(200102)22:2<79::AID-BEM1009>3.0.CO;2-7] [PMID: 11180252]

[56] Zhang S, Wei W, Zhang J, Mao Y, Liu S. Effect of static magnetic field on growth of *Escherichia coli* and relative response model of series piezoelectric quartz crystal. Analyst (Lond) 2002; 127(3): 373-7. [http://dx.doi.org/10.1039/b109617f] [PMID: 11996362]

[57] Piatti E, Albertini MC, Baffone W, *et al.* Antibacterial effect of a magnetic field on *Serratia marcescens* and related virulence to *Hordeum vulgare* and *Rubus fruticosus* callus cells. Comp Biochem Physiol B Biochem Mol Biol 2002; 132(2): 359-65. [http://dx.doi.org/10.1016/S1096-4959(02)00065-9] [PMID: 12031461]

[58] Triampo W, Doungchawee G, Triampo D, Wong-Ekkabut J, Tang IM. Effects of static magnetic field on growth of leptospire, *Leptospira interrogans serovar canicola*: immunoreactivity and cell division. J Biosci Bioeng 2004; 98(3): 182-6. [http://dx.doi.org/10.1016/S1389-1723(04)00263-4] [PMID: 16233687]

[59] Gao W, Liu Y, Zhou J, Pan H. Effects of a strong static magnetic field on bacterium *Shewanella oneidensis*: an assessment by using whole genome microarray. Bioelectromagnetics 2005; 26(7): 558-63. [http://dx.doi.org/10.1002/bem.20133] [PMID: 16037957]

[60] Morrow AC, Dunstan RH, King BV, Roberts TK. Metabolic effects of static magnetic fields on *Streptococcus pyogenes*. Bioelectromagnetics 2007; 28(6): 439-45. [http://dx.doi.org/10.1002/bem.20332] [PMID: 17486599]

[61] Lefèvre CT, Song T, Yonnet JP, Wu LF. Characterization of bacterial magnetotactic behaviors by using a magnetospectrophotometry assay. Appl Environ Microbiol 2009; 75(12): 3835-41. [http://dx.doi.org/10.1128/AEM.00165-09] [PMID: 19376916]

[62] Pósfai M, Lefèvre CT, Trubitsyn D, Bazylinski DA, Frankel RB. Phylogenetic significance of composition and crystal morphology of magnetosome minerals. Front Microbiol 2013; 4: 344. [http://dx.doi.org/10.3389/fmicb.2013.00344] [PMID: 24324461]

[63] Le Bars D, Gozariu M, Cadden SW. Animal models of nociception. Pharmacol Rev 2001; 53(4): 597-652. [PMID: 11734620]

[64] Yaksh TL. Spinal systems and pain processing: development of novel analgesic drugs with mechanistically defined models. Trends Pharmacol Sci 1999; 20(8): 329-37. [http://dx.doi.org/10.1016/S0165-6147(99)01370-X] [PMID: 10431212]

[65] Zimmermann M. Ethical guidelines for investigations of experimental pain in conscious animals. Pain 1983; 16(2): 109-10. [http://dx.doi.org/10.1016/0304-3959(83)90201-4] [PMID: 6877845]

[66] Houpt TA, Pittman DW, Barranco JM, Brooks EH, Smith JC. Behavioral effects of high-strength static

magnetic fields on rats. J Neurosci 2003; 23(4): 1498-505.
[PMID: 12598638]

[67] Satow Y, Satake H, Matsunami K. Effect of long exposure to large static magnetic field on the recovery process of bullfrog sciatic nerve activity. Proc Jpn Acad Ser B 1990; 66: 151-5.
[http://dx.doi.org/10.2183/pjab.66.151]

[68] Rosen AD. Magnetic field influence on acetylcholine release at the neuromuscular junction. Am J Physiol 1992; 262(6 Pt 1): C1418-22.
[PMID: 1616009]

[69] Satow Y, Matsunami K, Kawashima T, Satake H, Huda K. A strong constant magnetic field affects muscle tension development in bullfrog neuromuscular preparations. Bioelectromagnetics 2001; 22(1): 53-9.
[http://dx.doi.org/10.1002/1521-186X(200101)22:1<53::AID-BEM6>3.0.CO;2-5] [PMID: 11122493]

[70] Rosen AD. Mechanism of action of moderate-intensity static magnetic fields on biological systems. Cell Biochem Biophys 2003; 39(2): 163-73.
[http://dx.doi.org/10.1385/CBB:39:2:163] [PMID: 14515021]

[71] Chase R. Behavior and its neural control in gastropod molluscs. New York, NY, USA: Oxford University Press 2002.

[72] Balaban PM, Bravarenko NI, Kuznetzov AN. Influence of a stationary magnetic field on bioelectric properties of snail neurons. Bioelectromagnetics 1990; 11(1): 13-25.
[http://dx.doi.org/10.1002/bem.2250110104] [PMID: 2346504]

[73] Nikolić L, Kartelija G, Nedeljković M. Effect of static magnetic fields on bioelectric properties of the Br and N1 neurons of snail *Helix pomatia.* Comp Biochem Physiol A Mol Integr Physiol 2008; 151(4): 657-63.
[http://dx.doi.org/10.1016/j.cbpa.2008.08.006] [PMID: 18760374]

[74] Prato FS, Kavaliers M, Thomas AW. Extremely low frequency magnetic fields can either increase or decrease analgaesia in the land snail depending on field and light conditions. Bioelectromagnetics 2000; 21(4): 287-301.
[http://dx.doi.org/10.1002/(SICI)1521-186X(200005)21:4<287::AID-BEM5>3.0.CO;2-N] [PMID: 10797457]

[75] Saksida LM, Galea LA, Kavaliers M. Antinociceptive effects of the enkephalinase inhibitor, SCH 34826, in the snail, *Cepaea nemoralis*. Peptides 1993; 14(4): 763-5.
[http://dx.doi.org/10.1016/0196-9781(93)90110-3] [PMID: 8234022]

[76] Kavaliers M, Hirst M, Teskey GC. A functional role for an opiate system in snail thermal behavior. Science 1983; 220(4592): 99-101.
[http://dx.doi.org/10.1126/science.6298941] [PMID: 6298941]

[77] Thomas AW, Kavaliers M, Prato FS, Ossenkopp KP. Pulsed magnetic field induced "analgesia" in the land snail, Cepaea nemoralis, and the effects of mu, δ, and κ opioid receptor agonists/antagonists. Peptides 1997; 18(5): 703-9.
[http://dx.doi.org/10.1016/S0196-9781(97)00004-1] [PMID: 9213364]

[78] Prato FS, Kavaliers M, Carson JL. Behavioral responses to magnetic fields by land snails are

dependent on both magnetic field direction and light. Proc Biol Sci 1996; 263: 1437-42. [http://dx.doi.org/10.1098/rspb.1996.0209]

[79] Kavaliers M. Evidence for opioid and non-opioid forms of stress-induced analgesia in the snail, *Cepaea nemoralis*. Brain Res 1987; 410(1): 111-5. [http://dx.doi.org/10.1016/S0006-8993(87)80029-X] [PMID: 3580888]

[80] Kavaliers M. Novelty-induced opioid analgesia in the terrestrial snail, *Cepaea nemoralis*. Physiol Behav 1988; 42(1): 29-32. [http://dx.doi.org/10.1016/0031-9384(88)90255-7] [PMID: 2838852]

[81] Kavaliers M, Ossenkopp KP, Lipa SM. Day-night rhythms in the inhibitory effects of 60 Hz magnetic fields on opiate-mediated 'analgesic' behaviors of the land snail, *Cepaea nemoralis*. Brain Res 1990; 517(1-2): 276-82. [http://dx.doi.org/10.1016/0006-8993(90)91038-I] [PMID: 2375996]

[82] Kavaliers M, Ossenkopp KP. Magnetic fields inhibit opioid-mediated 'analgesic' behaviours of the terrestrial snail, Cepaea nemoralis. J Comp Physiol A 1988; 162(4): 551-8. [http://dx.doi.org/10.1007/BF00612520] [PMID: 2452251]

[83] Del Seppia C, Ghione S, Luschi P, Ossenkopp KP, Choleris E, Kavaliers M. Pain perception and electromagnetic fields. Neurosci Biobehav Rev 2007; 31(4): 619-42. [http://dx.doi.org/10.1016/j.neubiorev.2007.01.003] [PMID: 17374395]

[84] Cancela L, Volosin M, Molina VA. Opioid involvement in the adaptive change of 5-HT1 receptors induced by chronic restraint. Eur J Pharmacol 1990; 176(3): 313-9. [http://dx.doi.org/10.1016/0014-2999(90)90025-2] [PMID: 2139414]

[85] Adey WR. Biological effects of electromagnetic fields. J Cell Biochem 1993; 51(4): 410-6. [http://dx.doi.org/10.1002/jcb.2400510405] [PMID: 8388394]

[86] Yeh SR, Yang JW, Lee YT, Tsai LY. Static magnetic field expose enhances neurotransmission in crayfish nervous system. Int J Radiat Biol 2008; 84(7): 561-7. [http://dx.doi.org/10.1080/09553000802203622] [PMID: 18661372]

[87] Edwards DH, Kravitz EA. Serotonin, social status and aggression. Curr Opin Neurobiol 1997; 7(6): 812-9. [http://dx.doi.org/10.1016/S0959-4388(97)80140-7] [PMID: 9464985]

[88] Elliott CJ, Susswein AJ. Comparative neuroethology of feeding control in molluscs. J Exp Biol 2002; 205(Pt 7): 877-96. [PMID: 11916985]

[89] Tops M, Russo S, Boksem MA, Tucker DM. Serotonin: modulator of a drive to withdraw. Brain Cogn 2009; 71(3): 427-36. [http://dx.doi.org/10.1016/j.bandc.2009.03.009] [PMID: 19423206]

[90] Lissmann HW. The mechanism of locomotion in gastropod molluscs; kinetics. J Exp Biol 1945; 21: 58-69. [PMID: 21012714]

[91] Miller-Pérez C, Sánchez-Islas E, Pellicer F, Rodríguez-Manzo G, Cruz SL, León-Olea M. Role of nociceptin/orphanin FQ and the pseudopeptide [Phe1Ψ(CH2NH)Gly2]-nociceptin(1-13)-NH2 and

their interaction with classic opioids in the modulation of thermonociception in the land snail Helix aspersa. Eur J Pharmacol 2008; 581(1-2): 77-85.
[http://dx.doi.org/10.1016/j.ejphar.2007.11.039] [PMID: 18096155]

[92] Achaval M, Penha MAP, Swarowsky A, *et al.* The terrestrial Gastropoda Megalobulimus abbreviatus as a useful model for nociceptive experiments: effects of morphine and naloxone on thermal avoidance behavior. Braz J Med Biol Res 2005; 38(1): 73-80.
[http://dx.doi.org/10.1590/S0100-879X2005000100012] [PMID: 15665992]

[93] Kavaliers M, Hirst M. Naloxone-reversible stress-induced feeding and analgesia in the slug Limax maximus. Life Sci 1986; 38(3): 203-9.
[http://dx.doi.org/10.1016/0024-3205(86)90304-8] [PMID: 3941593]

[94] Kavaliers M. Evolutionary and comparative aspects of nociception. Brain Res Bull 1988; 21(6): 923-31.
[http://dx.doi.org/10.1016/0361-9230(88)90030-5] [PMID: 2906273]

[95] Waldhoer M, Bartlett SE, Whistler JL. Opioid receptors. Annu Rev Biochem 2004; 73: 953-90.
[http://dx.doi.org/10.1146/annurev.biochem.73.011303.073940] [PMID: 15189164]

[96] Rosen AD. Inhibition of calcium channel activation in GH3 cells by static magnetic fields. Biochim Biophys Acta 1996; 1282(1): 149-55.
[http://dx.doi.org/10.1016/0005-2736(96)00053-3] [PMID: 8679652]

[97] Rosen AD. Effect of a 125 mT static magnetic field on the kinetics of voltage activated Na+ channels in GH3 cells. Bioelectromagnetics 2003; 24(7): 517-23.
[http://dx.doi.org/10.1002/bem.10124] [PMID: 12955757]

[98] Stefano GB, Salzet M. Invertebrate opioid precursors: evolutionary conservation and the significance of enzymatic processing. Int Rev Cytol 1999; 187: 261-86.
[PMID: 10212982]

[99] Elekes K, Stefano GB, Carpenter DO. Enkephalin-like immunoreactive neurons in the central nervous system of gastropods (*Helix pomatia, Lymnaea stagnalis, Aplysia californica*): a comparative immunocytochemical study. Cell Tissue Res 1993; 272: 329-41.
[http://dx.doi.org/10.1007/BF00302738]

[100] Sonetti D, Mola L, Casares F, Bianchi E, Guarna M, Stefano GB. Endogenous morphine levels increase in molluscan neural and immune tissues after physical trauma. Brain Res 1999; 835(2): 137-47.
[http://dx.doi.org/10.1016/S0006-8993(99)01534-6] [PMID: 10415368]

[101] Stefano GB, Vadász I, Hiripi L. Methionine enkephalin inhibits the bursting activity of the Br-type neuron in *Helix pomatia L.* Experientia 1980; 36(6): 666-7.
[http://dx.doi.org/10.1007/BF01970127] [PMID: 6252038]

[102] Rózsa KS, Solntseva EJ. Modulation of cholinergic transmission by opiate peptide and FMRFamide on identified neurons of *Helix pomatia L.* (Gastropoda, Mollusca). Acta Physiol Hung 1986; 67(4): 429-33.
[PMID: 3019078]

[103] Pivovarov AS. Differently directed modulation of cholinoreceptor plasticity of RPa3 and LPa3

neurons by opiate μ and κ agonists in the common snail. Zh Vyssh Nerv Deiat Im I P Pavlova 1993; 43: 826-36.
[PMID: 8212886]

[104] Burrowes WR, Assanah P, Stefano GB. Behavioral effects of opiates on the land snail *Helix aspersa.* Life Sci 1983; 33 (Suppl. 1): 381-4.
[http://dx.doi.org/10.1016/0024-3205(83)90522-2] [PMID: 6664219]

[105] Norekian TP, Sakharov DA. Mechanoreception in the pteropod mollusk *Clione limachina*: tactile inputs are blocked by opiate antagonist. Sens Syst 1991; 5: 5-11.

[106] Hernádi L, Vehovszky A, Győri J, Hiripi L. Neuronal background of activation of estivated snails, with special attention to the monoaminergic system: a biochemical, physiological, and neuroanatomical study. Cell Tissue Res 2008; 331(2): 539-53.
[http://dx.doi.org/10.1007/s00441-007-0522-3] [PMID: 17973120]

[107] Vehovszky A, Walker RJ. An analysis of the 5-hydroxytryptamine (serotonin) receptor subtypes of central neurones of *Helix aspersa.* Comp Biochem Physiol C Comp Pharmacol Toxicol 1991; 100(3): 463-76.
[http://dx.doi.org/10.1016/0742-8413(91)90025-O] [PMID: 1687543]

[108] Dyakonova VE, Elofsson R, Carlberg M, Sakharov DA. Complex avoidance behaviour and its neurochemical regulation in the land snail *Cepaea nemoralis.* Gen Pharmacol 1995; 26(4): 773-7.
[http://dx.doi.org/10.1016/0306-3623(94)00263-M] [PMID: 7635251]

[109] D'iakonova TL. Interaction of opioid peptides and monoamines in the mechanism of pulmonate mollusk respiratory behavior: analysis on isolated neurons. Dokl Akad Nauk SSSR 1998; 308: 1264-9.
[PMID: 2612353]

[110] Dyakonova V, Carlberg M, Sakharov D, Elofsson R. Anatomical basis for interactions of enkephalins with other transmitters in the CNS of a snail. J Comp Neurol 1995; 361(1): 38-47.
[http://dx.doi.org/10.1002/cne.903610104] [PMID: 8550880]

[111] Banks ML, Rice KC, Negus SS. Antinociceptive interactions between Mu-opioid receptor agonists and the serotonin uptake inhibitor clomipramine in rhesus monkeys: role of Mu agonist efficacy. J Pharmacol Exp Ther 2010; 335(2): 497-505.
[http://dx.doi.org/10.1124/jpet.110.169276] [PMID: 20675432]

[112] Gatch MB, Negus SS, Mello NK. Antinociceptive effects of monoamine reuptake inhibitors administered alone or in combination with mu opioid agonists in rhesus monkeys. Psychopharmacology 1998; 135(1): 99-106.
[http://dx.doi.org/10.1007/s002130050490] [PMID: 9489939]

[113] Kalyuzhny AE, Arvidsson U, Wu W, Wessendorf MW. mu-Opioid and δ-opioid receptors are expressed in brainstem antinociceptive circuits: studies using immunocytochemistry and retrograde tract-tracing. J Neurosci 1996; 16(20): 6490-503.
[PMID: 8815927]

[114] Swarowsky A, Monteiro AF, Xavier LL, Zancan DM, Achaval M. Serotonergic immunoreactivity in the pedal ganglia of the pulmonate snail Megalobulimus abbreviatus after thermal stimulus: A semi-quantitative analysis. Comp Biochem Physiol A Mol Integr Physiol 2005; 141(2): 230-8.
[http://dx.doi.org/10.1016/j.cbpb.2005.05.045] [PMID: 15979914]

[115] Grauer SM, Tao R, Auerbach SB. Morphine induces an increase in extracellular serotonin in the rat diencephalon. Brain Res 1992; 599(2): 277-82. [http://dx.doi.org/10.1016/0006-8993(92)90402-U] [PMID: 1283972]

[116] Hernádi L, Elekes K. Topographyic organization of serotonergic neurons in the cerebral ganglia and their peripheral projection patterns in the head areas of the snail *Helix pomatia*. J Comp Neurol 1999; 411(2): 274-87. [http://dx.doi.org/10.1002/(SICI)1096-9861(19990823)411:2<274::AID-CNE8>3.0.CO;2-9] [PMID: 10404253]

[117] Hernádi L, Elekes K. S-Rózsa K. Distribution of serotonin containing neuron sin the central nervous system of the snail *Helix pomatia*: Comparison of immunocytochemical and 5,6-dihydroxytryptamine labelling. Cell Tissue Res 1989; 257: 313-23. [http://dx.doi.org/10.1007/BF00261835]

[118] Balaban PM. Cellular mechanisms of behavioral plasticity in terrestrial snail. Neurosci Biobehav Rev 2002; 26(5): 597-630. [http://dx.doi.org/10.1016/S0149-7634(02)00022-2] [PMID: 12367592]

[119] Marinesco S, Carew TJ. Serotonin release evoked by tail nerve stimulation in the CNS of aplysia: characterization and relationship to heterosynaptic plasticity. J Neurosci 2002; 22(6): 2299-312. [PMID: 11896169]

[120] Hernádi L, Kárpáti L, Győri J, Vehovszky A, Hiripi L. Humoral serotonin and dopamine modulate the feeding in the snail, *Helix pomatia.* Acta Biol Hung 2008; 59 (Suppl. 2): 39-46. [http://dx.doi.org/10.1556/ABiol.59.2008.Suppl.6] [PMID: 18652370]

[121] Spoont MR. Modulatory role of serotonin in neural information processing: implications for human psychopathology. Psychol Bull 1992; 112(2): 330-50. [http://dx.doi.org/10.1037/0033-2909.112.2.330] [PMID: 1454898]

[122] Levenson J, Byrne JH, Eskin A. Levels of serotonin in the hemolymph of *Aplysia* are modulated by light/dark cycles and sensitization training. J Neurosci 1999; 19(18): 8094-103. [PMID: 10479709]

[123] Jokela K, Saunders RD. Physiologic and dosimetric considerations for limiting electric fields induced in the body by movement in a static magnetic field. Health Phys 2011; 100(6): 641-53. [http://dx.doi.org/10.1097/HP.0b013e318202ec7e] [PMID: 22004933]

[124] Crozier S, Trakic A, Wang H, Liu F. Numerical study of currents in workers induced by body-motion around high-ultrahigh field magnets. J Magn Reson Imaging 2007; 26(5): 1261-77. [http://dx.doi.org/10.1002/jmri.21160] [PMID: 17969138]

[125] Shellock FG, Crues JV. MR procedures: biologic effects, safety, and patient care. Radiology 2004; 232(3): 635-52. [http://dx.doi.org/10.1148/radiol.2323030830] [PMID: 15284433]

[126] Nolte CM, Pittman DW, Kalevitch B, Henderson R, Smith JC. Magnetic field conditioned taste aversion in rats. Physiol Behav 1998; 63(4): 683-8. [http://dx.doi.org/10.1016/S0031-9384(97)00526-X] [PMID: 9523915]

[127] Snyder DJ, Jahng JW, Smith JC, Houpt TA. c-Fos induction in visceral and vestibular nuclei of the rat

brain stem by a 9.4 T magnetic field. Neuroreport 2000; 11(12): 2681-5.
[http://dx.doi.org/10.1097/00001756-200008210-00015] [PMID: 10976943]

[128] Kavaliers M, Ossenkopp KP, Hirst M. Magnetic fields abolish the enhanced nocturnal analgesic response to morphine in mice. Physiol Behav 1984; 32(2): 261-4.
[http://dx.doi.org/10.1016/0031-9384(84)90139-2] [PMID: 6538981]

[129] Choleris E, Del Seppia C, Thomas AW, *et al.* Shielding, but not zeroing of the ambient magnetic field reduces stress-induced analgesia in mice. Proc Biol Sci 2002; 269(1487): 193-201.
[http://dx.doi.org/10.1098/rspb.2001.1866] [PMID: 11798436]

[130] Del Seppia C, Mezzasalma L, Choleris E, Luschi P, Ghione S. Effects of magnetic field exposure on open field behaviour and nociceptive responses in mice. Behav Brain Res 2003; 144(1-2): 1-9.
[http://dx.doi.org/10.1016/S0166-4328(03)00042-1] [PMID: 12946589]

[131] Shupak NM, Hensel JM, Cross-Mellor SK, Kavaliers M, Prato FS, Thomas AW. Analgesic and behavioral effects of a 100 microT specific pulsed extremely low frequency magnetic field on control and morphine treated CF-1 mice. Neurosci Lett 2004; 354(1): 30-3.
[http://dx.doi.org/10.1016/j.neulet.2003.09.063] [PMID: 14698475]

[132] Davis HP, Mizumori SJ, Allen H, Rosenzweig MR, Bennett EL, Tenforde TS. Behavioral studies with mice exposed to DC and 60-Hz magnetic fields. Bioelectromagnetics 1984; 5(2): 147-64.
[http://dx.doi.org/10.1002/bem.2250050204] [PMID: 6732872]

[133] Levine RL, Bluni TD. Magnetic field effects on spatial discrimination learning in mice. Physiol Behav 1994; 55(3): 465-7.
[http://dx.doi.org/10.1016/0031-9384(94)90101-5] [PMID: 8190762]

[134] Levine RL, Dooley JK, Bluni TD. Magnetic field effects on spatial discrimination and melatonin levels in mice. Physiol Behav 1995; 58(3): 535-7.
[http://dx.doi.org/10.1016/0031-9384(95)00094-Y] [PMID: 8587962]

[135] Tsuji Y, Nakagawa M, Suzuki Y. Five-tesla static magnetic fields suppress food and water consumption and weight gain in mice. Ind Health 1996; 34(4): 347-57.
[http://dx.doi.org/10.2486/indhealth.34.347] [PMID: 8908845]

[136] Lockwood DR, Kwon B, Smith JC, Houpt TA. Behavioral effects of static high magnetic fields on unrestrained and restrained mice. Physiol Behav 2003; 78(4-5): 635-40.
[http://dx.doi.org/10.1016/S0031-9384(03)00040-4] [PMID: 12782218]

[137] Choleris E, Thomas AW, Kavaliers M, Prato FS. A detailed ethological analysis of the mouse open field test: effects of diazepam, chlordiazepoxide and an extremely low frequency pulsed magnetic field. Neurosci Biobehav Rev 2001; 25(3): 235-60.
[http://dx.doi.org/10.1016/S0149-7634(01)00011-2] [PMID: 11378179]

[138] Innis NK, Ossenkopp KP, Prato FS, Sestini E. Behavioral effects of exposure to nuclear magnetic resonance imaging: II. Spatial memory tests. Magn Reson Imaging 1986; 4(4): 281-4.
[http://dx.doi.org/10.1016/0730-725X(86)91037-4] [PMID: 3669943]

[139] Ossenkopp KP, Innis NK, Prato FS, Sestini E. Behavioral effects of exposure to nuclear magnetic resonance imaging: I. Open-field behavior and passive avoidance learning in rats. Magn Reson Imaging 1986; 4(4): 275-80.

[http://dx.doi.org/10.1016/0730-725X(86)91036-2] [PMID: 3669942]

[140] Messmer JM, Porter JH, Fatouros P, Prasad U, Weisberg M. Exposure to magnetic resonance imaging does not produce taste aversion in rats. Physiol Behav 1987; 40(2): 259-61. [http://dx.doi.org/10.1016/0031-9384(87)90217-4] [PMID: 3628535]

[141] Grzesik J, Bortel M, Duda D, *et al.* Influence of a static magnetic field on the reproductive function, certain biochemical indices and behaviour of rats. Pol J Occup Med 1988; 1(4): 329-39. [PMID: 2979568]

[142] Hong CZ, Huestis P, Thompson R, Yu J. Learning ability of young rats is unaffected by repeated exposure to a static electromagnetic field in early life. Bioelectromagnetics 1988; 9(3): 269-73. [http://dx.doi.org/10.1002/bem.2250090308] [PMID: 3178901]

[143] Nakagawa M, Matsuda Y. A strong static-magnetic field alters operant responding by rats. Bioelectromagnetics 1988; 9(1): 25-37. [http://dx.doi.org/10.1002/bem.2250090103] [PMID: 3345212]

[144] Weiss J, Herrick RC, Taber KH, Contant C, Plishker GA. Bio-effects of high magnetic fields: a study using a simple animal model. Magn Reson Imaging 1992; 10(4): 689-94. [http://dx.doi.org/10.1016/0730-725X(92)90021-Q] [PMID: 1501539]

[145] Trzeciak HI, Grzesik J, Bortel M, *et al.* Behavioral effects of long-term exposure to magnetic fields in rats. Bioelectromagnetics 1993; 14(4): 287-97. [http://dx.doi.org/10.1002/bem.2250140402] [PMID: 8216385]

[146] Houpt TA, Cassell JA, Riccardi C, DenBleyker MD, Hood A, Smith JC. Rats avoid high magnetic fields: dependence on an intact vestibular system. Physiol Behav 2007; 92(4): 741-7. [http://dx.doi.org/10.1016/j.physbeh.2007.05.062] [PMID: 17585969]

[147] Houpt TA, Cassell JA, Riccardi C, Kwon B, Smith JC. Suppression of drinking by exposure to a high-strength static magnetic field. Physiol Behav 2007; 90(1): 59-65. [http://dx.doi.org/10.1016/j.physbeh.2006.08.027] [PMID: 17055009]

[148] Saunders R. Static magnetic fields: animal studies. Prog Biophys Mol Biol 2005; 87(2-3): 225-39. [http://dx.doi.org/10.1016/j.pbiomolbio.2004.09.001] [PMID: 15556661]

[149] Martin LJ, Koren SA, Persinger MA. Influence of a complex magnetic field application in rats upon thermal nociceptive thresholds: the importance of polarity and timing. Int J Neurosci 2004; 114(10): 1259-76. [http://dx.doi.org/10.1080/00207450490475689] [PMID: 15370185]

[150] Herz A. Opioid reward mechanisms: a key role in drug abuse? Can J Physiol Pharmacol 1998; 76(3): 252-8. [http://dx.doi.org/10.1139/y98-017] [PMID: 9673788]

[151] Tsuji M, Takeda H, Matsumiya T, Nagase H, Narita M, Suzuki T. The novel κ-opioid receptor agonist TRK-820 suppresses the rewarding and locomotor-enhancing effects of morphine in mice. Life Sci 2001; 68(15): 1717-25. [http://dx.doi.org/10.1016/S0024-3205(01)00957-2] [PMID: 11270618]

[152] Ito S, Mori T, Sawaguchi T. Dopamine-independent psychostimulant activity of a δ-agonist. Behav Pharmacol 2008; 19(2): 113-9.

[http://dx.doi.org/10.1097/FBP.0b013e3282f62c1b] [PMID: 18332675]

[153] Kavaliers M, Ossenkopp KP. Magnetic field inhibition of morphine-induced analgesia and behavioral activity in mice: evidence for involvement of calcium ions. Brain Res 1986; 379(1): 30-8. [http://dx.doi.org/10.1016/0006-8993(86)90252-0] [PMID: 3091191]

[154] Coggeshall RE, Lekan HA, White FA, Woolf CJ. A-fiber sensory input induces neuronal cell death in the dorsal horn of the adult rat spinal cord. J Comp Neurol 2001; 435(3): 276-82. [http://dx.doi.org/10.1002/cne.1029] [PMID: 11406811]

[155] Price DD. Psychological and neural mechanisms of the affective dimension of pain. Science 2000; 288(5472): 1769-72. [http://dx.doi.org/10.1126/science.288.5472.1769] [PMID: 10846154]

[156] Ji RR, Kohno T, Moore KA, Woolf CJ. Central sensitization and LTP: do pain and memory share similar mechanisms? Trends Neurosci 2003; 26(12): 696-705. [http://dx.doi.org/10.1016/j.tins.2003.09.017] [PMID: 14624855]

[157] Wiech K, Ploner M, Tracey I. Neurocognitive aspects of pain perception. Trends Cogn Sci 2008; 12(8): 306-13. [http://dx.doi.org/10.1016/j.tics.2008.05.005] [PMID: 18606561]

[158] Kavaliers M, Ossenkopp K. Effects of magnetic fields and electric fields in invertebrates and lower vertebrates. In: Carpenter D, Ayrapetyan S, Eds. Biological effects of electric and magnetic fields. New York, NY, USA: Academic Press 1994; pp. 205-40. [http://dx.doi.org/10.1016/B978-0-12-160261-1.50014-6]

[159] Wieraszko A. Dantrolene modulates the influence of steady magnetic fields on hippocampal evoked potentials *in vitro*. Bioelectromagnetics 2000; 21(3): 175-82. [http://dx.doi.org/10.1002/(SICI)1521-186X(200004)21:3<175::AID-BEM4>3.0.CO;2-3] [PMID: 10723017]

[160] Maggi CA. Tachykinins and calcitonin gene-related peptide (CGRP) as co-transmitters released from peripheral endings of sensory nerves. Prog Neurobiol 1995; 45(1): 1-98. [http://dx.doi.org/10.1016/0301-0082(94)E0017-B] [PMID: 7716258]

[161] Szolcsányi J. Forty years in capsaicin research for sensory pharmacology and physiology. Neuropeptides 2004; 38(6): 377-84. [http://dx.doi.org/10.1016/j.npep.2004.07.005] [PMID: 15567473]

[162] Szállási A, Cruz F, Geppetti P. TRPV1: a therapeutic target for novel analgesic drugs? Trends Mol Med 2006; 12(11): 545-54. [http://dx.doi.org/10.1016/j.molmed.2006.09.001] [PMID: 16996800]

[163] Thomas AW, Kavaliers M, Prato FS, Ossenkopp KP. Antinociceptive effects of a pulsed magnetic field in the land snail, Cepaea nemoralis. Neurosci Lett 1997; 222(2): 107-10. [http://dx.doi.org/10.1016/S0304-3940(97)13359-6] [PMID: 9111740]

[164] Shupak NM, McKay JC, Nielson WR, Rollman GB, Prato FS, Thomas AW. Exposure to a specific pulsed low-frequency magnetic field: a double-blind placebo-controlled study of effects on pain ratings in rheumatoid arthritis and fibromyalgia patients. Pain Res Manag 2006; 11(2): 85-90. [PMID: 16770449]

[165] Choleris E, Thomas AW, Ossenkopp K, Kavaliers M, Valsecchi P, Prato FS. Sex differences in conditioned taste aversion and in the effects of exposure to a specific pulsed magnetic field in deer mice Peromyscus maniculatus. Physiol Behav 2000; 71(3-4): 237-49.
[http://dx.doi.org/10.1016/S0031-9384(00)00323-1] [PMID: 11150555]

[166] Morris CE, Skalak TC. Acute exposure to a moderate strength static magnetic field reduces edema formation in rats. Am J Physiol Heart Circ Physiol 2008; 294(1): H50-7.
[http://dx.doi.org/10.1152/ajpheart.00529.2007] [PMID: 17982018]

[167] Ammari M, Jeljeli M, Maaroufi K, Roy V, Sakly M, Abdelmelek H. Static magnetic field exposure affects behavior and learning in rats. Electromagn Biol Med 2008; 27(2): 185-96.
[http://dx.doi.org/10.1080/15368370802072158] [PMID: 18568936]

[168] Łopuch S. A magnetic field effect on learning in male golden hamsters. Behav Processes 2009; 81(1): 133-5.
[http://dx.doi.org/10.1016/j.beproc.2008.12.014] [PMID: 19150395]

[169] Bao X, Shi Y, Huo X, Song T. A possible involvement of β-endorphin, substance P, and serotonin in rat analgesia induced by extremely low frequency magnetic field. Bioelectromagnetics 2006; 27(6): 467-72.
[http://dx.doi.org/10.1002/bem.20232] [PMID: 16622860]

[170] Rogachefsky RA, Altman RD, Markov MS, Cheung HS. Use of a permanent magnetic field to inhibit the development of canine osteoarthritis. Bioelectromagnetics 2004; 25(4): 260-70.
[http://dx.doi.org/10.1002/bem.10192] [PMID: 15114635]

[171] Bölcskei K, Helyes Z, Szabó A, *et al.* Investigation of the role of TRPV1 receptors in acute and chronic nociceptive processes using gene-deficient mice. Pain 2005; 117(3): 368-76.
[http://dx.doi.org/10.1016/j.pain.2005.06.024] [PMID: 16150543]

[172] Tjølsen A, Berge OG, Hunskaar S, Rosland JH, Hole K. The formalin test: an evaluation of the method. Pain 1992; 51(1): 5-17.
[http://dx.doi.org/10.1016/0304-3959(92)90003-T] [PMID: 1454405]

[173] Helyes Z, Szabó A, Németh J, *et al.* Antiinflammatory and analgesic effects of somatostatin released from capsaicin-sensitive sensory nerve terminals in a Freund's adjuvant-induced chronic arthritis model in the rat. Arthritis Rheum 2004; 50(5): 1677-85.
[http://dx.doi.org/10.1002/art.20184] [PMID: 15146439]

[174] Szállási A, Joó F, Blumberg PM. Duration of desensitization and ultrastructural changes in dorsal root ganglia in rats treated with resiniferatoxin, an ultrapotent capsaicin analog. Brain Res 1989; 503(1): 68-72.
[http://dx.doi.org/10.1016/0006-8993(89)91705-8] [PMID: 2611660]

[175] Jones BJ, Roberts DJ. The quantiative measurement of motor inco-ordination in naive mice using an acelerating rotarod. J Pharm Pharmacol 1968; 20(4): 302-4.
[http://dx.doi.org/10.1111/j.2042-7158.1968.tb09743.x] [PMID: 4384609]

[176] Sándor K, Elekes K, Szabó A, *et al.* Analgesic effects of the somatostatin sst4 receptor selective agonist J-2156 in acute and chronic pain models. Eur J Pharmacol 2006; 539(1-2): 71-5.
[http://dx.doi.org/10.1016/j.ejphar.2006.03.082] [PMID: 16697366]

[177] Poole S, Cunha FQ, Selkirk S, Lorenzetti BB, Ferreira SH. Cytokine-mediated inflammatory hyperalgesia limited by interleukin-10. Br J Pharmacol 1995; 115(4): 684-8.
[http://dx.doi.org/10.1111/j.1476-5381.1995.tb14987.x] [PMID: 7582491]

[178] Doi Y, Minami T, Nishizawa M, Mabuchi T, Mori H, Ito S. Central nociceptive role of prostacyclin (IP) receptor induced by peripheral inflammation. Neuroreport 2002; 13(1): 93-6.
[http://dx.doi.org/10.1097/00001756-200201210-00022] [PMID: 11924902]

[179] Wende VC, Margoli S. Analgesic test based upon experimentally induced acute abdominal pain in rats. Fed Proc 1956; 15: 494.

[180] Witkin LB, Heubner CF, Galdi F, O'Keefe E, Spitaletta P, Plummer AJ. Pharmacology of 2-amin--indane hydrochloride (Su-8629): a potent non-narcotic analgesic. J Pharmacol Exp Ther 1961; 133: 400-8.
[PMID: 13831371]

[181] Collier HO, Dinneen LC, Johnson CA, Schneider C. The abdominal constriction response and its suppression by analgesic drugs in the mouse. Br Pharmacol Chemother 1968; 32(2): 295-310.
[http://dx.doi.org/10.1111/j.1476-5381.1968.tb00973.x] [PMID: 4230818]

[182] Gyires K, Torma Z. The use of the writhing test in mice for screening different types of analgesics. Arch Int Pharmacodyn Ther 1984; 267(1): 131-40.
[PMID: 6721621]

[183] Lloyd E, Ed. Handbook. Statistics. Handbook of applicable mathematics. Chichester, UK: Wiley 1984.

[184] Kirson ED, Gurvich Z, Schneiderman R, *et al.* Disruption of cancer cell replication by alternating electric fields. Cancer Res 2004; 64(9): 3288-95.
[http://dx.doi.org/10.1158/0008-5472.CAN-04-0083] [PMID: 15126372]

[185] Miranda HF, Lopez J, Sierralta F, Correa A, Pinardi G. NSAID antinociception measured in a chemical and a thermal assay in mice. Pain Res Manag 2001; 6(4): 190-6.
[PMID: 11854764]

[186] Hansen G, Crooks LE, Davis P, *et al. In vivo* imaging of the rat anatomy with nuclear magnetic resonance. Radiology 1980; 136(3): 695-700.
[http://dx.doi.org/10.1148/radiology.136.3.7403549] [PMID: 7403549]

[187] Pirko I, Fricke ST, Johnson AJ, Rodriguez M, Macura SI. Magnetic resonance imaging, microscopy, and spectroscopy of the central nervous system in experimental animals. NeuroRx 2005; 2(2): 250-64.
[http://dx.doi.org/10.1602/neurorx.2.2.250] [PMID: 15897949]

[188] Lukasik VM, Gillies RJ. Animal anaesthesia for *in vivo* magnetic resonance. NMR Biomed 2003; 16(8): 459-67.
[http://dx.doi.org/10.1002/nbm.836] [PMID: 14696002]

[189] Prasad N, Bushong SC, Thornby JI, Bryan RN, Hazlewood CF, Harrell JE. Effect of nuclear magnetic resonance on chromosomes of mouse bone marrow cells. Magn Reson Imaging 1984; 2(1): 37-9.
[http://dx.doi.org/10.1016/0730-725X(84)90123-1] [PMID: 6530917]

[190] Teskey GC, Ossenkopp KP, Prato FS, Sestini E. Survivability and long-term stress reactivity levels following repeated exposure to nuclear magnetic resonance imaging procedures in rats. Physiol Chem Phys Med NMR 1987; 19(1): 43-9.

[PMID: 3039549]

[191] Shivers RR, Kavaliers M, Teskey GC, Prato FS, Pelletier RM. Magnetic resonance imaging temporarily alters blood-brain barrier permeability in the rat. Neurosci Lett 1987; 76(1): 25-31. [http://dx.doi.org/10.1016/0304-3940(87)90186-8] [PMID: 3587744]

[192] Kwong-Hing A, Sandhu HS, Prato FS, Frappier JR, Kavaliers M. Effects of magnetic resonance imaging (MRI) on the formation of mouse dentin and bone. J Exp Zool 1989; 252(1): 53-9. [http://dx.doi.org/10.1002/jez.1402520108] [PMID: 2809534]

[193] Prato FS, Frappier JR, Shivers RR, *et al.* Magnetic resonance imaging increases the blood-brain barrier permeability to 153-gadolinium diethylenetriaminepentaacetic acid in rats. Brain Res 1990; 523(2): 301-4. [http://dx.doi.org/10.1016/0006-8993(90)91502-8] [PMID: 2400915]

[194] Rofsky NM, Pizzarello DJ, Duhaney MO, Falick AK, Prendergast N, Weinreb JC. Effect of magnetic resonance exposure combined with gadopentetate dimeglumine on chromosomes in animal specimens. Acad Radiol 1995; 2(6): 492-6. [http://dx.doi.org/10.1016/S1076-6332(05)80405-2] [PMID: 9419596]

[195] High WB, Sikora J, Ugurbil K, Garwood M. Subchronic *in vivo* effects of a high static magnetic field (9.4 T) in rats. J Magn Reson Imaging 2000; 12(1): 122-39. [http://dx.doi.org/10.1002/1522-2586(200007)12:1<122::AID-JMRI14>3.0.CO;2-C] [PMID: 10931572]

[196] Ossenkopp KP, Kavaliers M, Prato FS, Teskey GC, Sestini E, Hirst M. Exposure to nuclear magnetic resonance imaging procedure attenuates morphine-induced analgesia in mice. Life Sci 1985; 37(16): 1507-14. [http://dx.doi.org/10.1016/0024-3205(85)90182-1] [PMID: 4046745]

[197] Prato FS, Ossenkopp KP, Kavaliers M, Sestini E, Teskey GC. Attenuation of morphine induced analgesia in mice by exposure to magnetic resonance imaging: separate effects of the static, radiofrequency and time-varying magnetic fields. J Magn Reson Imaging 1987; 5(1): 9-14. [http://dx.doi.org/10.1016/0730-725X(87)90478-4]

[198] Moelker A, Maas RA, Lethimonnier F, Pattynama PM. Interventional MR imaging at 1.5 T: quantification of sound exposure. Radiology 2002; 224(3): 889-95. [http://dx.doi.org/10.1148/radiol.2243010978] [PMID: 12202729]

[199] Sesay M, Tauzin-Fin P, Verdonck O, Paolantoni J, Maurette P. Acoustic noise during magnetic resonance imaging (MRI): its interference with anesthesia alarm sounds. Annual Meeting of the American Society of Anaesthesiologists 2007.

[200] Smith KC, Comite SL, Balasubramanian S, Carver A, Liu JF. Vibration anesthesia: a noninvasive method of reducing discomfort prior to dermatologic procedures. Dermatol Online J 2004; 10(2): 1. [PMID: 15530291]

[201] Charlton J, Ed. IASP. Core curriculum for professional education in pain. Seattle, WA, USA: International Association for the Study of Pain Press 2005.

[202] Kaplan M, Jackson B, Sparer R. Escape behavior under continuous reinforcement as a function of aversive light intensity. J Exp Anal Behav 1965; 8(5): 321-3.

[http://dx.doi.org/10.1901/jeab.1965.8-321] [PMID: 14342369]

[203] Pinel JP, Mumby DG, Dastur FN, Pinel JG. Rat (Rattus norvegicus) defensive behavior in total darkness: risk-assessment function of defensive burying. J Comp Psychol 1994; 108(2): 140-7. [http://dx.doi.org/10.1037/0735-7036.108.2.140] [PMID: 8026165]

[204] Stern S, Laties VG. 60 Hz electric fields and incandescent light as aversive stimuli controlling the behavior of rats responding under concurrent schedules of reinforcement. Bioelectromagnetics 1998; 19(4): 210-21. [http://dx.doi.org/10.1002/(SICI)1521-186X(1998)19:4<210::AID-BEM3>3.0.CO;2-4] [PMID: 9581964]

[205] de Jongh R, Groenink L, van Der Gugten J, Olivier B. The light-enhanced startle paradigm as a putative animal model for anxiety: effects of chlordiazepoxide, flesinoxan and fluvoxamine. Psychopharmacology 2002; 159(2): 176-80. [http://dx.doi.org/10.1007/s002130100914] [PMID: 11862346]

[206] Takao K, Miyakawa T. Light/dark transition test for mice. J Vis Exp 2006; 13(1): 104. [PMID: 18704188]

[207] Garcia AM, Cardenas FP, Morato S. Effect of different illumination levels on rat behavior in the elevated plus-maze. Physiol Behav 2005; 85(3): 265-70. [http://dx.doi.org/10.1016/j.physbeh.2005.04.007] [PMID: 15927214]

[208] Dacke M, Nilsson DE, Scholtz CH, Byrne M, Warrant EJ. Animal behaviour: insect orientation to polarized moonlight. Nature 2003; 424(6944): 33. [http://dx.doi.org/10.1038/424033a] [PMID: 12840748]

[209] Cain SW, Chou T, Ralph MR. Circadian modulation of performance on an aversion-based place learning task in hamsters. Behav Brain Res 2004; 150(1-2): 201-5. [http://dx.doi.org/10.1016/j.bbr.2003.07.001] [PMID: 15033293]

[210] Schenck JF. Safety of strong, static magnetic fields. J Magn Reson Imaging 2000; 12(1): 2-19. [http://dx.doi.org/10.1002/1522-2586(200007)12:1<2::AID-JMRI2>3.0.CO;2-V] [PMID: 10931560]

[211] Collins CM. Numerical field calculations considering the human subject for engineering and safety assurance in MRI. NMR Biomed 2009; 22(9): 919-26. [http://dx.doi.org/10.1002/nbm.1251] [PMID: 18384179]

[212] Crozier S, Liu F. Numerical evaluation of the fields induced by body motion in or near high-field MRI scanners. Prog Biophys Mol Biol 2005; 87(2-3): 267-78. [http://dx.doi.org/10.1016/j.pbiomolbio.2004.08.002] [PMID: 15556665]

[213] Dawson TW, Caputa K, Stuchly MA, Kavet R. Comparison of electric fields induced in humans and rodents by 60-Hz contact currents. IEEE Trans Biomed Eng 2003; 50(6): 744-53. [http://dx.doi.org/10.1109/TBME.2003.812165] [PMID: 12814241]

[214] IPCS. International Programme on Chemical Safety: Magnetic fields: Health and safety guide. 1987. Available at http://www.inchem.org/documents/hsg/hsg/hsg027.htm.

[215] International Commission on Non-Ionizing Radiation Protection. Guidelines on limits of exposure to static magnetic fields. Health Phys 1994; 66(1): 100-6. Available at http://www.icnirp.de/documents/static.pdf.

[PMID: 8253572]

[216] Kangarlu A, Robitaille PM. Biological effects and health implications in magnetic resonance imaging. Concepts Magn Reson 2000; 12: 321-59.
[http://dx.doi.org/10.1002/1099-0534(2000)12:5<321::AID-CMR4>3.0.CO;2-J]

[217] Zhao H, Crozier S, Liu F. Finite difference time domain (FDTD) method for modeling the effect of switched gradients on the human body in MRI. Magn Reson Med 2002; 48(6): 1037-42.
[http://dx.doi.org/10.1002/mrm.10313] [PMID: 12465114]

[218] Tenforde TS. Magnetically induced electric fields and currents in the circulatory system. Prog Biophys Mol Biol 2005; 87(2-3): 279-88.
[http://dx.doi.org/10.1016/j.pbiomolbio.2004.08.003] [PMID: 15556666]

[219] Vecchia P. Exposure of humans to electromagnetic fields. Standards and regulations. Ann Ist Super Sanita 2007; 43(3): 260-7.
[PMID: 17938457]

[220] Wood AW. Extremely low frequency (ELF) electric and magnetic field exposure limits: rationale for basic restrictions used in the development of an Australian standard. Bioelectromagnetics 2008; 29(6): 414-28.
[http://dx.doi.org/10.1002/bem.20412] [PMID: 18381600]

[221] Formica D, Silvestri S. Biological effects of exposure to magnetic resonance imaging: an overview. Biomed Eng Online 2004; 3(1): 12.
[http://dx.doi.org/10.1186/1475-925X-3-11] [PMID: 15104797]

[222] Bencsik M, Bowtell R, Bowley R. Electric fields induced in the human body by time-varying magnetic field gradients in MRI: numerical calculations and correlation analysis. Phys Med Biol 2007; 52(9): 2337-53.
[http://dx.doi.org/10.1088/0031-9155/52/9/001] [PMID: 17440238]

[223] Gandhi OP, Chen XB. Specific absorption rates and induced current densities for an anatomy-based model of the human for exposure to time-varying magnetic fields of MRI. Magn Reson Med 1999; 41 (4): 816-23.
[http://dx.doi.org/10.1002/(SICI)1522-2594(199904)41:4<816::AID-MRM22>3.0.CO;2-5] [PMID: 10332859]

[224] Center for fMRI. Safety guidelines for conducting magnetic resonance imaging (MRI) experiments involving human subjects 2007. Available at http://fmriserver.ucsd.edu/pdf/center_safety_ policies.pdf.

[225] Kangarlu A, Burgess RE, Zhu H, *et al.* Cognitive, cardiac, and physiological safety studies in ultra high field magnetic resonance imaging. Magnetic Resonance Imaging 17 1999; 10: 1407-16.
[http://dx.doi.org/10.1016/S0730-725X(99)00086-7]

[226] van Rongen E, Saunders RD, van DET, Repacholi MH. Static fields: biological effects and mechanisms relevant to exposure limits. Health Phys 2007; 92(6): 584-90.
[http://dx.doi.org/10.1097/01.HP.0000232776.94463.c4] [PMID: 17495659]

[227] Prato FS, Desjardins-Holmes D, Keenliside LD, McKay JC, Robertson JA, Thomas AW. Light alters nociceptive effects of magnetic field shielding in mice: intensity and wavelength considerations. J R Soc Interface 2009; 6(30): 17-28.

[http://dx.doi.org/10.1098/rsif.2008.0156] [PMID: 18583276]

[228] Chappell MA, Garland T Jr, Rezende EL Jr, Gomes FR. Voluntary running in deer mice: speed, distance, energy costs and temperature effects. J Exp Biol 2004; 207(Pt 22): 3839-54. [http://dx.doi.org/10.1242/jeb.01213] [PMID: 15472015]

[229] Marton D, László J, Giber J, Rüdenauer FG. EFSA - A new evaluation method of the depth resolution in depth profiling of multilayer structures. Vacuum 1985; 35(12): 523-6. [http://dx.doi.org/10.1016/0042-207X(85)90308-2]

[230] Cason AM, Kwon B, Smith JC, Houpt TA. Labyrinthectomy abolishes the behavioral and neural response of rats to a high-strength static magnetic field. Physiol Behav 2009; 97(1): 36-43. [http://dx.doi.org/10.1016/j.physbeh.2009.01.018] [PMID: 19419674]

[231] Atkinson IC, Renteria L, Burd H, Pliskin NH, Thulborn KR. Safety of human MRI at static fields above the FDA 8 T guideline: sodium imaging at 9.4 T does not affect vital signs or cognitive ability. J Magn Reson Imaging 2007; 26(5): 1222-7. [http://dx.doi.org/10.1002/jmri.21150] [PMID: 17969172]

[232] Okano H, Ohkubo C. Elevated plasma nitric oxide metabolites in hypertension: synergistic vasodepressor effects of a static magnetic field and nicardipine in spontaneously hypertensive rats. Clin Hemorheol Microcirc 2006; 34(1-2): 303-8. [PMID: 16543650]

[233] Hinman MR. Comparative effect of positive and negative static magnetic fields on heart rate and blood pressure in healthy adults. Clin Rehabil 2002; 16(6): 669-74. [http://dx.doi.org/10.1191/0269215502cr538oa] [PMID: 12392343]

[234] Strekalova T, Spanagel R, Bartsch D, Henn FA, Gass P. Stress-induced anhedonia in mice is associated with deficits in forced swimming and exploration. Neuropsychopharmacology 2004; 29(11): 2007-17. [http://dx.doi.org/10.1038/sj.npp.1300532] [PMID: 15266352]

[235] Van Loo PL, Mol JA, Koolhaas JM, Van Zutphen BF, Baumans V. Modulation of aggression in male mice: influence of group size and cage size. Physiol Behav 2001; 72(5): 675-83. [http://dx.doi.org/10.1016/S0031-9384(01)00425-5] [PMID: 11336999]

[236] Tysdale DM, Lipa SM, Ossenkopp KP, Kavaliers M. Inhibitory effects of 60-Hz magnetic fields on opiate-induced "analgesia" in the land snail, *Cepaea nemoralis*, under natural conditions. Physiol Behav 1991; 49(1): 53-6. [http://dx.doi.org/10.1016/0031-9384(91)90229-H] [PMID: 1850141]

[237] Falone S, Mirabilio A, Carbone MC, *et al.* Chronic exposure to 50Hz magnetic fields causes a significant weakening of antioxidant defence systems in aged rat brain. Int J Biochem Cell Biol 2008; 40(12): 2762-70. [http://dx.doi.org/10.1016/j.biocel.2008.05.022] [PMID: 18585472]

[238] Cason AM, Denbleyker M, Ferrence K, Smith JC, Houpt TA. Sex and estrous cycle differences in the behavioral effects of high-strength static magnetic fields: Role of ovarian steroids. Am J Physiol Regul Integr Comp Physiol 2006; 290(3): R659-667. [PMID: 16223851]

[239] Houpt TA, Cassell JA, Hood A, *et al.* Repeated exposure attenuates the behavioral response of rats to static high magnetic fields. Physiol Behav 2010; 99(4): 500-8. [http://dx.doi.org/10.1016/j.physbeh.2009.12.024] [PMID: 20045422]

[240] Liu T, Wang S, He L, Ye K. Anxiogenic effect of chronic exposure to extremely low frequency magnetic field in adult rats. Neurosci Lett 2008; 434(1): 12-7. [http://dx.doi.org/10.1016/j.neulet.2008.01.019] [PMID: 18258364]

[241] Malmivuo J, Plonsey R. Bioelectromagnetism. New York, NY, USA: Oxford University Press 1995.

[242] Del Seppia C, Luschi P, Ghione S, Crosio E, Choleris E, Papi F. Exposure to a hypogeomagnetic field or to oscillating magnetic fields similarly reduce stress-induced analgesia in C57 male mice. Life Sci 2000; 66(14): 1299-306. [http://dx.doi.org/10.1016/S0024-3205(00)00437-9] [PMID: 10755465]

[243] Betancur C, Dell'Omo G, Alleva E. Magnetic field effects on stress-induced analgesia in mice: modulation by light. Neurosci Lett 1994; 182(2): 147-50. [http://dx.doi.org/10.1016/0304-3940(94)90784-6] [PMID: 7715799]

[244] Prato FS, Kavaliers M, Cullen AP, Thomas AW. Light-dependent and -independent behavioral effects of extremely low frequency magnetic fields in a land snail are consistent with a parametric resonance mechanism. Bioelectromagnetics 1997; 18(3): 284-91. [http://dx.doi.org/10.1002/(SICI)1521-186X(1997)18:3<284::AID-BEM13>3.0.CO;2-P] [PMID: 9096848]

[245] Martin WR, Eades CG, Thompson JA, Huppler RE, Gilbert PE. The effects of morphine- and nalorphine- like drugs in the nondependent and morphine-dependent chronic spinal dog. J Pharmacol Exp Ther 1976; 197(3): 517-32. [PMID: 945347]

[246] Zadina JE, Hackler L, Ge LJ, Kastin AJ. A potent and selective endogenous agonist for the μ-opiate receptor. Nature 1997; 386(6624): 499-502. [http://dx.doi.org/10.1038/386499a0] [PMID: 9087409]

[247] Martin-Schild S, Zadina JE, Gerall AA, Vigh S, Kastin AJ. Localization of endomorphin-2-like immunoreactivity in the rat medulla and spinal cord. Peptides 1997; 18(10): 1641-9. [http://dx.doi.org/10.1016/S0196-9781(97)00320-3] [PMID: 9437728]

[248] Pierce TL, Grahek MD, Wessendorf MW. Immunoreactivity for endomorphin-2 occurs in primary afferents in rats and monkey. Neuroreport 1998; 9(3): 385-9. [http://dx.doi.org/10.1097/00001756-199802160-00005] [PMID: 9512376]

[249] Barr GA, Zadina JE. Maturation of endomorphin-2 in the dorsal horn of the medulla and spinal cord of the rat. Neuroreport 1999; 10(18): 3857-60. [http://dx.doi.org/10.1097/00001756-199912160-00025] [PMID: 10716223]

[250] Gutstein HB, Bronstein DM, Akil H. β-endorphin processing and cellular origins in rat spinal cord. Pain 1992; 51(2): 241-7. [http://dx.doi.org/10.1016/0304-3959(92)90265-D] [PMID: 1336592]

[251] Cabot PJ, Carter L, Gaiddon C, *et al.* Immune cell-derived β-endorphin. Production, release, and control of inflammatory pain in rats. J Clin Invest 1997; 100(1): 142-8.

[http://dx.doi.org/10.1172/JCI119506] [PMID: 9202066]

[252] Mousa SA, Machelska H, Schäfer M, Stein C. Immunohistochemical localization of endomorphin-1 and endomorphin-2 in immune cells and spinal cord in a model of inflammatory pain. J Neuroimmunol 2002; 126(1-2): 5-15.
[http://dx.doi.org/10.1016/S0165-5728(02)00049-8] [PMID: 12020952]

[253] Rittner HL, Brack A, Machelska H, *et al.* Opioid peptide-expressing leukocytes: identification, recruitment, and simultaneously increasing inhibition of inflammatory pain. Anesthesiology 2001; 95 (2): 500-8.
[http://dx.doi.org/10.1097/00000542-200108000-00036] [PMID: 11506126]

[254] Smith EM. Opioid peptides in immune cells. Adv Exp Med Biol 2003; 521: 51-68.
[PMID: 12617564]

[255] Brack A, Rittner HL, Machelska H, Beschmann K, Sitte N, Schafer M. Mobilization of opioid-containing polymorphonuclear cells by hematopoetic growth factors and influence on inflammatory pain. Anesthesiology 2004; 101: 204-11.
[http://dx.doi.org/10.1097/00000542-200407000-00031] [PMID: 15220792]

[256] Wu J, Su G, Ma L, *et al.* The role of c-AMP-dependent protein kinase in spinal cord and post synaptic dorsal column neurons in a rat model of visceral pain. Neurochem Int 2007; 50(5): 710-8.
[http://dx.doi.org/10.1016/j.neuint.2007.01.006] [PMID: 17320244]

[257] Thán M, Kocsis P, Tihanyi K, *et al.* Concerted action of antiepileptic and antidepressant agents to depress spinal neurotransmission: Possible use in the therapy of spasticity and chronic pain. Neurochem Int 2007; 50(4): 642-52.
[http://dx.doi.org/10.1016/j.neuint.2006.12.008] [PMID: 17280740]

[258] Lecca D, Abbracchio MP. Deorphanisation of G protein-coupled receptors: A tool to provide new insights in nervous system pathophysiology and new targets for psycho-active drugs. Neurochem Int 2008; 52(3): 339-51.
[http://dx.doi.org/10.1016/j.neuint.2007.08.002] [PMID: 17884255]

[259] Sindrup SH, Jensen TS. Efficacy of pharmacological treatments of neuropathic pain: an update and effect related to mechanism of drug action. Pain 1999; 83(3): 389-400.
[http://dx.doi.org/10.1016/S0304-3959(99)00154-2] [PMID: 10568846]

[260] Raji AR, Bowden RE. Effects of high-peak pulsed electromagnetic field on the degeneration and regeneration of the common peroneal nerve in rats. J Bone Joint Surg Br 1983; 65(4): 478-92.
[PMID: 6603461]

[261] Vallbona C, Hazlewood CF, Jurida G. Response of pain to static magnetic fields in postpolio patients: a double-blind pilot study. Arch Phys Med Rehabil 1997; 78(11): 1200-3.
[http://dx.doi.org/10.1016/S0003-9993(97)90332-4] [PMID: 9365349]

[262] Man D, Man B, Plosker H. The influence of permanent magnetic field therapy on wound healing in suction lipectomy patients: a double-blind study. Plast Reconstr Surg 1999; 104(7): 2261-6.
[http://dx.doi.org/10.1097/00006534-199912000-00051] [PMID: 11149796]

[263] Holcomb RR, Worthington WB, McCullough BA, McLean MJ. Static magnetic field therapy for pain in the abdomen and genitals. Pediatr Neurol 2000; 23(3): 261-4.

[http://dx.doi.org/10.1016/S0887-8994(00)00180-6] [PMID: 11033291]

[264] Alfano AP, Taylor AG, Foresman PA, *et al.* Static magnetic fields for treatment of fibromyalgia: a randomized controlled trial. J Altern Complement Med 2001; 7(1): 53-64. [http://dx.doi.org/10.1089/107555301300004538] [PMID: 11246937]

[265] Segal NA, Toda Y, Huston J, *et al.* Two configurations of static magnetic fields for treating rheumatoid arthritis of the knee: a double-blind clinical trial. Arch Phys Med Rehabil 2001; 82(10): 1453-60. [http://dx.doi.org/10.1053/apmr.2001.24309] [PMID: 11588753]

[266] Brown CS, Ling FW, Wan JY, Pilla AA. Efficacy of static magnetic field therapy in chronic pelvic pain: a double-blind pilot study. Am J Obstet Gynecol 2002; 187(6): 1581-7. [http://dx.doi.org/10.1067/mob.2002.128026] [PMID: 12501067]

[267] Weintraub MI, Wolfe GI, Barohn RA, *et al.* Magnetic Research Group. Static magnetic field therapy for symptomatic diabetic neuropathy: a randomized, double-blind, placebo-controlled trial. Arch Phys Med Rehabil 2003; 84(5): 736-46. [http://dx.doi.org/10.1016/S0003-9993(03)00106-0] [PMID: 12736891]

[268] Wolsko PM, Eisenberg DM, Simon LS, *et al.* Double-blind placebo-controlled trial of static magnets for the treatment of osteoarthritis of the knee: results of a pilot study. Altern Ther Health Med 2004; 10(2): 36-43. [PMID: 15055092]

[269] Collacott EA, Zimmerman JT, White DW, Rindone JP. Bipolar permanent magnets for the treatment of chronic low back pain: a pilot study. JAMA 2000; 283(10): 1322-5. [http://dx.doi.org/10.1001/jama.283.10.1322] [PMID: 10714732]

[270] Carter R, Aspy CB, Mold J. The effectiveness of magnet therapy for treatment of wrist pain attributed to carpal tunnel syndrome. J Fam Pract 2002; 51(1): 38-40. [PMID: 11927062]

[271] Chaloupka EC, Kang J, Mastrangelo MA. The effect of flexible magnets on hand muscle strength: a randomized, double-blind study. J Strength Cond Res 2002; 16(1): 33-7. [PMID: 11834104]

[272] Reeser JC, Smith DT, Fischer V, *et al.* Static magnetic fields neither prevent nor diminish symptoms and signs of delayed onset muscle soreness. Arch Phys Med Rehabil 2005; 86(3): 565-70. [http://dx.doi.org/10.1016/j.apmr.2004.04.025] [PMID: 15759245]

[273] Cepeda MS, Carr DB, Sarquis T, Miranda N, Garcia RJ, Zarate C. Static magnetic therapy does not decrease pain or opioid requirements: a randomized double-blind trial. Anesth Analg 2007; 104(2): 290-4. [http://dx.doi.org/10.1213/01.ane.0000230613.25754.08] [PMID: 17242082]

[274] Wróbel MP, Szymborska-Kajanek A, Wystrychowski G, *et al.* Impact of low frequency pulsed magnetic fields on pain intensity, quality of life and sleep disturbances in patients with painful diabetic polyneuropathy. Diabetes Metab 2008; 34(4 Pt 1): 349-54. [http://dx.doi.org/10.1016/j.diabet.2008.02.003] [PMID: 18585071]

[275] Kavaliers M, Ossenkopp KP. Magnetic fields differentially inhibit mu, δ, κ and σ opiate-induced

analgesia in mice. Peptides 1986; 7(3): 449-53.
[http://dx.doi.org/10.1016/0196-9781(86)90013-6] [PMID: 3022253]

[276] Kavaliers M, Ossenkopp KP. Stress-induced opioid analgesia and activity in mice: inhibitory influences of exposure to magnetic fields. Psychopharmacology (Berl) 1986; 89(4): 440-3.
[http://dx.doi.org/10.1007/BF02412118] [PMID: 3092274]

[277] Seltzer Z, Dubner R, Shir Y. A novel behavioral model of neuropathic pain disorders produced in rats by partial sciatic nerve injury. Pain 1990; 43(2): 205-18.
[http://dx.doi.org/10.1016/0304-3959(90)91074-S] [PMID: 1982347]

[278] Bassett CA. Beneficial effects of electromagnetic fields. J Cell Biochem 1993; 51(4): 387-93.
[http://dx.doi.org/10.1002/jcb.2400510402] [PMID: 8496242]

[279] Yang J, Sadler TR, Givrad TK, Maarek JM, Holschneider DP. Changes in brain functional activation during resting and locomotor states after unilateral nigrostriatal damage in rats. Neuroimage 2007; 36 (3): 755-73.
[http://dx.doi.org/10.1016/j.neuroimage.2007.03.010] [PMID: 17481921]

[280] Willis WD Jr. Is central sensitization of nociceptive transmission in the spinal cord a variety of long-term potentiation? Neuroreport 1997; 8(16): 3427-30.
[PMID: 9480005]

[281] Woolf CJ, Salter MW. Neuronal plasticity: increasing the gain in pain. Science 2000; 288(5472): 1765-9.
[http://dx.doi.org/10.1126/science.288.5472.1765] [PMID: 10846153]

[282] Campbell J, Basbaum A, Dray A, Dubner A, Dworkin R, Sang C, Eds. IASP. Emerging strategies for the treatment of neuropathic pain. Seattle, WA, USA: International Association for the Study of Pain Press 2006.

[283] Bus SA, Maas M, Lindeboom R. Reproducibility of foot structure measurements in neuropathic diabetic patients using magnetic resonance imaging. J Magn Reson Imaging 2006; 24(1): 25-32.
[http://dx.doi.org/10.1002/jmri.20601] [PMID: 16736473]

[284] Larroque G, Kamba C, Blin D, Lopez FM, Cyteval C. Imagerie ostéo-articulaire du pied diabétique. J Radiol 2006; 87(5): 541-7.
[http://dx.doi.org/10.1016/S0221-0363(06)74035-5] [PMID: 16733410]

[285] Weintraub MI, Cole SP. Pulsed magnetic field therapy in refractory neuropathic pain secondary to peripheral neuropathy: electrodiagnostic parameters--pilot study. Neurorehabil Neural Repair 2004; 18(1): 42-6.
[http://dx.doi.org/10.1177/0888439003261024] [PMID: 15035963]

[286] Oztaş B, Kalkan T, Tuncel H. Influence of 50 Hz frequency sinusoidal magnetic field on the blood-brain barrier permeability of diabetic rats. Bioelectromagnetics 2004; 25(5): 400-2.
[http://dx.doi.org/10.1002/bem.20030] [PMID: 15197766]

[287] Chebotar'ova LL, Chebotar'ov HIe. [Use of low-power electromagnetic therapy in diabetic polyneuropathy]. Fiziol Zh 2003; 49(2): 85-90.
[PMID: 12945120]

[288] Chen Y. Magnets on ears helped diabetics. Am J Chin Med 2002; 30(1): 183-5.

[http://dx.doi.org/10.1142/S0192415X02000193] [PMID: 12067093]

[289] Szor JK, Holewinski P. Double blind placebo-controlled study of ulcer care - Static magnets in chronic leg ulcer healing. Ostomy/Wound Manage 2002; 48(2): 24-9.
[PMID: 15382410]

[290] Khan GM, Chen SR, Pan HL. Role of primary afferent nerves in allodynia caused by diabetic neuropathy in rats. Neuroscience 2002; 114(2): 291-9.
[http://dx.doi.org/10.1016/S0306-4522(02)00372-X] [PMID: 12204199]

[291] Hunskaar S, Berge OG, Hole K. A modified hot-plate test sensitive to mild analgesics. Behav Brain Res 1986; 21(2): 101-8.
[http://dx.doi.org/10.1016/0166-4328(86)90088-4] [PMID: 3755945]

[292] Tjølsen A, Rosland JH, Berge OG, Hole K. The increasing-temperature hot-plate test: an improved test of nociception in mice and rats. J Pharmacol Methods 1991; 25(3): 241-50.
[http://dx.doi.org/10.1016/0160-5402(91)90014-V] [PMID: 2056753]

[293] Chen SR, Khan GM, Pan HL. Antiallodynic effect of intrathecal neostigmine is mediated by spinal nitric oxide in a rat model of diabetic neuropathic pain. Anesthesiology 2001; 95(4): 1007-12.
[http://dx.doi.org/10.1097/00000542-200110000-00033] [PMID: 11605898]

[294] Konermann G, Mönig H. [Effect of static magnetic fields on the prenatal development of the mouse]. Radiologe 1986; 26(10): 490-7.
[PMID: 3786703]

[295] Yan QC, Tomita N, Ikada Y. Effects of static magnetic field on bone formation of rat femurs. Med Eng Phys 1998; 20(6): 397-402.
[http://dx.doi.org/10.1016/S1350-4533(98)00051-4] [PMID: 9796945]

[296] Tablado L, Soler C, Núñez M, Núñez J, Pérez-Sánchez F. Development of mouse testis and epididymis following intrauterine exposure to a static magnetic field. Bioelectromagnetics 2000; 21(1): 19-24.
[http://dx.doi.org/10.1002/(SICI)1521-186X(200001)21:1<19::AID-BEM4>3.0.CO;2-1] [PMID: 10615088]

[297] Hashish AH, El-Missiry MA, Abdelkader HI, Abou-Saleh RH. Assessment of biological changes of continuous whole body exposure to static magnetic field and extremely low frequency electromagnetic fields in mice. Ecotoxicol Environ Saf 2008; 71(3): 895-902.
[http://dx.doi.org/10.1016/j.ecoenv.2007.10.002] [PMID: 17996303]

[298] Rossi S, D'Amico M, Capuano A, Romano M, Petronella P, Di Filippo C. Hyperglycemia in streptozotocin-induced diabetes leads to persistent inflammation and tissue damage following uveitis due to reduced levels of ciliary body heme oxygenase-1. Mediators Inflamm 2006; 2006(4): 60285.
[PMID: 17047293]

[299] Lu L, Zhang Q, Pu LJ, *et al.* Elevation of tumor necrosis factor-α, interleukin-1β and interleukin-6 levels in aortic intima of Chinese Guizhou minipigs with streptozotocin-induced diabetes. Chin Med J (Engl) 2007; 120(6): 479-84.
[PMID: 17439741]

[300] Harb G, Toreson J, Dufour J, Korbutt G. Acute exposure to streptozotocin but not human

proinflammatory cytokines impairs neonatal porcine islet insulin secretion *in vitro* but not *in vivo*. Xenotransplantation 2007; 14(6): 580-90.
[http://dx.doi.org/10.1111/j.1399-3089.2007.00427.x] [PMID: 17991146]

[301] Bi Y, Sun WP, Chen X, *et al.* Effect of early insulin therapy on nuclear factor kappaB and cytokine gene expressions in the liver and skeletal muscle of high-fat diet, streptozotocin-treated diabetic rats. Acta Diabetol 2008; 45(3): 167-78.
[http://dx.doi.org/10.1007/s00592-008-0038-7] [PMID: 18500427]

[302] Ehses JA, Lacraz G, Giroix MH, *et al.* IL-1 antagonism reduces hyperglycemia and tissue inflammation in the type 2 diabetic GK rat. Proc Natl Acad Sci USA 2009; 106(33): 13998-4003.
[http://dx.doi.org/10.1073/pnas.0810087106] [PMID: 19666548]

[303] Chater S, Abdelmelek H, Pequignot JM, Sakly M, Rhouma KB. Effects of sub-acute exposure to static magnetic field on hematologic and biochemical parameters in pregnant rats. Electromagn Biol Med 2006; 25(3): 135-44.
[http://dx.doi.org/10.1080/15368370600860135] [PMID: 16954116]

[304] Lin SL, Chang WJ, Lin YS, *et al.* Static magnetic field attenuates mortality rate of mice by increasing the production of IL-1 receptor antagonist. Int J Radiat Biol 2009; 85(7): 633-40.
[http://dx.doi.org/10.1080/09553000902993908] [PMID: 19557603]

[305] Johnson MS, Ryals JM, Wright DE. Diabetes-induced chemogenic hypoalgesia is paralleled by attenuated stimulus-induced fos expression in the spinal cord of diabetic mice. J Pain 2007; 8(8): 637-49.
[http://dx.doi.org/10.1016/j.jpain.2007.04.004] [PMID: 17532267]

[306] Kamei J, Ohsawa M, Miyata S, Endo K, Hayakawa H. Effects of cytidine 5′-diphosphocholine (CDP-choline) on the thermal nociceptive threshold in streptozotocin-induced diabetic mice. Eur J Pharmacol 2008; 598(1-3): 32-6.
[http://dx.doi.org/10.1016/j.ejphar.2008.09.012] [PMID: 18834878]

[307] Xu S, Okano H, Ohkubo C. Acute effects of whole-body exposure to static magnetic fields and 50-Hz electromagnetic fields on muscle microcirculation in anesthetized mice. Bioelectrochemistry 2001; 53 (1): 127-35.
[http://dx.doi.org/10.1016/S0302-4598(00)00120-3] [PMID: 11206920]

[308] Ichioka S, Minegishi M, Iwasaka M, *et al.* Skin temperature changes induced by strong static magnetic field exposure. Bioelectromagnetics 2003; 24(6): 380-6.
[http://dx.doi.org/10.1002/bem.10115] [PMID: 12929156]

[309] Okano H, Ohkubo C. Anti-pressor effects of whole body exposure to static magnetic field on pharmacologically induced hypertension in conscious rabbits. Bioelectromagnetics 2003; 24(2): 139-47.
[http://dx.doi.org/10.1002/bem.10092] [PMID: 12524681]

[310] McLean MJ, Engström S, Holcomb RR, Sanchez D. A static magnetic field modulates severity of audiogenic seizures and anticonvulsant effects of phenytoin in DBA/2 mice. Epilepsy Res 2003; 55(1-2): 105-16.
[http://dx.doi.org/10.1016/S0920-1211(03)00109-8] [PMID: 12948620]

[311] Veliks V, Ceihnere E, Svikis I, Aivars J. Static magnetic field influence on rat brain function detected

by heart rate monitoring. Bioelectromagnetics 2004; 25(3): 211-5.
[http://dx.doi.org/10.1002/bem.10186] [PMID: 15042630]

[312] Taniguchi N, Kanai S, Kawamoto M, Endo H, Higashino H. Study on application of static magnetic field for adjuvant arthritis rats. Evid Based Complement Alternat Med 2004; 1(2): 187-91.
[http://dx.doi.org/10.1093/ecam/neh024] [PMID: 15480444]

[313] Onodera H, Jin Z, Chida S, Suzuki Y, Tago H, Itoyama Y. Effects of 10-T static magnetic field on human peripheral blood immune cells. Radiat Res 2003; 159(6): 775-9.
[http://dx.doi.org/10.1667/0033-7587(2003)159[0775:EOTSMF]2.0.CO;2] [PMID: 12751960]

[314] Yang H, Wright JR Jr. Human beta cells are exceedingly resistant to streptozotocin *in vivo*. Endocrinology 2002; 143(7): 2491-5.
[PMID: 12072379]

[315] Okamoto H. Recent advances in physiological and pathological significance of tryptophan-NAD+ metabolites: lessons from insulin-producing pancreatic beta-cells. Adv Exp Med Biol 2003; 527: 243-52.
[PMID: 15206738]

[316] Girard S, Kadhim H, Roy M, *et al.* Role of perinatal inflammation in cerebral palsy. Pediatr Neurol 2009; 40(3): 168-74.
[http://dx.doi.org/10.1016/j.pediatrneurol.2008.09.016] [PMID: 19218029]

[317] Romero R, Espinoza J, Kusanovic JP, *et al.* The preterm parturition syndrome. Int J Obstet Gynecol 2006; 113 (Suppl. 3): 17-42.
[http://dx.doi.org/10.1111/j.1471-0528.2006.01120.x]

[318] Holst D, Garnier Y. Preterm birth and inflammation-The role of genetic polymorphisms. Eur J Obstet Gynecol Reprod Biol 2008; 141(1): 3-9.
[http://dx.doi.org/10.1016/j.ejogrb.2008.07.020] [PMID: 18783866]

[319] Goldenberg RL, Culhane JF. Prepregnancy health status and the risk of preterm delivery. Arch Pediatr Adolesc Med 2005; 159(1): 89-90.
[http://dx.doi.org/10.1001/archpedi.159.1.89] [PMID: 15630064]

[320] Lindström TM, Bennett PR. 15-Deoxy-delta12,14-prostaglandin j2 inhibits interleukin-1beta-induced nuclear factor-κb in human amnion and myometrial cells: mechanisms and implications. J Clin Endocrinol Metab 2005; 90(6): 3534-43.
[http://dx.doi.org/10.1210/jc.2005-0055] [PMID: 15755849]

[321] Christiaens I, Zaragoza DB, Guilbert L, Robertson SA, Mitchell BF, Olson DM. Inflammatory processes in preterm and term parturition. J Reprod Immunol 2008; 79(1): 50-7.
[http://dx.doi.org/10.1016/j.jri.2008.04.002] [PMID: 18550178]

[322] Whitelaw DA, Hall D, Kotze T. Pregnancy in systemic lupus erythematosus: a retrospective study from a developing community. Clin Rheumatol 2008; 27(5): 577-80.
[http://dx.doi.org/10.1007/s10067-007-0749-0] [PMID: 17909740]

[323] Parry S, Strauss JF III. Premature rupture of the fetal membranes. N Engl J Med 1998; 338(10): 663-70.
[http://dx.doi.org/10.1056/NEJM199803053381006] [PMID: 9486996]

[324] Medzhitov R, Preston-Hurlburt P, Janeway CA Jr. A human homologue of the Drosophila Toll protein signals activation of adaptive immunity. Nature 1997; 388(6640): 394-7.
[http://dx.doi.org/10.1038/41131] [PMID: 9237759]

[325] Thaxton JE, Nevers TA, Sharma S. TLR-mediated preterm birth in response to pathogenic agents. Infect Dis Obstet Gynecol 2010; 2010: 378472.

[326] Locksmith G, Duff P. Infection, antibiotics, and preterm delivery. Semin Perinatol 2001; 25(5): 295-309.
[http://dx.doi.org/10.1053/sper.2001.27163] [PMID: 11707017]

[327] Boehm K, Raak C, Vollmar HC, Ostermann T. An overview of 45 published database resources for complementary and alternative medicine. Health Info Libr J 2010; 27(2): 93-105.
[http://dx.doi.org/10.1111/j.1471-1842.2010.00888.x] [PMID: 20565550]

[328] Vallbona C, Richards T. Evolution of magnetic therapy from alternative to traditional medicine. Phys Med Rehabil Clin N Am 1999; 10(3): 729-54.
[PMID: 10516987]

[329] Barth MM, Smith MP, Pedrosa I, Lenkinski RE, Rofsky NM. Body MR imaging at 3.0 T: understanding the opportunities and challenges. Radiographics 2007; 27(5): 1445-62.
[http://dx.doi.org/10.1148/rg.275065204] [PMID: 17848702]

[330] Colletti P. Magnetic resonance procedures and pregnancy. In: Shellock F, Ed. Magnetic Resonance Procedures: Health effects and safety. Boca Raton, FL, USA: CRC Press 2001; pp. 149-82.

[331] Salminen A, Paananen R, Vuolteenaho R, *et al.* Maternal endotoxin-induced preterm birth in mice: fetal responses in toll-like receptors, collectins, and cytokines. Pediatr Res 2008; 63(3): 280-6.
[http://dx.doi.org/10.1203/PDR.0b013e318163a8b2] [PMID: 18287966]

[332] Giamberardino MA. Women and visceral pain: are the reproductive organs the main protagonists? Mini-review at the occasion of the "European Week Against Pain in Women 2007". Eur J Pain 2008; 12(3): 257-60.
[http://dx.doi.org/10.1016/j.ejpain.2007.11.007] [PMID: 18249016]

[333] Dinarello CA. Interleukin-1, interleukin-1 receptors and interleukin-1 receptor antagonist. Int Rev Immunol 1998; 16(5-6): 457-99.
[http://dx.doi.org/10.3109/08830189809043005] [PMID: 9646173]

[334] Sakurai T, Terashima S, Miyakoshi J. Enhanced secretion of prostaglandin E2 from osteoblasts by exposure to a strong static magnetic field. Bioelectromagnetics 2008; 29(4): 277-83.
[http://dx.doi.org/10.1002/bem.20392] [PMID: 18163441]

[335] Breunig A, Schneider FA, Jonas I, Nagursky H, Decker K. [The effect of static magnetic fields on prostaglandin synthesis in L-929 and 3T3 mouse fibroblasts. An *in-vitro* study]. Fortschr Kieferorthop 1993; 54(5): 218-28.
[http://dx.doi.org/10.1007/BF02341468] [PMID: 8244218]

[336] Saito K, Suzuki H, Suzuki K. Teratogenic effects of static magnetic field on mouse fetuses. Reprod Toxicol 2006; 22(1): 118-24.
[http://dx.doi.org/10.1016/j.reprotox.2005.08.003] [PMID: 16257173]

[337] Yip YP, Capriotti C, Talagala SL, Yip JW. Effects of MR exposure at 1.5 T on early embryonic development of the chick. J Magn Reson Imaging 1994; 4(5): 742-8.
[http://dx.doi.org/10.1002/jmri.1880040518] [PMID: 7981520]

[338] Möller HE, von Cramon DY. Survey of risks related to static magnetic fields in ultra high field MRI. Rofo 2008; 180(4): 293-301.
[http://dx.doi.org/10.1055/s-2008-1027227] [PMID: 18370347]

[339] Häfeli U. The history of magnetism in medicine. In: Andrä W, Nowak H, Eds. Magnetism in medicine. Weinheim, Germany: Wiley 2007.
[http://dx.doi.org/10.1055/s-2008-1027227]

[340] Weinberger A, Nyska A, Giler S. Treatment of experimental inflammatory synovitis with continuous magnetic field. Isr J Med Sci 1996; 32(12): 1197-201.
[PMID: 9007153]

[341] Capodaglio P, Vicenzi G. [Efficacy of a chair with magnets in the prevention of musculo-skeletal disorders caused by prolonged sitting]. G Ital Med Lav Ergon 2000; 22(4): 332-6.
[PMID: 11284158]

[342] Suomi R, Koceja DM. Effect of magnetic insoles on postural sway measures in men and women during a static balance test. Percept Mot Skills 2001; 92(2): 469-76.
[http://dx.doi.org/10.2466/pms.2001.92.2.469] [PMID: 11361310]

[343] Simoncini L, Giuriati L, Giannini S. Clinical evaluation of the effective use of magnetic fields in podology. Chir Organi Mov 2001; 86(3): 243-7.
[PMID: 12025189]

[344] Hulme J, Robinson V, DeBie R, Wells G, Judd M, Tugwell P. Electromagnetic fields for the treatment of osteoarthritis. Cochrane Database Syst Rev 2002; 1(1): CD003523.
[PMID: 11869668]

[345] Linovitz RJ, Pathria M, Bernhardt M, *et al.* Combined magnetic fields accelerate and increase spine fusion: a double-blind, randomized, placebo controlled study. Spine 2002; 27(13): 1383-9.
[http://dx.doi.org/10.1097/00007632-200207010-00002] [PMID: 12131732]

[346] Smania N, Corato E, Fiaschi A, Pietropoli P, Aglioti SM, Tinazzi M. Therapeutic effects of peripheral repetitive magnetic stimulation on myofascial pain syndrome. Clin Neurophysiol 2003; 114(2): 350-8.
[http://dx.doi.org/10.1016/S1388-2457(02)00367-X] [PMID: 12559244]

[347] Engström S, Markov MS, McLean MJ, Holcomb RR, Markov JM. Effects of non-uniform static magnetic fields on the rate of myosin phosphorylation. Bioelectromagnetics 2002; 23(6): 475-9.
[http://dx.doi.org/10.1002/bem.10035] [PMID: 12210566]

[348] Salvatore JR, Harrington J, Kummet T. Phase I clinical study of a static magnetic field combined with anti-neoplastic chemotherapy in the treatment of human malignancy: initial safety and toxicity data. Bioelectromagnetics 2003; 24(7): 524-7.
[http://dx.doi.org/10.1002/bem.10149] [PMID: 12955758]

[349] Hong CZ, Shellock FG. Short-term exposure to a 1.5 tesla static magnetic field does not affect somato-sensory-evoked potentials in man. Magnetic Resonance Imaging 8 1990; 1: 64-9.

[350] Mayrovitz HN, Groseclose EE, King D. No effect of 85 mT permanent magnets on laser-Doppler measured blood flow response to inspiratory gasps. Bioelectromagnetics 2005; 26(4): 331-5. [http://dx.doi.org/10.1002/bem.20096] [PMID: 15832329]

[351] Harlow T, Greaves C, White A, Brown L, Hart A, Ernst E. Randomised controlled trial of magnetic bracelets for relieving pain in osteoarthritis of the hip and knee. BMJ 2004; 329(7480): 1450-4. [http://dx.doi.org/10.1136/bmj.329.7480.1450] [PMID: 15604181]

[352] Richmond SJ. Magnet therapy for the relief of pain and inflammation in rheumatoid arthritis (CAMBRA): a randomised placebo-controlled crossover trial. Trials 2008; 9: 53. [http://dx.doi.org/10.1186/1745-6215-9-53] [PMID: 18789135]

[353] Pacini S, Gulisano M, Peruzzi B, *et al.* Effects of 0.2 T static magnetic field on human skin fibroblasts. Cancer Detect Prev 2003; 27(5): 327-32. [http://dx.doi.org/10.1016/S0361-090X(03)00124-7] [PMID: 14585318]

[354] Takashima Y, Miyakoshi J, Ikehata M, Iwasaka M, Ueno S, Koana T. Genotoxic effects of strong static magnetic fields in DNA-repair defective mutants of *Drosophila melanogaster*. J Radiat Res (Tokyo) 2004; 45(3): 393-7. [http://dx.doi.org/10.1269/jrr.45.393] [PMID: 15613784]

[355] Salerno S, La Mendola C, Lo Casto A, *et al.* Reversible effect of MR and ELF magnetic fields (0.5 T and 0.5 mT) on human lymphocyte activation patterns. Int J Radiat Biol 2006; 82(2): 77-85. [http://dx.doi.org/10.1080/09553000600589131] [PMID: 16546906]

[356] Ghibelli L, Cerella C, Cordisco S, *et al.* NMR exposure sensitizes tumor cells to apoptosis. Apoptosis 2006; 11(3): 359-65. [http://dx.doi.org/10.1007/s10495-006-4001-1] [PMID: 16528477]

[357] Tenuzzo B, Chionna A, Panzarini E, *et al.* Biological effects of 6 mT static magnetic fields: a comparative study in different cell types. Bioelectromagnetics 2006; 27(7): 560-77. [http://dx.doi.org/10.1002/bem.20252] [PMID: 16724329]

[358] Schwenzer NF, Bantleon R, Maurer B, *et al.* *In vitro* evaluation of magnetic resonance imaging at 3.0 tesla on clonogenic ability, proliferation, and cell cycle in human embryonic lung fibroblasts. Invest Radiol 2007; 42(4): 212-7. [http://dx.doi.org/10.1097/01.rli.0000255831.40115.83] [PMID: 17351426]

[359] Amara S, Douki T, Ravanat JL, *et al.* Influence of a static magnetic field (250 mT) on the antioxidant response and DNA integrity in THP1 cells. Phys Med Biol 2007; 52(4): 889-98. [http://dx.doi.org/10.1088/0031-9155/52/4/002] [PMID: 17264359]

[360] Okano H, Onmori R, Tomita N, Ikada Y. Effects of a moderate-intensity static magnetic field on VEGF-A stimulated endothelial capillary tubule formation *in vitro*. Bioelectromagnetics 2006; 27(8): 628-40. [http://dx.doi.org/10.1002/bem.20246] [PMID: 16838273]

[361] Güerci A, Zúñiga L, Marcos R. Construction and validation of a dose-response curve using the comet assay to determine human radiosensitivity to ionizing radiation. J Toxicol Environ Health A 2011; 74 (15-16): 1087-93. [http://dx.doi.org/10.1080/15287394.2011.582318] [PMID: 21707432]

[362] Singh NP, McCoy MT, Tice RR, Schneider EL. A simple technique for quantitation of low levels of DNA damage in individual cells. Exp Cell Res 1988; 175(1): 184-91. [http://dx.doi.org/10.1016/0014-4827(88)90265-0] [PMID: 3345800]

[363] Norimura T, Imada H, Kunugita N, Yoshida N, Nikaido M. Effects of strong magnetic fields on cell growth and radiation response of human T-lymphocytes in culture. J UOEH 1993; 15(2): 103-12. [PMID: 8316709]

[364] Gorczyńska E. The process of myelopoiesis in guinea pigs under conditions of a static magnetic field. Acta Physiol Pol 1987; 38(5): 425-32. [PMID: 3452975]

[365] Capstick M, McRobbie D, Hand J, *et al.* An investigation into occupational exposure to electromagnetic fields for personnel working with and around medical magnetic resonance imaging equipment. 2008.

[366] Takatsuji T, Sasaki MS, Takekoshi H. Effect of static magnetic field on the induction of chromosome aberrations by 4.9 MeV protons and 23 MeV alpha particles. J Radiat Res (Tokyo) 1989; 30(3): 238-46. [http://dx.doi.org/10.1269/jrr.30.238] [PMID: 2553938]

[367] Dini L, Dwikat M, Panzarini E, Vergallo C, Tenuzzo B. Morphofunctional study of 12--tetradecanoyl-13-phorbol acetate (TPA)-induced differentiation of U937 cells under exposure to a 6 mT static magnetic field. Bioelectromagnetics 2009; 30(5): 352-64. [http://dx.doi.org/10.1002/bem.20474] [PMID: 19189300]

[368] Dini L, Panzarini E. The influence of a 6 mT static magnetic field on apoptotic cell phagocytosis depends on monocyte/macrophage differentiation. Exp Biol Med (Maywood) 2010; 235(12): 1432-41. [http://dx.doi.org/10.1258/ebm.2010.010122] [PMID: 21127341]

[369] Tenuzzo B, Vergallo C, Dini L. Effect of 6mT static magnetic field on the bcl-2, bax, p53 and hsp70 expression in freshly isolated and *in vitro* aged human lymphocytes. Tissue Cell 2009; 41(3): 169-79. [http://dx.doi.org/10.1016/j.tice.2008.09.004] [PMID: 19054536]

[370] Pagliara P, Lanubile R, Dwikat M, Abbro L, Dini L. Differentiation of monocytic U937 cells under static magnetic field exposure. Eur J Histochem 2005; 49(1): 75-86. [http://dx.doi.org/10.4081/930] [PMID: 15823797]

[371] Dini L, Abbro L. Bioeffects of moderate-intensity static magnetic fields on cell cultures. Micron 2005; 36(3): 195-217. [http://dx.doi.org/10.1016/j.micron.2004.12.009] [PMID: 15725590]

[372] Chionna A, Dwikat M, Panzarini E, *et al.* Cell shape and plasma membrane alterations after static magnetic fields exposure. Eur J Histochem 2003; 47(4): 299-308. [PMID: 14706925]

[373] Chionna A, Tenuzzo B, Panzarini E, Dwikat MB, Abbro L, Dini L. Time dependent modifications of Hep G2 cells during exposure to static magnetic fields. Bioelectromagnetics 2005; 26(4): 275-86. [http://dx.doi.org/10.1002/bem.20081] [PMID: 15832333]

[374] Dini L, Vergallo C. Environmental factors affecting phagocytosis of dying cells: smoking and static magnetic fields. In: Krysko D, Vandenabeele P, Eds. Phagocytosis of dying cells: from molecular

mechanisms to human diseases. Heidelberg, Germany: Springer 2009; pp. 409-38.
[http://dx.doi.org/10.1007/978-1-4020-9293-0_15]

[375] Luferova NB, Konchugova TV, Gysakova EV. [The theoretical aspects of modern magnetobiology and magnetotherapy]. Vopr Kurortol Fizioter Lech Fiz Kult 2011; 3(3): 52-5.
[PMID: 21834472]

[376] Salerno S, Lo Casto A, Caccamo N, *et al.* Static magnetic fields generated by a 0.5 T MRI unit affects *in vitro* expression of activation markers and interleukin release in human peripheral blood mononuclear cells (PBMC). Int J Radiat Biol 1999; 75(4): 457-63.
[http://dx.doi.org/10.1080/095530099140384] [PMID: 10331851]

[377] Aldinucci C, Garcia JB, Palmi M, *et al.* The effect of strong static magnetic field on lymphocytes. Bioelectromagnetics 2003; 24(2): 109-17.
[http://dx.doi.org/10.1002/bem.10071] [PMID: 12524677]

[378] Sontag W. Release of mediators by DMSO-differentiated HL-60 cells exposed to electric interferential current and the requirement of biochemical prestimulation. Int J Radiat Biol 2001; 77(6): 723-34.
[http://dx.doi.org/10.1080/09553000110046376] [PMID: 11403712]

[379] Wang Z, Sarje A, Che PL, Yarema KJ. Moderate strength (0.23-0.28 T) static magnetic fields (SMF) modulate signaling and differentiation in human zembryonic cells. BMC Genomics 2009; 10(356): 1-23.
[http://dx.doi.org/10.1186/1471-2164-10-356] [PMID: 19653909]

[380] Lee JW, Kim MS, Kim YJ, Choi YJ, Lee Y, Chung HW. Genotoxic effects of 3 T magnetic resonance imaging in cultured human lymphocytes. Bioelectromagnetics 2011; 32(7): 535-42.
[http://dx.doi.org/10.1002/bem.20664] [PMID: 21412810]

[381] Nichols TW Jr. Mitochondria of mice and men: moderate magnetic fields in obesity and fatty liver. Med Hypotheses 2012; 79(3): 287-93.
[http://dx.doi.org/10.1016/j.mehy.2012.05.006] [PMID: 22743025]

[382] Lin SL, Tsai RY, Tai YH, *et al.* Ultra-low dose naloxone upregulates interleukin-10 expression and suppresses neuroinflammation in morphine-tolerant rat spinal cords. Behav Brain Res 2010; 207(1): 30-6.
[http://dx.doi.org/10.1016/j.bbr.2009.09.034] [PMID: 19799935]

[383] Cunha FQ, Teixeira MM, Ferreira SH. Pharmacological modulation of secondary mediator systems--cyclic AMP and cyclic GMP--on inflammatory hyperalgesia. Br J Pharmacol 1999; 127(3): 671-8.
[http://dx.doi.org/10.1038/sj.bjp.0702601] [PMID: 10401557]

[384] Chao PK, Lu KT, Lee YL, *et al.* Early systemic granulocyte-colony stimulating factor treatment attenuates neuropathic pain after peripheral nerve injury. PLoS One 2012; 7(8): e43680.
[http://dx.doi.org/10.1371/journal.pone.0043680] [PMID: 22937076]

[385] Gmitrov J, Ohkubo C, Okano H. Effect of 0.25 T static magnetic field on microcirculation in rabbits. Bioelectromagnetics 2002; 23(3): 224-9.
[http://dx.doi.org/10.1002/bem.10007] [PMID: 11891752]

[386] Hong CZ, Lin JC, Bender LF, Schaeffer JN, Meltzer RJ, Causin P. Magnetic necklace: its therapeutic effectiveness on neck and shoulder pain. Arch Phys Med Rehabil 1982; 63(10): 462-6.

[PMID: 7138256]

[387] Lin JC, Singleton GW, Schaeffer JN, Hong CZ, Meltzer RJ. Geophysical variables and behavior: XXVII. Magnetic necklace: its therapeutic effectiveness on neck and shoulder pain: 2. Psychological assessment. Psychol Rep 1985; 56(2): 639-49. [http://dx.doi.org/10.2466/pr0.1985.56.2.639] [PMID: 4001267]

[388] Schwartz JL. Influence of a constant magnetic field on nervous tissues: I. Nerve conduction velocity studies. IEEE Trans Biomed Eng 1978; 25(5): 467-73. [http://dx.doi.org/10.1109/TBME.1978.326353] [PMID: 700716]

[389] Schwartz JL. Influence of a constant magnetic field on nervous tissues: II. Voltage-clamp studies. IEEE Trans Biomed Eng 1979; 26(4): 238-43. [http://dx.doi.org/10.1109/TBME.1979.326508] [PMID: 437805]

[390] Wikswo JP, Barach JP. An estimate of the steady magnetic field strength required to influence nerve conduction. IEEE Trans Biomed Eng 1980; 27(12): 722-3. [http://dx.doi.org/10.1109/TBME.1980.326598] [PMID: 7461647]

[391] Rosen AD, Lubowsky J. Magnetic field influence on central nervous system function. Exp Neurol 1987; 95(3): 679-87. [http://dx.doi.org/10.1016/0014-4886(87)90308-6] [PMID: 3817086]

[392] Rosen AD, Lubowsky J. Modification of spontaneous unit discharge in the lateral geniculate body by a magnetic field. Exp Neurol 1990; 108(3): 261-5. [http://dx.doi.org/10.1016/0014-4886(90)90132-C] [PMID: 2351213]

[393] Rosen AD. A proposed mechanism for the action of strong static magnetic fields on biomembranes. Int J Neurosci 1993; 73(1-2): 115-9. [http://dx.doi.org/10.3109/00207459308987217] [PMID: 7510673]

[394] Kuipers NT, Sauder CL, Ray CA. Influence of static magnetic fields on pain perception and sympathetic nerve activity in humans. J Appl Physiol 2007; 102(4): 1410-5. [http://dx.doi.org/10.1152/japplphysiol.00734.2006] [PMID: 17194733]

[395] Eckert WA III, Julius D, Basbaum AI. Differential contribution of TRPV1 to thermal responses and tissue injury-induced sensitization of dorsal horn neurons in laminae I and V in the mouse. Pain 2006; 126(1-3): 184-97. [http://dx.doi.org/10.1016/j.pain.2006.06.032] [PMID: 16945484]

[396] Mandadi S, Numazaki M, Tominaga M, Bhat MB, Armati PJ, Roufogalis BD. Activation of protein kinase C reverses capsaicin-induced calcium-dependent desensitization of TRPV1 ion channels. Cell Calcium 2004; 35(5): 471-8. [http://dx.doi.org/10.1016/j.ceca.2003.11.003] [PMID: 15003856]

[397] Mandadi S, Tominaga T, Numazaki M, *et al.* Increased sensitivity of desensitized TRPV1 by PMA occurs through PKCepsilon-mediated phosphorylation at S800. Pain 2006; 123(1-2): 106-16. [http://dx.doi.org/10.1016/j.pain.2006.02.016] [PMID: 16564619]

[398] Apkarian AV, Gelnar PA, Krauss BR, Szeverenyi NM. Cortical responses to thermal pain depend on stimulus size: a functional MRI study. J Neurophysiol 2000; 83(5): 3113-22. [PMID: 10805705]

[399] Apkarian AV, Stea RA, Bolanowski SJ. Heat-induced pain diminishes vibrotactile perception: a touch gate. Somatosens Mot Res 1994; 11(3): 259-67.
[http://dx.doi.org/10.3109/08990229409051393] [PMID: 7887057]

[400] Eisenberg DM, Kessler RC, Foster C, Norlock FE, Calkins DR, Delbanco TL. Unconventional medicine in the United States. Prevalence, costs, and patterns of use. N Engl J Med 1993; 328(4): 246-52.
[http://dx.doi.org/10.1056/NEJM199301283280406] [PMID: 8418405]

[401] Jeske AJ, Blanton PL. Selection of local anesthetics in dentistry: clinical impression *versus* scientific assessment. J Am Coll Dent 2006; 73(3): 21-4.
[PMID: 17477214]

[402] Tenforde T, Budinger T. Biological effects and physical safety aspects of NMR imaging and *in vivo* spectroscopy. In: Thomas S, Dixon R, Eds. NMR in medicine: Instrumentation and clinical applications. New York, NY, USA: American Association of Physicists in Medicine 1986; pp. 493-548.

[403] ASTM. American Society for Testing and Materials: Standard test method for measurement of magnetically induced displacement force on medical devices in the magnetic resonance environment (F2052-02) and Standard test method for measurement of magnetically induced torque on passive implants in the magnetic resonance environment (F2213-04). West Conshohocken, PA, USA 2003.

[404] Linder-Aronson A, Forsberg CM, Rygh P, Lindskog S. Tissue response to space closure in monkeys: a comparison of orthodontic magnets and superelastic coil springs. Eur J Orthod 1996; 18(6): 581-8.
[http://dx.doi.org/10.1093/ejo/18.6.581] [PMID: 9009422]

[405] Bondemark L, Kurol J, Larsson A. Long-term effects of orthodontic magnets on human buccal mucosa--a clinical, histological and immunohistochemical study. Eur J Orthod 1998; 20(3): 211-8.
[http://dx.doi.org/10.1093/ejo/20.3.211] [PMID: 9699399]

[406] Bondemark L, Kurol J, Wisten A. Extent and flux density of static magnetic fields generated by orthodontic samarium-cobalt magnets. Am J Orthod Dentofacial Orthop 1995; 107(5): 488-96.
[http://dx.doi.org/10.1016/S0889-5406(95)70116-8] [PMID: 7733058]

[407] Yao W, Zhao Y, Li BY, Chao YL, Du L. [Effect of simulating static magnetic field of magnetic attachment on osteoblastic morphology and surface ultrastructure]. Zhonghua Kou Qiang Yi Xue Za Zhi 2008; 43(1): 48-9.
[PMID: 18380977]

[408] Xu C, Fan Z, Chao YL, Du L, Zhang FQ. [The research for magnetic attachments producing static magnetic fields to influence on cytoskeletons of human periodontal ligament cells]. Sichuan Da Xue Xue Bao Yi Xue Ban 2007; 38(4): 681-4.
[PMID: 17718441]

[409] Shen JF, Du L, Chao YL, Xu C. [Effects of static magnetic field on the activity of superoxide dismutase of human gingival fibroblasts]. Sichuan Da Xue Xue Bao Yi Xue Ban 2007; 38(2): 276-8.
[PMID: 17441348]

[410] Xu C, Chao YL, Du L, Yang L. [Measurements of the flux densities of static magnetic fields generated by two types of dental magnetic attachments and their retentive forces]. Sichuan Da Xue Xue Bao Yi

Xue Ban 2004; 35(3): 412-5.
[PMID: 15181852]

[411] Vickers ER, Cousins MJ. Neuropathic orofacial pain part 1--prevalence and pathophysiology. Aust Endod J 2000; 26(1): 19-26.
[http://dx.doi.org/10.1111/j.1747-4477.2000.tb00146.x] [PMID: 11359293]

[412] Ghione S, Seppia CD, Mezzasalma L, Bonfiglio L. Effects of 50 Hz electromagnetic fields on electroencephalographic alpha activity, dental pain threshold and cardiovascular parameters in humans. Neurosci Lett 2005; 382(1-2): 112-7.
[http://dx.doi.org/10.1016/j.neulet.2005.02.072] [PMID: 15911132]

[413] Ropohl A, Hiller M, Elstner S, Sperling W, Kornhuber J. Dental pain during repetitive transcranial magnetic stimulation. Letters to the Editor/European Psychiatry 2004; 19: 454-8.
[http://dx.doi.org/10.1016/j.eurpsy.2004.05.007]

[414] Altman DG, Schulz KF, Moher D, *et al.* CONSORT GROUP (Consolidated Standards of Reporting Trials). The revised CONSORT statement for reporting randomized trials: explanation and elaboration. Ann Intern Med 2001; 134(8): 663-94.
[http://dx.doi.org/10.7326/0003-4819-134-8-200104170-00012] [PMID: 11304107]

[415] Foucher JR, Gounot D, Pham BT, Marrer C, Dufour A. 'Magnetized' brains are slower - The cognitive effects of fMRI. Nat Preced 2008.
[http://dx.doi.org/10.1038/npre.2008.2443.1]

[416] Gupta A, Weeks AR, Richie SM. Simulation of elevated T-waves of an ECG inside a static magnetic field (MRI). IEEE Trans Biomed Eng 2008; 55(7): 1890-6.
[http://dx.doi.org/10.1109/TBME.2008.919868] [PMID: 18595808]

[417] Petrikas AZh, Ziuz'kov DI, Piekalnits I. [Teeth electroexcitability in periodontitis]. Stomatologia (Mosk) 2005; 84(2): 23-6.
[PMID: 15798748]

[418] Hsieh CH, Lee MC, Tsai-Wu JJ, *et al.* Deleterious effects of MRI on chondrocytes. Osteoarthritis Cartilage 2008; 16(3): 343-51.
[http://dx.doi.org/10.1016/j.joca.2007.07.001] [PMID: 17804262]

[419] Chen CY, Fu TC, Hu CF, Hsu CC, Chen CL, Chen CK. Influence of magnetic knee wraps on joint proprioception in individuals with osteoarthritis: a randomized controlled pilot trial. Clin Rehabil 2011; 25(3): 228-37.
[http://dx.doi.org/10.1177/0269215510382849] [PMID: 20980352]

[420] Jaberi FM, Keshtgar S, Tavakkoli A, *et al.* A moderate-intensity static magnetic field enhances repair of cartilage damage in rabbits. Arch Med Res 2011; 42(4): 268-73.
[http://dx.doi.org/10.1016/j.arcmed.2011.06.004] [PMID: 21820604]

[421] Klepetko W, Moritz A, Holle J, Laczkovics A. [The problem of scars in heart surgery with special reference to the use of static magnetic fields]. Wien Klin Wochenschr 1984; 96(5): 185-90.
[PMID: 6375145]

[422] Eccles NK, Hollinworth H. A pilot study to determine whether a static magnetic device can promote chronic leg ulcer healing. J Wound Care 2005; 14(2): 64-7.

[http://dx.doi.org/10.12968/jowc.2005.14.2.26731] [PMID: 15739653]

[423] Nursal TZ, Bal N, Anarat R, *et al.* Effects of a static magnetic field on wound healing: results in experimental rat colon anastomoses. Am J Surg 2006; 192(1): 76-81. [http://dx.doi.org/10.1016/j.amjsurg.2006.01.024] [PMID: 16769280]

[424] Henry SL, Concannon MJ, Yee GJ. The effect of magnetic fields on wound healing - Experimental study and review of the literature. Eplasty 2008; 8: 93-9. [PMID: 18725953]

[425] Shen JG, Chen WS, Wang CX, Jiang T, Dong LQ. [Effect of static magnetic field on deep wound healing of SD rats]. Zhongguo Gu Shang 2009; 22(5): 371-4. [PMID: 19522401]

[426] Jing D, Shen G, Cai J, *et al.* Effects of 180 mT static magnetic fields on diabetic wound healing in rats. Bioelectromagnetics 2010; 31(8): 640-8. [http://dx.doi.org/10.1002/bem.20592] [PMID: 20607739]

[427] Boutron I, Moher D, Altman DG, Schulz KF, Ravaud P, Consort G. Methods and Processes of the CONSORT Group: Example of an extension for trials assessing nonpharmacologic treatments. Ann Intern Med 2008; 148(4 W): 60-6. and 295-309 *ibid.* [http://dx.doi.org/10.7326/0003-4819-148-4-200802190-00008-w1]

[428] Fillingim RB, King CD, Ribeiro-Dasilva MC, Williams BR, Riley JL III. Sex, gender, and pain: A review of recent clinical and experimental findings. J of Pain 2009; 10: 447-85. and *references ibid.* [http://dx.doi.org/10.1016/j.jpain.2008.12.001]

[429] Brocklehurst B, McLauchlan KA. Free radical mechanism for the effects of environmental electromagnetic fields on biological systems. Int J Radiat Biol 1996; 69(1): 3-24. [http://dx.doi.org/10.1080/095530096146147] [PMID: 8601753]

[430] Timmel CR, Till U, Brocklehurst B, McLauchlan KA, Hore PJ. Effects of weak magnetic fields on free radical recombination reactions. Mol Phys 1998; 95: 71-89. [http://dx.doi.org/10.1080/00268979809483134]

[431] Timmel CR, Henbest KB. A study of spin chemistry in weak magnetic fields. Philos Trans A Math Phys Eng Sci 2004; 362(1825): 2573-89. [http://dx.doi.org/10.1098/rsta.2004.1459] [PMID: 15539359]

[432] Woodward JR. Radical pairs in solution. Prog React Kinet Mech 2002; 27: 165-207. [http://dx.doi.org/10.3184/007967402103165388]

[433] Rodgers CT. Magnetic field effects in chemical systems. Pure Appl Chem 2009; 81: 19-43. [http://dx.doi.org/10.1351/PAC-CON-08-10-18]

[434] Rodgers CT, Hore PJ. Chemical magnetoreception in birds: the radical pair mechanism. Proc Natl Acad Sci USA 2009; 106(2): 353-60. [http://dx.doi.org/10.1073/pnas.0711968106] [PMID: 19129499]

[435] Kanis JA, Johnell O. The burden of osteoporosis. J Endocrinol Invest 1999; 22(8): 583-8. [http://dx.doi.org/10.1007/BF03343614] [PMID: 10532244]

[436] Kroeling P, Gross A, Goldsmith CH, *et al.* Electrotherapy for neck pain. Cochrane Database Syst Rev 2009; 8(4): CD004251.

[PMID: 19821322]

[437] Weintraub MI, Cole SP. A randomized controlled trial of the effects of a combination of static and dynamic magnetic fields on carpal tunnel syndrome. Pain Med 2008; 9(5): 493-504. [http://dx.doi.org/10.1111/j.1526-4637.2007.00324.x] [PMID: 18777606]

[438] Khoromi S, Blackman MR, Kingman A, *et al.* Low intensity permanent magnets in the treatment of chronic lumbar radicular pain. J Pain Symptom Manage 2007; 34(4): 434-45. [http://dx.doi.org/10.1016/j.jpainsymman.2006.12.008] [PMID: 17618081]

[439] Kotani H, Kawaguchi H, Shimoaka T, *et al.* Strong static magnetic field stimulates bone formation to a definite orientation *in vitro* and *in vivo.* J Bone Miner Res 2002; 17(10): 1814-21. [http://dx.doi.org/10.1359/jbmr.2002.17.10.1814] [PMID: 12369785]

[440] Qiu LH, Zhong M, Tang XN, Wang ZY. [Effect of static magnetic field on bone morphogenetic protein 2 and collagen type I of osteoblast cell]. Shanghai Kou Qiang Yi Xue 2007; 16(1): 33-5. [PMID: 17377697]

[441] Hsu SH, Chang JC. The static magnetic field accelerates the osteogenic differentiation and mineralization of dental pulp cells. Cytotechnology 2010; 62(2): 143-55. [http://dx.doi.org/10.1007/s10616-010-9271-3] [PMID: 20464482]

[442] Papadopulos MA, Hörler I, Gerber H, Rahn BA, Rakosi T. [The effect of static magnetic fields on osteoblast activity: an *in-vitro* study]. Fortschr Kieferorthop 1992; 53(4): 218-22. [http://dx.doi.org/10.1007/BF02327638] [PMID: 1526613]

[443] Denaro V, Cittadini A, Barnaba SA, *et al.* Static electromagnetic fields generated by corrosion currents inhibit human osteoblast differentiation. Spine 2008; 33(9): 955-9. [http://dx.doi.org/10.1097/BRS.0b013e31816c90b8] [PMID: 18427315]

[444] Xu S, Okano H, Tomita N, Ikada Y. Recovery effects of a 180 mT static magnetic field on bone mineral density of osteoporotic lumbar vertebrae in ovariectomized rats. Evidence-based Complementary and Alternative Medicine 2011; 2011: 620984. [http://dx.doi.org/10.1155/2011/620984]

[445] Xu S, Tomita N, Ikeuchi K, Ikada Y. Recovery of small-sized blood vessels in ischemic bone under static magnetic field. Evid Based Complement Alternat Med 2007; 4(1): 59-63. [http://dx.doi.org/10.1093/ecam/nel055] [PMID: 17342242]

[446] Xu S, Tomita N, Ohata R, Yan Q, Ikada Y. Static magnetic field effects on bone formation of rats with an ischemic bone model. Biomed Mater Eng 2001; 11(3): 257-63. [PMID: 11564908]

[447] Bruce GK, Howlett CR, Huckstep RL. Effect of a static magnetic field on fracture healing in a rabbit radius. Preliminary results. Clin Orthop Relat Res 1987; (222): 300-6. [PMID: 3621734]

[448] Aydin N, Bezer M. The effect of an intramedullary implant with a static magnetic field on the healing of the osteotomised rabbit femur. Int Orthop 2011; 35(1): 135-41. [http://dx.doi.org/10.1007/s00264-009-0932-9] [PMID: 20062989]

[449] Qiu LH, Qin K, Zhong M, Wang ZY. [Effect of static magnetic field on bone morphogenetic protein-2 in periodontal membrane of experimental periodontitis rat]. Hua Xi Kou Qiang Yi Xue Za Zhi 2005;

23(4): 319-21.
[PMID: 16178195]

[450] Darendeliler MA, Darendeliler A, Sinclair PM. Effects of static magnetic and pulsed electromagnetic fields on bone healing. Int J Adult Orthodon Orthognath Surg 1997; 12(1): 43-53.
[PMID: 9456617]

[451] Taniguchi N, Kanai S. Efficacy of static magnetic field for locomotor activity of experimental osteopenia. Evid Based Complement Alternat Med 2007; 4(1): 99-105.
[http://dx.doi.org/10.1093/ecam/nel067] [PMID: 17342247]

[452] Costantino C, Pogliacomi F, Passera F, Concari G. Treatment of wrist and hand fractures with natural magnets: preliminary report. Acta Biomed 2007; 78(3): 198-203.
[PMID: 18330079]

[453] Brkovic-Popovic S, Stamenkovic D, Stanisic-Sinobad D, Rakocevic Z, Zelic O. [The influence of continuous magnetic field on periodontal tissues under overdentures]. Srp Arh Celok Lek 2009; 137(7-8): 363-70.
[http://dx.doi.org/10.2298/SARH0908363B] [PMID: 19764589]

[454] Schulz KF, Altman DG, Moher DBV. CONSORT. CONSORT 2010 statement: updated guidelines for reporting parallel group randomised trials. BMJ 2010; 340: c332.
[http://dx.doi.org/10.1136/bmj.c332] [PMID: 20332509]

[455] Huskisson EC. Measurement of pain. Lancet 1974; 2(7889): 1127-31.
[http://dx.doi.org/10.1016/S0140-6736(74)90884-8] [PMID: 4139420]

[456] Ostelo RW, Deyo RA, Stratford P, *et al.* Interpreting change scores for pain and functional status in low back pain: towards international consensus regarding minimal important change. Spine 2008; 33(1): 90-4.
[http://dx.doi.org/10.1097/BRS.0b013e31815e3a10] [PMID: 18165753]

[457] Kallmes DF, Comstock BA, Heagerty PJ, *et al.* A randomized trial of vertebroplasty for osteoporotic spinal fractures. N Engl J Med 2009; 361(6): 569-79.
[http://dx.doi.org/10.1056/NEJMoa0900563] [PMID: 19657122]

[458] László JF, Solténszky J, Pórszász R, Kónya A. The effect of whole-body, repetitive, inhomogeneous static magnetic field-exposure on the symptoms of experimental autoimmune encephalomyelitis in mice. J Complement Integr Med 2014; 11(1): 19-25.
[http://dx.doi.org/10.1515/jcim-2013-0055] [PMID: 24425581]

[459] Csillag A, Kumar BV, Szabó K, *et al.* Exposure to inhomogeneous static magnetic field beneficially affects allergic inflammation in a murine model. J R Soc Interface 2014; 11(95): 20140097.
[http://dx.doi.org/10.1098/rsif.2014.0097] [PMID: 24647908]

[460] Juhász M, Nagy VL, Székely H, Kocsis D, Tulassay Z, László JF. Influence of inhomogeneous static magnetic field-exposure on patients with erosive gastritis: a randomized, self- and placebo-controlled, double-blind, single centre, pilot study. J R Soc Interface 2014; 11(98): 20140601.
[http://dx.doi.org/10.1098/rsif.2014.0601] [PMID: 25008086]

[461] Chekhun VF, Demash DV, Nalieskina LA. Evaluation of biological effects and possible mechanisms of action of static magnetic field. Fiziol Zh 2012; 58(3): 85-94.

[PMID: 22946317]

[462] Bacri J, Cebers A, Bourdon A, *et al.* Transient grating in a ferrofluid under magnetic field: Effect of magnetic interactions on the diffusion coefficient of translation. Phys Rev E Stat Phys Plasmas Fluids Relat Interdiscip Topics 1995; 52(4): 3936-42. [http://dx.doi.org/10.1103/PhysRevE.52.3936] [PMID: 9963866]

[463] Miyake T, Inatomi Y, Kuribayashi K. Measurement of diffusion coefficient in liquid metal under static magnetic field. Jpn J Appl Phys 2002; 41(L): 811. [http://dx.doi.org/10.1143/JJAP.41.L811]

[464] Hürlimann MD. Diffusion and relaxation effects in general stray field NMR experiments. J Magn Reson 2001; 148(2): 367-78. [http://dx.doi.org/10.1006/jmre.2000.2263] [PMID: 11237644]

[465] Lia Z, Donga J, Zenga X, Lua C, Dinga W, Renb Z. Influence of strong static magnetic field on intermediate phase growth in Mg-Al diffusion couple. J Alloys Compd 2007; 440(1-2): 132-6. [http://dx.doi.org/10.1016/j.jallcom.2006.09.032]

[466] Eguchi Y, Ogiue-Ikeda M, Ueno S. Control of orientation of rat Schwann cells using an 8-T static magnetic field. Neurosci Lett 2003; 351(2): 130-2. [http://dx.doi.org/10.1016/S0304-3940(03)00719-5] [PMID: 14583398]

[467] Umeno A, Ueno S. Quantitative analysis of adherent cell orientation influenced by strong magnetic fields. IEEE Trans Nanobioscience 2003; 2(1): 26-8. [http://dx.doi.org/10.1109/TNB.2003.810157] [PMID: 15382419]

[468] Kim S, Im WS, Kang L, Lee ST, Chu K, Kim BI. The application of magnets directs the orientation of neurite outgrowth in cultured human neuronal cells. J Neurosci Methods 2008; 174(1): 91-6. [http://dx.doi.org/10.1016/j.jneumeth.2008.07.005] [PMID: 18682261]

[469] Yip YP, Capriotti C, Yip JW. Effects of MR exposure on axonal outgrowth in the sympathetic nervous system of the chick. J Magn Reson Imaging 1995; 5(4): 457-62. [http://dx.doi.org/10.1002/jmri.1880050416] [PMID: 7549211]

[470] Sipka S, Szöllosi I, Batta G, *et al.* Decreased chemotaxis of human peripheral phagocytes exposed to a strong static magnetic field. Acta Physiol Hung 2004; 91(1): 59-65. [http://dx.doi.org/10.1556/APhysiol.91.2004.1.4] [PMID: 15334831]

[471] Ohata R, Tomita N, Ikada Y. Effect of a static magnetic field on ion transport in a cellulose membrane. J Colloid Interface Sci 2004; 270(2): 413-6. [http://dx.doi.org/10.1016/j.jcis.2003.09.035] [PMID: 14697708]

[472] Scorei RI, Cimpoiaşu VM, Popa R. TD-^{1}HNMR measurements show enantioselective dissociation of ribose and glucose in the presence of $H_2^{(17)}O$. Astrobiology 2007; 7(5): 733-44. [http://dx.doi.org/10.1089/ast.2006.0076] [PMID: 17963473]

[473] Alexander A, Dwivedi S, Ajazuddin , *et al.* Approaches for breaking the barriers of drug permeation through transdermal drug delivery. J Control Release 2012; 164(1): 26-40. [http://dx.doi.org/10.1016/j.jconrel.2012.09.017] [PMID: 23064010]

[474] Murthy SN. Magnetophoresis: an approach to enhance transdermal drug diffusion. Pharmazie 1999; 54(5): 377-9.

[PMID: 10368832]

[475] Plouffe B, Lewis L, Murthy S. Computational design optimization for microfluidic magnetophoresis. Biomicrofluidics 2011; 5: 13413.
[http://dx.doi.org/10.1063/1.3668225] ; and erratum in: Biomicrofluidics 2011; 5(4): 49901.

[476] Kimball GC. The growth of yeast in a magnetic field. J Bacteriol 1938; 35(2): 109-22.
[PMID: 16560087]

[477] Galland P, Pazur A. Magnetoreception in plants. J Plant Res 2005; 118(6): 371-89.
[http://dx.doi.org/10.1007/s10265-005-0246-y] [PMID: 16283069]

[478] Ahmad M, Galland P, Ritz T, Wiltschko R, Wiltschko W. Magnetic intensity aVects cryptochrome-dependent responses. Planta 2007; 225: 615-24.
[http://dx.doi.org/10.1007/s00425-006-0383-0] [PMID: 16955271]

[479] Kimura T, Takahashi K, Suzuki Y, *et al.* The effect of high strength static magnetic fields and ionizing radiation on gene expression and DNA damage in *Caenorhabditis elegans.* Bioelectromagnetics 2008; 29(8): 605-14.
[http://dx.doi.org/10.1002/bem.20425] [PMID: 18512716]

[480] Hung YC, Lee JH, Chen HM, Huang GS. Effects of static magnetic fields on the development and aging of *Caenorhabditis elegans.* J Exp Biol 2010; 213(Pt 12): 2079-85.
[http://dx.doi.org/10.1242/jeb.039768] [PMID: 20511522]

[481] Lee CH, Chen HM, Yeh LK, Hong MY, Huang GS. Dosage-dependent induction of behavioral decline in *Caenorhabditis elegans* by long-term treatment of static magnetic fields. J Radiat Res (Tokyo) 2012; 53(1): 24-32.
[http://dx.doi.org/10.1269/jrr.11057] [PMID: 22302042]

[482] Lee CH, Hung YC, Huang GS. Static magnetic field accelerates aging and development in nematode. Commun Integr Biol 2010; 3(6): 528-9.
[http://dx.doi.org/10.4161/cib.3.6.12749] [PMID: 21331230]

[483] Moisescu C, Ardelean II, Benning L. The effect and role of environmental conditions on magnetosome synthesis. Front Microbiol 2014; 5(49): 1-25. and *references ibid.*
[http://dx.doi.org/10.3389/fmicb.2014.00049]

[484] Langendorff O. Untersuchungen am ulberlebenden Saugetierherzen. Pflugers Arch 1895; 61: 291-332.
[http://dx.doi.org/10.1007/BF01812150]

[485] Mészáros K. Magnetic field elicits hypotension mediated by platelet activating factor in rats injected with iron beads. Biochem Biophys Res Commun 1991; 180(1): 315-22.
[http://dx.doi.org/10.1016/S0006-291X(05)81294-X] [PMID: 1930228]

[486] Janssen B, De Celle T, Debets J, Brouns A, Callahan M, Smith T. Effects of anesthetics on systemic hemodynamics in mice. Am J Physiol Heart Circ Physiol 2004; 287(H): 1618-24.
[http://dx.doi.org/10.1152/ajpheart.01192.2003]

[487] Wang X, Sun Z. RNAi silencing of brain klotho potentiates cold-induced elevation of blood pressure *via* the endothelin pathway. Physiol Genomics 2010; 41(2): 120-6.
[http://dx.doi.org/10.1152/physiolgenomics.00192.2009] [PMID: 20086041]

[488] Swoap S, Overton J, Garber G. Effect of ambient temperature on cardiovascular parameters in rats and mice: a comparative approach. Am J Physiol Regul Integr Comp Physiol 2004; 287(R): 391-6.
[http://dx.doi.org/10.1152/ajpregu.00731.2003]

[489] Feng M, DiPetrillo K. Non-invasive blood pressure measurement in mice. Methods Mol Biol 2009; 573: 45-55.
[PMID: 19763921]

[490] Gábor M. Mouse ear inflammation models and their pharmacological applications. Budapest, Hungary: Akadémia Press 2000.

[491] Tofani S, Cintorino M, Barone D, *et al.* Increased mouse survival, tumor growth inhibition and decreased immunoreactive p53 after exposure to magnetic fields. Bioelectromagnetics 2002; 23(3): 230-8.
[http://dx.doi.org/10.1002/bem.10010] [PMID: 11891753]

[492] Mevissen M, Stamm A, Buntenkötter S, Zwingelberg R, Wahnschaffe U, Löscher W. Effects of magnetic fields on mammary tumor development induced by 7,12-dimethylbenz(a)anthracene in rats. Bioelectromagnetics 1993; 14(2): 131-43.
[http://dx.doi.org/10.1002/bem.2250140206] [PMID: 8494555]

[493] Gray JR, Frith CH, Parker JD. *In vivo* enhancement of chemotherapy with static electric or magnetic fields. Bioelectromagnetics 2000; 21(8): 575-83.
[http://dx.doi.org/10.1002/1521-186X(200012)21:8<575::AID-BEM3>3.0.CO;2-F] [PMID: 11102947]

[494] Nobuto H, Sugita T, Kubo T, *et al.* Evaluation of systemic chemotherapy with magnetic liposomal doxorubicin and a dipole external electromagnet. Int J Cancer 2004; 109(4): 627-635 .
[http://dx.doi.org/10.1002/ijc.20035] [PMID: 14991586]

[495] Flipo D, Fournier M, Benquet C, *et al.* Increased apoptosis, changes in intracellular Ca2+, and functional alterations in lymphocytes and macrophages after *in vitro* exposure to static magnetic field. J Toxicol Environ Health A 1998; 54(1): 63-76.
[http://dx.doi.org/10.1080/009841098159033] [PMID: 9588349]

[496] Strieth S, Strelczyk D, Eichhorn ME, *et al.* Static magnetic fields induce blood flow decrease and platelet adherence in tumor microvessels. Cancer Biol Ther 2008; 7(6): 814-9.
[http://dx.doi.org/10.4161/cbt.7.6.5837] [PMID: 18340115]

[497] Halicka HD, Darzynkiewicz Z, Teodori L. Attenuation of constitutive ATM activation and H2AX phosphorylation in human leukemic TK6 cells by their exposure to static magnetic field. Cell Cycle 2009; 8(19): 3238-40.
[http://dx.doi.org/10.4161/cc.8.19.9598] [PMID: 19755848]

[498] Coots A, Shi R, Rosen AD. Effect of a 0.5-T static magnetic field on conduction in guinea pig spinal cord. J Neurol Sci 2004; 222(1-2): 55-7.
[http://dx.doi.org/10.1016/j.jns.2004.04.010] [PMID: 15240196]

[499] Colbert AP, Markov MS, Carlson N, Gregory WL, Carlson H, Elmer PJ. Static magnetic field therapy for carpal tunnel syndrome: a feasibility study. Arch Phys Med Rehabil 2010; 91(7): 1098-104.
[http://dx.doi.org/10.1016/j.apmr.2010.02.013] [PMID: 20599049]

[500] Okano H, Ino H, Osawa Y, Osuga T, Tatsuoka H. The effects of moderate-intensity gradient static

magnetic fields on nerve conduction. Bioelectromagnetics 2012; 33(6): 518-26. [http://dx.doi.org/10.1002/bem.21717] [PMID: 22430817]

[501] Hinch R, Lindsay KA, Noble D, Rosenberg JR. The effects of static magnetic field on action potential propagation and excitation recovery in nerve. Prog Biophys Mol Biol 2005; 87(2-3): 321-8. [http://dx.doi.org/10.1016/j.pbiomolbio.2004.08.013] [PMID: 15556668]

[502] Shellock FG, Schaefer DJ, Crues JV. Exposure to a 1.5-T static magnetic field does not alter body and skin temperatures in man. Magn Reson Med 1989; 11(3): 371-5. [http://dx.doi.org/10.1002/mrm.1910110311] [PMID: 2779423]

[503] Mayrovitz HN, Groseclose EE. Effects of a static magnetic field of either polarity on skin microcirculation. Microvasc Res 2005; 69(1-2): 24-7. [http://dx.doi.org/10.1016/j.mvr.2004.11.002] [PMID: 15797257]

[504] Pawluk W. Miracle of magnetics. Natural Health and Longevity Resource Center. 1995. Available at http://all-natural.com/magnetic.html.

[505] Maki M. Biomedical engineering study demonstrates the healing value of magnets.2008. Available at http://virginia.edu/uvatoday/newsRelease.php?id=3573#).

[506] Hermans J. Q magnet therapy for a shin bruise with a child. 2010. Available at http://qmagnets.com/blog/condition-testimonies/bruise-healing-after-one-day.html.

[507] Havill J. Faster recovery for soft tissue injury - Grade III calf tear. 2012. Available at http://qmagnets.com/blog/sport/faster-recovery-for-soft-tissue-injury-grade-iii-calf-tear-2.html.

[508] Keenan MA, Stabin MG, Segars WP, Fernald MJ. RADAR realistic animal model series for dose assessment. J Nucl Med 2010; 51(3): 471-6. [http://dx.doi.org/10.2967/jnumed.109.070532] [PMID: 20197451]

SUBJECT INDEX

Made in the USA
Las Vegas, NV
03 November 2026

57425160R00226